THE
PATIENT-
PHYSICIAN
RELATION

The Patient as Partner, Part 2

Medical Ethics Series

DAVID H. SMITH AND ROBERT M. VEATCH, EDITORS

THE

PATIENT-
PHYSICIAN
RELATION

The Patient as Partner, Part 2

Robert M. Veatch

Indiana
University
Press
BLOOMINGTON AND INDIANAPOLIS

The paper used in this publication meets the minimum requirements of American National Standard for Information Sciences—Permanence of Paper for Printed Library Materials, ANSI Z39.48-1984.

 ™

Manufactured in the United States of America

Library of Congress Cataloging-in-Publication Data

Veatch, Robert M.
  The patient-physician relation : the patient as partner, part 2 / Robert M. Veatch.
    p.   cm. -- (Medical ethics series)
  A sequel to the author's earlier book: The patient as partner.
  Includes bibliographical references.
  ISBN 0-253-36207-5 (alk. paper)
  1. Physician and patient. 2. Medical ethics.
  1. Veatch, Robert M. Patient as partner.
  II. Title. III. Series.
  [DNLM: 1. Consumer Participation. 2. Decision Making.
  3. Ethics, Medical. 4. Physician-Patient Relations. W 50 V394p]
  R727.3.V38 1991
  174'.2—dc20
  DNLM/DLC
  for Library of Congress   90-4261
                                                           CIP

1 2 3 4 5 95 94 93 92 91

Contents

Part IV. Special Problem Areas

Part V. The Future of the Partnership

Cases

PREFACE

The health professional and lay person are increasingly seen as active partners pursuing interests that, to a limited degree, converge. For many years I have sensed that the more traditional model of the physician/patient relation was eroding. In that model, a physician dedicated to the patient's medical welfare would benevolently make decisions for his or her good. Then it seemed obvious that the physician could know what was good even for an unfamiliar patient. There was a naive sense that never would the patient's other, nonmedical interests make pursuit of the medical good undesirable; never would patients' rights conflict with their medical good; and never would the interests or rights of others conflict with those of the patient.

It is now apparent that these assumptions are terribly implausible. A new understanding of the lay-professional relation is needed. I see a partnership based on a complex social contract. As I acknowledged in my earlier volume, *The Patient as Partner*, I began using the title for the David Barap Brim lecture on Ethical Issues in Clinical Cancer Research given at Johns Hopkins Oncology Center in 1982. It attracted enough attention that I adopted it as the title for a collection of essays outlining the implications of the partnership model for medical ethics. That volume was limited to exploring this new understanding of the lay-professional relation for research medicine, for the relation between investigator and research subject. At the time I indicated that a second volume was in order, one devoted to the application of the partnership model to the physician/patient relation in clinical medicine. This volume delivers on that promise.

Many of the essays contained herein have been published previously, but often in obscure locations and frequently divorced from the overarching medical ethical theory that provides their foundation. What appears here is presented as a more systematic discussion of the implications of the partnership model for clinical medicine. Those essays published previously have been edited, combined, and revised in an attempt to present a systematic picture. Several entirely new chapters have been written for this volume. Others have been modified to varying degrees.

Much of the underlying theory has been presented elsewhere, first in my more theoretical volume, *A Theory of Medical Ethics*, and then to provide the foundation for *The Patient as Partner*. In order to orient the reader of this volume, many of the main aspects of that theory are summarized here in chapters 2 and 6. Those familiar with the earlier works need not dwell on those summaries. The application of the theory to the clinical medical context is my aim here. We shall see that basic ethical theory has radical, sometimes surprising, implications for some areas of health care that have not received adequate attention. We shall see that a partnership in medical decisionmaking has implications not only for the ethically obvious cases of abortion and euthanasia, but also for broken arm treatments, hernia surgery, and malpractice.

The preparation of this manuscript has involved a thorough reworking and updating of materials. It would not have been possible without the capable assistance of many people, including research assistance from Carol Mason and Lil Nicolai and administrative support from Denise Brooks, Michelle Lewis, Mary Jane Bingham, and Irene McDonald.

ACKNOWLEDGMENTS

Chapter 1 is adapted from "Models for Ethical Medicine in a Revolutionary Age," *Hastings Center Report* 2 (No. 3, June 1972):5–7. Reproduced by permission. © The Hastings Center.

Chapter 2 is extensively rewritten, incorporating some material from "Medical Ethics: Professional or Universal," *Harvard Theological Review* 65 (No. 4, October 1972):531–539. Reproduced by permission.

Chapter 3 is adapted from "The Physician as Stranger: The Ethics of the Anonymous Patient-Physician Relationship," in *The Clinical Encounter: The Moral Fabric of the Patient-Physician Relationship*, edited by Earl E. Shelp (Dordrecht, Holland: D. Reidel Publishing Co., 1983), pp. 187–207.

Chapter 4 is based on "Bringing Nonmedical Values into Practical Medicine," *Medical Ethics for Physicians* 3 (No. 1, January 1988):6–7, and on "Doctor's Orders," *Journal of the American Medical Association* 254 (December 27, 1985):3468, copyright 1985, American Medical Association.

Chapter 5 "The Concept of 'Medical Indications,'" has not been published previously.

Chapter 6 was prepared for this volume.

Chapter 7 is adapted from "Informed Consent: The Emerging Principles," *U.S. Pharmacist* 6 (March 1981):78–80.

Chapter 8 "Malpractice in the Contract Mode," has not been published previously.

Chapter 9 first appeared as "The Ethics of Generic Drug Use," *U.S. Pharmacist* 7 (March 1982):62–64.

Chapter 10 was originally published as "Drug Research in Humans: The Ethics of Nonrandomized Trials," *Clinical Pharmacy* 8 (1989):366–370. © 1989, American Society of Hospital Pharmacists, Inc. All rights reserved. Reprinted with permission. (R9207)

Chapter 11 is based in part on "Ethics of Drug Use for Non-approved Uses," *U.S. Pharmacist* 8 (July 1983):69–72.

Chapter 12 is based on "When Should the Patient Know?" *Barrister* 8 (1981): 6–8, 17–20, copyright 1981, American Bar Association, reprinted by permission of the American Bar Association.

Chapter 13 is a revised and expanded version of "An Unexpected Chromosome: The Physician's Dilemma," *Hastings Center Report* 2 (No. 1, February 1972):8–9. Reproduced by permission. © The Hastings Center.

Chapter 14 is based on "The Ethics of Dispensing Placebos," *U.S. Pharmacist* 5 (September 1980):70–72.

Chapter 15 is adapted from "Record-Breaking Problems," *Hospital Physician* 12 (November 1976):38–39.

Chapter 16 incorporates material from "Case Studies in Bioethics: The Homosexual Husband and Physician Confidentiality," *Hastings Center Report* 7 (April 1977):16–17. Reproduced by permission. © The Hastings Center.

Chapter 17, "Patients' Duties and Physicians' Rights," has not been published previously.

Chapter 18 is adapted from "Autonomy's Temporary Triumph," *Hastings Center Report* 14 (No. 5, October 1984):38–40. Reproduced by permission. © The Hastings Center.

Chapter 19 is a revised version of "DRGs and the Ethical Reallocation of Resources," *Hastings Center Report* 16 (No. 3, June 1986):32–40. Reproduced by permission. © The Hastings Center.

Chapter 20 incorporates portions of "Justice and the Economics of Terminal Illness," *Hastings Center Report* 18 (August/September 1988): 34–40. Reproduced by permission. © The Hastings Center, as well as parts of "Age-based Allocation: Discrimination or Justice?" *Medical Ethics for the Physician* 3 (July 1988):1–2, 4, copyright The KSF Group, 630 Ninth Avenue, Suite 901, New York, NY 10036.

Chapter 21 is based on "Voluntary Risks to Health: The Ethical Issues," *Journal of the American Medical Association* 243 (January 4, 1980):50–55, copyright 1980, American Medical Association.

Chapter 22 is based on testimony before the Subcommittee on Investigations and Oversight of the Committee on Science and Technology, U.S. House of Representatives, Ninety-eighth Congress, April 14, 1983 (Washington D.C.: U.S. Government Printing Office, 1983), pp. 341–349, and on "From Fae to Schroeder: The Ethics of Allocating High Technology," *Spectrum: Journal of the Association of Adventist Forums* 16 (No. 1, April 1985):15–18.

Chapter 23 is based on "The Technical Criteria Fallacy: The Case of Spina Bifida." *Hastings Center Report* 7 (August 1977):15–16. Reproduced by permission. © The Hastings Center.

Chapter 24 is based on "Limits of Guardian Treatment Refusal: A Reasonableness Standard," *American Journal of Law and Medicine* 9 (No. 4, Winter 1984):427–468.

Chapter 25 "'Do Not Resuscitate' Orders: An Ethical Analysis," has not been published previously.

Chapter 26 is adapted in part from "The Ethics of Institutional Ethics Committees" in *Institutional Ethics Committees and Health Care Decision Making*, edited by Ronald E. Cranford and A. Edward Doudera (Ann Arbor, Mich: American Society of Law & Medicine, 1984), pp. 35–50. It also incorporates portions of "Ethics Committees: Are They Legitimate?" in *Ethics Committee Newsletter* (Boston: American Society of Law & Medicine, November 1983), and "Advice and Consent," *Hastings*

Center Report 19 (January/February 1989):20–22, reproduced by permission. © The Hastings Center.

Chapter 27 "Medical Ethics and the Demise of Modern Medicine," was written as the summarizing and concluding chapter to this volume. Other versions appear as "Contemporary Bioethics and the Demise of Modern Medicine," *Bioethics News* 8 (January 1989):6–21, and in *Prescriptions: The Dissemination of Medical Authority,* edited by Gayle L. Ormiston and Raphael Sassower (New York: Greenwood Press, 1990), pp. 23–29.

THE PATIENT-PHYSICIAN RELATION:

The Patient as Partner, Part 2

Introduction

MEDICAL ETHICS AND THE PATIENT-PHYSICIAN RELATION

Medical ethics is sometimes taken to be the same as the ethics of physicians. That is a mistake. In fact, the very notion of the ethics of physicians is ambiguous. Sometimes it refers to ethical stances articulated by physicians or by physician groups such as the American Medical Association. These stances might address what physicians believe to be the morally appropriate conduct in their relationships with patients. They might also address the conduct of physicians in other relations such as among colleagues or with other health professionals. They might even address nonmedical matters such as physician views on war or race relations.

MEDICAL ETHICS AND PHYSICIAN ETHICS

Ethical stances articulated by physicians constitute only one aspect of medical ethics. Also included are the ethical positions of others pertaining to the medical sphere. Religious groups, philosophers, participants in public policy formation, and ordinary lay people have views about what is right or wrong in medicine, sometimes including what constitutes ethically appropriate physician behavior (for example, the position of the Catholic church about whether physicians should actively kill dying patients for mercy could be called "physician ethics," even though it is not articulated by physicians). The church may take a medical ethical stance about the morality of its members' use of contraceptives. A philosopher may develop an argument over whether a woman should offer to become a surrogate mother. A legislator may propose a bill to fund transplants for children dying of liver failure or to control Medicare expenditures for the terminally ill elderly. All of these involve medical ethics although they do not directly involve moral stances about physician conduct. Some—such as the use of over-the-counter contraceptives—may never affect the physician. Medical ethics is far broader than ethics articulated by physicians or ethical positions about how physicians ought to act.

THE ROLE OF PATIENT

One of the most significant aspects of medical ethics is the ethics of people in the role of patient. Patients are not simply sick people. They are

1

people in an active relation with a health professional, normally a physician. The term *patient* is not a good one. Etymologically it implies suffering, with the connotation of passivity. But patients can be passive no longer. Especially in recent times, persons interacting with physicians are frequently rather healthy. They are coming in for a physical examination, for immunizations, or for medical services that do not imply illness—for prenatal visits and child-birth, for employment or insurance physicals, or for follow-up on some old medical problem. Other patients have illnesses, but they are chronic and stable. The cancer patient in remission, the patient in the cardiology exercise program following a myocardial infarction, and the chronic dialysis patient are examples. None of these persons is really sick to the extent of being incapable of participating actively in an ongoing patient-physician relation. Moreover, for those patients who are really so debilitated that they are incapable of active participation, someone else—a next of kin, parent, or court-appointed surrogate—often interacts with the physician with the ca-pacity for active partnership in the decisionmaking process.

It would be nice if we had a new term for the lay person in the health care relation. Some people, especially nurses, are now using the term *client*, but that also implies subordination. A client is a vassal or a dependent. To some people it also implies too commercial a role. Certainly *customer* has these negative connotations.

If patients (or their surrogates) are capable of functioning as active moral agents in communication with health professionals, they, like their physi-cians, ought to be thought of as having moral duties and rights. They ought to be viewed as partners in the moral enterprise of the patient-physician relation. The ethics of that relation is thus very important. But medical ethics also involves such aspects as the ethics of health policy and public action in the medical arena, the ethics of lay decisionmaking outside the patient role, and the ethics of research medicine involving studies on animals and with humans who are not patients.

Research involving persons who are patients as well as research subjects suggests a bridge between research and clinical medicine and their ethics. In *The Patient as Partner* I developed a theory of the ethics of the lay-profes-sional relationship in the context of medical research. At that time I promised that the exploration of this relation in clinical medicine would have to await another volume. This work fulfills that promise, focusing explicitly on the interaction of a person in the patient role with a physician or other health professional for the purpose of pursuing medical objectives that are the patient's and not primarily the physician's.

THE PATIENT AS PARTNER

In *The Patient as Partner* I proposed that the relationship between physician/medical researcher and patient/research subject should be viewed as a partnership, as a complex relation in which each has an agenda. The patient/subject might want to gain potential benefits of an untested therapy to which he or she has no access outside the research protocol, or perhaps to gain ancillary benefits—compensation, an interesting experience, or a feeling of moral worthiness from contributing to society. The researcher might want to contribute to medical knowledge or gain the glory of publishing a scientific article or the money that comes from the grant for the research. While these agendas are not by any means the same, they do have some common features. I argued that there is often sufficient convergence that an agreement—a contract or covenant—can be established permitting each to accomplish things that could not be achieved without the cooperation of the other. As a result, I suggested that the researcher/subject relationship should be structured as a contractual compromise, with neither party getting from the relation all of the things he or she would like. The subject may not be able to get exactly the medication she wants on the schedule she wants, but the researcher may not be able to get exactly the protocol and participants she wants either. The researchers may have to compromise not only in recruiting subjects, but in actually designing the research. The relation is rightfully the result of an active bargaining process, with each pursuing interests (including altruistic interests). The outcome is an active partnership mutually negotiated and agreed upon.

A MORAL THEORY OF THE
PATIENT-PHYSICIAN RELATION

In this volume I develop the same theme for the clinical patient-physician relation. If it is true that medical ethics involves the stances of lay people as well as health professionals, and that patients (or their surrogates) are often healthy enough to be substantially autonomous agents, then the patient-physician relation ought to be one in which both parties are active moral agents articulating their expectations of the interaction, their moral frameworks, and their moral commitments. The result should be a partnership grounded in a complex contractual relation of mutual promising and commitment. In this book I examine the dimensions of this moral partnership.

THE MORAL GROUNDING OF THE PARTNERSHIP

The contractual agreement and the partnership relation will necessarily have a moral foundation. That foundation was outlined in some detail in *The Patient as Partner*, but some additional aspects will be developed further here. Part I of this volume explores some foundational issues. It begins with a conceptual chapter that examines several alternative models for the patient-physician relation in contemporary medicine. It is quite fashionable today to challenge the model in which the physician is seen as authoritative, as a priest in secular garb, possessing secret knowledge and complex potions that can make the passive patient well again. That model is challenged here as well, but I go on to find equally offensive the diametrically opposed model of the physician as an engineer, a plumber, who will fix any problem at the patient's command. If the priestly model is offensive to the moral character and integrity of the patient, the engineering or plumber model is offensive to the character of the physician, who is also a human moral actor.

I go on to reject the idea of the physician and patient as equals with a complete convergence of interests. That model, in which I refer to the physician as a colleague or "pal" of the patient, simply does not take seriously the differences in ability, knowledge, power, and interests between the two parties. Instead I want to press the notion that a true partnership results when two persons of widely different backgrounds, find a point of mutual interest in which each can give to the other while retaining substantial autonomy. A covenant or contract spells out the obligations and expectations.

Having set the theme of partnership in chapter 1, I go on to explore the foundations and meaning of the moral terms of that relation. The central issue is the source of the norms for the relation. It should already be clear that there is no reason why the medical profession should be able to create them or even have a monopoly on articulating what they should be. If the relation is one of active partnership between two autonomous, intelligent actors, then each will have to contribute to articulating such norms. In chapter 2 I explore the way the contract metaphor provides alternative bases for the moral norms of the patient/physician relation. Here I reject the idea that the norms are generated de novo by two isolated individuals bargaining over the rules for the relation. Instead I turn to a much more moral contract, one with three stages including many more social dimensions. I suggest that the moral foundations of the patient-physician relation come, as all other moral norms do, from sources well beyond medicine—from sources understood and known through religious, philosophical, and rational methods, not merely from agreements among professionals or even from personal deals made by individual patients and their physicians.

Medical ethics in contemporary society, I argue in chapter 3, is shaped by the fact that medicine is normally practiced in a world where the physician is a stranger. In the typical encounter, physician and patient do not know each other very well. Even if they have met previously, they are not likely to share moral frameworks. They are unlikely to be of the same religion, social philosophy, socioeconomic and political persuasion, or moral instinct. This has radical implications for the patient-physician relation. It means that there is no basis for assuming prior to contractual agreement that the two parties are working with the same understanding of what constitutes the appropriate virtues for the relationship.

If I am right about the necessity of viewing the patient-physician relation as a partnership, then we are in for a very different future for medicine. In the next chapter I explore more fundamental conceptual matters. I suggest that ethical and other evaluative judgments are ubiquitous in the patient-physician relation, that they penetrate literally every decision that is made by either party. I illustrate the implications further in this and the following chapter, which examine two basic, but, I believe, misguided, concepts in medicine, the notions of "doctor's orders" and of "medical indications."

The Principles of Right Conduct

The normative ethical theory of right conduct presented in chapter 6 follows the theory developed in *The Patient as Partner* and more systematically in my *A Theory of Medical Ethics*. In *The Patient as Partner* I examined three major ethical principles: beneficence, autonomy, and justice. I made clear, however, that this list of principles is not exhaustive. A full list would include promise-keeping, veracity, avoiding killing, and what W. D. Ross recognized as duties deriving from previous relations with others, gratitude and reparation. It is now increasingly recognized that beneficence—that is, doing good—has been the dominant moral principle of traditional Hippocratic medical ethics. The physician's duty was to do what he thought would benefit the patient. Some have noticed that this ethic focuses on consequences, but in a way that differs from the dominant consequentialistic normative theory of the twentieth century, utilitarianism. While utilitarianism affirms the principle that an action is right if it does the greatest good for the greatest number, Hippocratic consequentialism counts as morally significant only consequences to the patient.

Much of the contemporary challenge to classical Hippocratism accepts the idea that there is more to ethics than simply maximizing good consequences in the individual act. But it pushes the point well beyond the Hippocratists. It insists that there are additional ethical moves that must be made. Some—the rule utilitarians—accept the grounding of ethics in consequences, but then offer some intermediary rules (sometimes called principles), which become the standards for assessing individual actions. Others—often called the deontologists—press for principles not on the grounds that they maximize consequences but as independent right-making characteristics of actions. Actions are right insofar as they respect autonomy, involve keeping promises, avoid falsehoods, avoid killing others, or distribute goods in morally just ways.

Virtually all of contemporary medical ethics incorporates some or all of these moves beyond mere maximizing of good consequences. In *The Patient as Partner* I argued that the informed consent movement in medical ethics can be understood adequately only as a manifestation of the principle of autonomy and its ascendance over Hippocratic beneficence. Likewise, the right of AIDS patients to experimental drugs such as AZT, even if granting access jeopardizes important medical research, can best be understood as a reconciliation of the principle of justice with the goal of maximizing social benefits. AIDS patients, as particularly disadvantaged members of the moral community, have special claims that override mere maximizing of the good.

The idea that nonconsequentialistic principles such as autonomy and justice take precedence over beneficence is an important feature of contemporary medical ethics. I go so far as to insist that there is an absolute lexical ordering of nonconsequentialistic principles over beneficence; that is, consequences do not count morally until these other principles have been satisfied. In *The Patient as Partner*, the lexical ordering of autonomy over producing good explained why persons were always given the right to consent (or refuse consent) to medical research no matter how much good would come from forcing people to be subjects against their will. In this volume it will help explain why competent, substantially autonomous patients have an absolute right of refusal of treatment even in cases where we can be quite certain that more good would be done for them if treatment were forced against their wishes.

CASUISTRY: THE ISSUES OF THE PATIENT-PHYSICIAN RELATION

Once we have an understanding of the principles of the patient-physician relation, including their meaning and justification, we can turn to the more obvious issues. In part II of this volume I examine the implications of the normative theory for conducting the day-to-day business of the individual patient-physician relation. There I examine some of the standard issues—informed consent, malpractice, truth-telling, and confidentiality. One of the more provocative implications of the partnership model is that responsibilities as well as rights extend to both parties. In the traditional Hippocratic model, in which the patient was a passive, uninformed recipient of the physician's largess, it made little sense to speak of the duties of the patient. Likewise, it was not normal to speak of the rights of physicians. The moral relationship was one-sided. In the partnership model, however, there is reciprocity. The final chapter in part II examines the duties of the patient and the rights of the professional in the contractual relation between the parties.

In an earlier day this might have been all there was to the ethics of the patient-physician relation. The moral relation was viewed as one involving only two parties. Today, however, we recognize that this individualist conception is inaccurate. There are always social dimensions to medical ethical decisions. In part III I examine these social relations, including problems of justice and the allocation of resources, transplantation, and death and dying.

We shall see that the partnership model has radical implications for every move that a physician makes. The patient as a partner will play a very different—a more active—role in deciding what counts as appropriate. The result is likely to be some behaviors very different from what the physician would have chosen.

In the final chapter, I put forward the bold thesis that contemporary medical ethics is so changing medicine that modern medicine—medicine as we have known it in the twentieth century—will be a thing of the past. It will be replaced by something I call contemporary or postmodern medicine, in which every move in the patient-physician interaction will be seen as requiring evaluative judgments—judgments that traditionally were made by the priestly physician but increasingly will be seen as more appropriate for the patient. This new medicine cannot simply lead to the often-proposed adjustment of having the physician give the patient the facts and then confer with the patient to incorporate his or her values into the treatment decision. That not only would make the physician a plumber, but it also would make the relationship unworkable. If in this new perspective values are ubiquitous, they penetrate even the process of conveying the so-called facts. They are logical necessities in deciding to make every clinical move.

If values were relevant only occasionally, in the ethically exotic cases, it would be fine to stop and confer with the patient, but if evaluation and conceptual framework shape every move made in medicine, then stopping for such a consultation becomes impossible. Something far more radical is in order.

The final chapter begins to explore some of that change. Just as the term *doctor's orders* is seen as a relic from a more authoritarian medicine, so many other terms in medicine will be challenged by the new order. The idea that certain drugs and treatments are the "drugs of choice," that safety and efficacy can be determined scientifically, will all be rejected. Even the notion that physicians should write prescriptions will be challenged. The very institutional structure of modern medicine will be called into question. The National Institutes of Health and the Food and Drug Administration, for example, will be given new tasks if we move to a postmodern medicine in which the patient is a partner in the decisionmaking process. Hospitals and other health care institutions that are thought of as operating without explicit moral, religious, and philosophical commitments will become an impossibility. I argue that soon we will have to pair up patients and physicians on the basis of their moral and philosophical frameworks, that hospitals will have to come to terms with the fact that they too have evaluative world views, and that patients will have to take a much more active part in the shaping of clinical practice.

The partnership model should not just be taken as a polite appeal for more respect and a more caring attitude on the part of health professionals. Far more, it is an appeal for a whole new basis for lay-professional relations, one that views patients and physicians as full, active partners negotiating a contract to pursue mutually shared objectives within a larger framework of cultural and subcultural commitments.

PART
I

The Foundations of the
Patient-Physician Relation

CHAPTER ONE

Models for Ethical Medicine in a Revolutionary Age

Most of the ethical questions in the practice of medicine come up in cases where the medical condition or desired procedure itself presents no moral problem. For the woman who spends five hours in the clinic waiting room with two screaming children waiting to be seen for the flu, the flu is not a special moral issue; her wait is. When medical students practice drawing blood from clinic patients in the cardiac care unit—when teaching material is treated as material—the moral problem is not really related to the patient's heart in the way it might be in a more exotic heart transplant. It is related to the whole relationship. Many more blood samples are drawn, however, than hearts transplanted. It is only by moving beyond the specific issues to more basic underlying ethical themes that the real ethical problems in medicine can be dealt with.

These themes are reflected in new possibilities for the relation between the patient and the physician, or, since important health care today is increasingly being delivered by other professionals such as nurses and pharmacists, between the lay person and the health care professional. Now, as never before, it is a matter of real controversy what the proper model should be for the relation between patient and professional. There are at least four options.

THE ENGINEERING MODEL

One of the impacts of the biological revolution has been to make physicians scientific. All too often they behave like applied scientists. The modern rhetoric is that scientists must be "pure." They must be factual and divorce themselves from all considerations of value. It has taken atomic bombs and Nazi medical research to show us the foolishness and danger of such a stance. In the first place the scientist, and certainly the applied scientist, just cannot logically be value-free. Choices must be made daily—in research design, in significance levels of statistical tests, and in perception of the "significant" observations from an infinite perceptual field—and each of these choices must be based on a frame of values. Even more so in an applied science such as medicine, choices based upon what is "significant," what is "valuable," must be made constantly. One response is to make the physician an engineer who will turn over to the patient the task of picking the values and setting the objectives of the medical relation. The physician becomes a plumber making repairs, connecting tubes, and flushing out clogged systems with no questions asked. In this model of the relation, the patient is simply presented with the facts and allowed to decide whether to use medical science to fix what he or she perceives to be a problem.

Physicians who think they can just present all the facts and let their patients make the choices are fooling themselves, even if it is morally sound and responsible to strive for objectivity when critical choices must be made. Even if physicians logically could eliminate all ethical and other value considerations from their decisionmaking, it would be morally outrageous for them to do so. Physicians who really believe abortion is murder, and yet agree to either perform one or refer to another physician, become moral automatons. Hopefully no physician would do so when confronted with a request for technical advice about murdering a postnatal human.

THE PRIESTLY MODEL

In proper moral revulsion to the model of the physician as a plumber, which completely excludes personal ethical judgments, some move to the opposite extreme, making the physician a new priest. Establishment sociologist of medicine Robert N. Wilson describes the physician-patient relationship as religious. "The doctor's office or the hospital room, for example," he says, "have somewhat the aura of a sanctuary"; "the patient must view his doctor in a manner far removed from the prosaic and the mundane."[1]

The priestly model leads to what I call the "as-a syndrome." The symptoms are verbal, but the disease is moral. The chief diagnostic sign is the phrase "speaking as a. . . ." In counseling a pregnant woman who has taken Thalidomide, a physician says, "The odds are against a normal baby, and speaking as a physician that is a risk you shouldn't take." One must ask what it is about medical training that lets this be said "as a physician" rather than as a friend or as a moral person or as a priest. The problem is one of generalization of expertise: transferring expertise in the technical aspects of a subject to expertise in moral advice.

The main ethical principle that summarizes this tradition is "Benefit and do no harm to the patient." It is reflected in the Hippocratic Oath, which is the foundation document for a medical ethics on the priestly model. Attacking the principle of doing no harm to the patient is a bit like attacking fatherhood. (Motherhood has not dominated the profession in the Western tradition.) But fatherhood has long been an alternative symbol for the priestly model; "Father" has traditionally been a personalistic metaphor for God and for the priest. Likewise, the classical medical sociology literature (the same literature using the religious images) uses the parent-child image as an analogy for the physician-patient relationship. It is this paternalism in the realm of values that is represented in the moral slogan "Benefit and do no harm to the patient." It takes the locus of decisionmaking away from the patient and places it in the hands of the professional. In doing so it destroys or at least minimizes the other moral themes essential to a more balanced ethical system. While a professional group may affirm this principle as adequate for a professional ethic, it is clear that society, more generally, has a much broader set of ethical norms. These norms, which I have discussed elsewhere[2] and will discuss more fully in later chapters of this volume, must include autonomy, fidelity, veracity, avoiding killing, and justice, as well as doing good and avoiding harm. If the professional group is affirming one norm while society affirms another for the same circumstances, then physicians are placed in the uncomfortable position of having to decide whether their loyalty is to the norms of their professional group or to those of the broader society.

THE COLLEGIAL MODEL

With the engineering model, physicians become plumbers without any moral integrity. With the priestly model, their moral authority so dominates the relationship that the patient's freedom and dignity are extinguished. In the effort to develop a more proper balance that would permit the other fundamental values and obligations to be preserved, some have suggested that the physician and the patient should see themselves as colleagues pursuing the common goal of eliminating illness and preserving the patient's health. When two individuals or groups are truly committed to common goals, then trust and confidence are justified and the collegial model is appropriate. It is a very pleasant, harmonious form of human interaction. There is an equality of dignity and respect, an equality of value contributions, lacking in the earlier models.

But social realism makes us ask the embarrassing question: Is there, in fact, any real basis for the assumption of mutual loyalty and goals, of common interest, that would permit this model to apply to the physician-patient relationship? There is some proleptic sign of such community in some elements of the radical health movement and free clinics, but for the most part we have to admit that ethnic, class, economic, and value differences make the assumption of common interest, which is necessary for the collegial model to function, a mere pipedream. What is needed is a more provisional model that permits equality in the realm of moral significance between patient and physician without making the utopian assumption of collegiality.

THE CONTRACTUAL MODEL

The model of social relationship that fits these conditions is that of the contract or covenant. The notion of contract should not be loaded with legalistic implications, but should be taken in its more symbolic form as in the traditional religious or marriage "contract" or "covenant."[3] Here two individuals or groups are interacting in such a way that there are obligations and expected benefits for both parties. These obligations and benefits are limited in scope, though, even if they are expressed in somewhat vague terms. The basic principles of autonomy, fidelity, veracity, avoiding killing, and justice are essential to a contractual relationship. The premise is trust and confidence, even though it is recognized that there is not a full mutuality of interests. Social sanctions institutionalize and stand behind the relationship, in case there is a violation of the contract, but for the most part the assumption is that there will be a faithful fulfillment of the obligations.

Only in the contractual model can there be a true sharing of ethical authority and responsibility. This avoids the moral abdication on the part of the physician in the engineering model and the moral abdication on the part of the patient in the priestly model. It also avoids the uncontrolled and false sense of equality in the collegial model. With the contractual relationship, physicians recognize that patients must maintain freedom of control over their own lives when significant choices are to be made. Should a physician not be able to live with his or her conscience under those terms, the contract is not made or is broken. This means there will have to be more open discussion of the moral premises underlying the medical decisions before and as they are made. With the contractual model, there is a sharing in which the patient has legitimate grounds for trusting that once the basic value framework for medical decisionmaking is mutually established, the myriad decisions regarding care that must be made daily will be made by the physician within that frame of reference.

In the contractual model, then, there is a real sharing of decisionmaking in such a way that both patients and physicians can be confident of retaining their moral integrity. In this context, the patient is ensured control of decisionmaking at the individual level without having to participate in every trivial decision. On the social level, community control of health care is made possible in the same way. The lay community is given and should be given the status of contractor, and thus is the locus of decisionmaking, but the day-to-day medical decisions can, with trust and confidence, rest with the medical community. If trust and confidence are broken, the contract is broken.

Medical ethics in the midst of the biological and social revolutions is dealing with a great number of new and difficult issues: in vitro fertilization, psychosurgery, happiness pills, brain death, and the military use of medical technology. But the real day-to-day ethical crises may not be nearly so exotic.

Whether the context is an exotic one or nothing more complicated medically than a routine physical exam, the selection of a model for the moral relationship between the professional and the lay communities will be decisive. This is the real framework for medical ethics in a revolutionary age. Understanding why the moral foundations of the relation ought to be seen as contractual and not simply generated by professionals is crucial to any development of a proper patient-physician relation. It is to this conflict between a professional source of ethics and a more universal, contractual source, and to a fuller explication of the nature of the contract, that we now turn.

CHAPTER TWO

Medical Ethics:
Professional or Universal?

I will impart a knowledge of the art to my own sons and those of
my teachers, and to disciples bound by stipulation and oath
according to the law of medicine, but to no others. I will follow
that system of regimen which, according to my ability and
judgment, I consider for the benefit of my patients, and abstain
from whatever harm or injustice.

—Hippocratic Oath

Act only on that maxim through which you can at the same time
will it should become a universal law.

—Immanuel Kant

From the first, professional ethics has been a hybrid. The scientific enterprise, which basically has universalistic tendencies, created a group with
special knowledge and interests; eventually it took on a separate identity as a
profession. Concern for the ethical point of view, which has the univer-
salizability of normative statements as its foundation, is particularized by
focusing on a specialized body of knowledge of a restricted professional
group.

In the fifth and fourth centuries, Greek science, including medical
science, was making its stand for rational autonomy and disciplined expertise
over against the folk tradition of magic, superstition, and mysticism. Hippocratic scientific medicine, at least in the earlier works of the corpus, stands
within this more scientific tradition. The Hippocratic author, attacking the
view that epilepsy was a "sacred disease," claimed: "It is not, in my opinion,
any more divine or more sacred than other diseases, but has a natural cause,
and its supposed divine origin is due to men's inexperience, and to their
wonder at its peculiar character."[1]

16

This special knowledge and experience distinguished the scientist from ordinary lay people. By the end of the fourth century, the scientist's role had come to be viewed as a special art, which in one significant trend gave rise to the quasi-religious oath that binds the Hippocratic physician to secrecy. His special knowledge is to be revealed to members of his brotherhood, his sons, the sons of his teachers, and disciples of the brotherhood, but to no others. Edelstein has shown that the Hippocratic Oath, in contrast to the earlier Hippocratic scientific writings, is heavily influenced by the Pythagorean cultic religio-scientific salvation quest.[2] Only upon the partial integration of the scientific enterprise with the religious calling could the professional Hippocratic physician combine the uniqueness of his rational, scientific pursuit with an ethical code that prescribes behavior that is uniquely normative for that profession. This setting apart of the professional scientist and the coupling of his intellectual, cognitive expertise with a unique set of normative patterns led Weber to his now-famous observation that the profession of science is a *Beruf,* a "calling," with all the religious overtones that that word carries. The very specialization that arose from the process of universalistic disenchantment of the world set apart a new priesthood with an inward calling to be pursued with passionate devotion.[3]

Neither the universalistic "pure science" model of the main body of the Hippocratic corpus nor the professional ethics model of the oath provides an adequate basis for dealing with the social and ethical dilemmas that arise in the practice of medicine. The "pure science" model maintains a necessary universal perspective—the recognition that certain phenomena are absolute in the sense of being independent of personal whim, cultural conditioning, or group affiliation—but does so at the expense of radically dichotomizing the scientific and the ethical. It provides the foundation for the application of pure science that I have referred to as the engineering model. The professional ethics model incorporates the necessary integration of the scientific and the ethical but at the same time particularizes or relativizes ethical responsibility by linking it with a particular group affiliation. It provides the basis for what I have called the priestly model. A medical ethic should be an integral component of a universal ethic, one which neither dichotomizes the ethical and the scientific nor makes ethical rightness dependent upon membership in a particular professional group. That, at any rate, is my contention.

Today there is a tremendous renewal of interest in the ethical responsibilities that arise out of the scientific enterprise. As medical ethics develops as a unique subspecialty, we must, from the outset, define its nature and limits. Two generations ago we knew what medical ethics was—a genteel code of etiquette among colleagues: do not advertise on billboards, do not air professional disputes in public, do show concern for the welfare of your patients. Today the definition is much less clear. Is the subject matter of medical ethics the personal moral requirements of the physician in relation to the patient, or does the concept include a social, political dimension that extends beyond personal ethics? Is medical ethics a subspecialty of ethics or of medicine or both? Is medical ethics something professional in scope in the sense that only members of the profession can define or articulate what the ethical norms are, or is it basically something more universal in the sense that lay people can also participate in specifying those norms? There is agreement only that it is more than a system of etiquette among professionals. I would like to explore here only one of these questions about the nature of the discipline of medical ethics: whether it is a "professional ethic," as is commonly assumed, or whether it is ultimately a specific application of a more universal system of ethical responsibility.

Whenever biological and medical scientists come together with philosophers, theologians, and ethicists to discuss matters of ethics and the life sciences, two basic problems emerge out of the particularistic perspectives of the disciplines involved. The first is the feeling on the part of the natural scientists that the philosophers and ethicists will claim to be experts in solving ethical dilemmas. This may be expressed as a hope that ethicists will provide clear answers to ethical dilemmas or the fear that they will think they are able to—depending on how well the natural scientists know their humanistic colleagues. At first glance it seems reasonable to assume that professionals devoting their lives to a discipline should have a peculiar expertise in that area. Why not so in the area of ethics? Most professional ethicists (at least those who do not have latent messianic tendencies) will claim that ethics is not like bridge-building; a professional ethicist cannot be expected to provide a simple answer to an ethical dilemma comparable to the one a civil engineer might give when asked whether a bridge will withstand the winter's wind. If ethics is a science at all, and I think it is, it is the science of describing ethical "events" and analyzing the implications of the use of various normative principles and ways of adjudicating ethical disputes. The ethicist, at least at this stage in the development of the discipline, has no inside track on prescribing specific courses of action in an ethical dilemma.

The second problem that emerges when ethicists and natural scientists come together to discuss questions of such ethical responsibility is the assumption, often by both parties, that the members of the relevant profession have a unique responsibility to specify the ethical norms for that professional context. In the words of Paul Ellwood, executive director of the American Rehabilitation Foundation, "Only the physician can determine what care is necessary, and only he can eliminate unneeded expense. He cannot be policed to do so, but must be motivated by professional ethics and by organizational arrangements which align his economic incentives with those of the consumer."[4]

What is the concept of "professional ethics" that is appealed to so frequently as the unique responsibility of a professional group, and why is it that professionals are thought to be in a better position than lay people, including ethicists, to make the ethical choices necessary to resolve problems in their field of technical competence?

TECHNICAL EXPERTISE AND ETHICAL DECISION-MAKING: THE FALLACY OF GENERALIZATION OF EXPERTISE

I want to take the second question first. It implies an error I referred to in chapter 1, the fallacy of generalization of expertise. Stated simply, it is the view that professionals with technical competence in a particular area also have some special expertise in the nontechnical values used to decide questions in their area.

An analysis of the structure of decisionmaking suggests that there are several components in the decisionmaking process.[5] These could be classified as secondary and primary. One secondary factor is psychological identification with certain groups. This component generates psychological predispositions on the part of decisionmakers to formulate problems in peculiar ways and identify with the interests of the reference groups. Another secondary factor is cultural identification with certain systems of meaning that generate cultural predispositions to use symbol systems, understand words, and interpret reality in characteristic patterns.

The primary factors in the decisionmaking process include, first, empirical data about the "relevant facts" in the situation and, second, a system for evaluating those facts to lead to an action such as deciding to use a medication. The secondary factors greatly influence the perception of the relevant facts as well as the system of evaluation. Further, the system of evaluation itself influences the selection of "relevant facts" and the perception of those facts. Even if we overlook these complications, however, it still is apparent that decisions must arise out of the interaction of "empirical," technical, "nonmoral facts" and the system of evaluation brought to bear on those facts.[6] Expertise in the technical component in no way necessarily conveys an expertise in the evaluation component.

We readily see the weakness of this illogical leap when it occurs in disciplines other than medicine. We would rightly be outraged if the government were to call upon Defense Department nuclear-bomb experts to decide whether it was moral to bomb an enemy city. In the first place, what we have called the secondary factors of psychological and cultural identification (such as loyalty to the military, military leaders, or the nationalistic enterprise, or acceptance of a particular technological world view) may bias measurements of the size of the bomb crater and the number of people killed and wounded. That is a preliminary problem, however—one which always hampers any scientific enterprise. Even if we were to assume that such experts were not in any way biased in their technical judgments, we must recognize that accurate determination of the nonmoral facts (crater size and casualty predictions) does not tell us whether it is moral to drop the bomb.

The same problem emerges when we attribute ethical expertise to medical professionals. One physician who is sensitive to the problem of generalization of expertise has observed that an abortion is no more a medical question than capital punishment through electrocution is a problem in electrical engineering.

A UNIVERSAL MEDICAL ETHIC

THE NOTION OF A UNIVERSAL ETHIC

An ethic can be called universal in the sense in which I am using the term if there is a single moral system, a single standard of reference for moral judgment, that should apply to everyone. For example, if one believed that to say an action was morally correct meant that a monotheistic god approved of that action, the holder of such a view would manifest a universalistic ethic. There would be a single standard of reference. If two monotheists were to engage in a dispute about morality, they would presumably agree that, at most, only one could be right, since God, which is the standard of reference, presumably does not consider a particular action moral and immoral at the same time. Since there is only one god in a monotheistic system, the ethical system is universal.

By contrast, if two parties in a moral dispute held that they lived in a polytheistic world in which each was loyal to a different god, their ethical system would be particularistic or relativistic if they agreed that each should judge an action right or wrong based on whether his god approved. One could hold that an action was right and the other that the same action was wrong simultaneously without contradiction.

There are other universal standards of morality besides a monotheistic god. If two people held that the standard of right and wrong was a universal natural law or reason, they could still view their ethical system as universal provided they agreed that there was only one natural law in the universe or only one rationality that provides a single definitive standard for determining whether a particular action is right or wrong. Just like the monotheists, if they were in a moral dispute, they would have to hold that both of them could not be right simultaneously in their judgments about a particular action.

A professional ethic is particularistic or relativistic to the extent that a claim is made that the normative standard for judging a professional's conduct is fundamentally distinct from the standard used for judging actions outside the profession. Sometimes the standard held out is the clinician's own conscience. Often, however, there will be acknowledgment of a higher standard. Individual members of the profession may be morally wrong even though they are acting according to individual conscience. The standard that a true professional ethic appeals to is more plausibly the consensus of the profession about what the norms of conduct are. Insofar as a professional ethic is one in which the profession itself is the professional's standard of reference, it is likely to be particularistic. Lay people presumably do not have access to that standard and must use some other.

UNIVERSAL, ROLE-SPECIFIC DUTIES

It should be clear, then, that not every normative code of behavior applied to a professional setting need be characterized as a particularistic "professional ethic." Suppose that a group of lay people and professionals held that the standard of reference for a moral system was reason (or universalistic natural law or the approval of a monotheistic god) and that by some method they had derived a set of principles for moral action based on this single universal standard. From that code they might, in turn, derive a set of moral norms or rules for persons acting in particular roles.

Imagine that from their single standard of reference they established two moral principles: fidelity and fairness. From these (and other principles of their system) they might derive moral rules for specific contexts. They might, for instance, explicate the notion of fidelity to determine that parents have special duties to their children—for example, to make sure they are given at least minimal nourishment even over and above other children who are equally needy. The same moral system derived from the same standard of reference might simultaneously explicate the principle of fairness to derive the rule that while in the role of relief agency manager, one should allocate food impartially. The relief agency manager, not being bound in a special relationship requiring the fidelity that obliges a parent, might be guided morally by the principle of fairness. Thus from a single universal system of ethics involving the principles of fidelity and fairness among others, special "role-specific" duties may be derived. It is not a contradiction to claim that one holds a universal ethic and that simultaneously there are special moral rules for people in special roles. The ethic remains universal provided that the special rules for parents and relief agency workers are viewed as being derived from a single universal source, that people in dispute about those rules ought, in principle, to be able to come to an agreement about the role-specific rules, and that if they continue to disagree, at least one of them must be wrong.

CHARACTERISTICS OF A PROFESSIONAL ETHIC

Sometimes what is called a professional ethic can be compatible with this notion of universalism. If, for example, the group of professionals and lay people referred to above held that there was a single standard of reference from which they could derive a set of ethical principles for assessing actions, their ethic would be universal. They might then reach further agreement on the moral rules for conduct in the role of physician or nurse or patient. The rules governing physicians, nurses, or other professionals might be referred to as a role-specific professional ethic. If the professional ethic were derived in this manner, it would be a universalist ethic.

Most professional ethical systems are not universalist in this way, however. Most incorporate some features that make them particularistic, including at least one of three claims: (1) professional groups themselves are the source of the moral norms that should be used in assessing professional conduct; (2) professional groups are the only ones who can know and articulate the proper moral norms for the professional role; or (3) professional groups are the only ones capable of adjudicating moral disputes. Each of these claims gives the professional group a special place in the ethics of professional conduct. Each has elements that make the professional ethic particularistic.

PROFESSIONAL GROUPS AS THE SOURCE OF MORAL NORMS

The most boldly particularistic claim is that professional groups actually generate the moral norms for their members. The holders of this position maintain that the ultimate standard of reference to decide what is right conduct in the professional role is the profession itself. If the physician wants to know whether it is wrong for a physician to perform an abortion or commit active mercy killing or sacrifice one patient for the good of another, the definitive standard of reference is what the profession says is right conduct.

The grounding of this claim is hard to determine. Some physicians have asserted that the "practice of medicine" has an internal morality and that the profession is the custodian of what is required by the practice. Some have argued, for example, that analysis of the concept of medicine reveals that its very nature requires a commitment to preservation of life which would make active killing even for mercy antithetical to the medical professional's role.

It is not clear yet whether this claim is particularistic. One of two claims may be made. On the one hand, medical professionals could declare that the profession is the only legitimate standard of reference in deciding what counts as morally appropriate conduct for physicians. If that were their claim, the medical ethic would remain universal. Lay people wanting to know the duty of the professional would simply have to ask the profession. That has the effect of placing nonprofessionals at the mercy of the profession in defining the professional role.

Some of the professional's potential actions have direct bearing on lay people. Physicians may maintain, for instance, that they have a professional obligation to treat patients against their will in order to preserve life. When asked the grounding of such a claim, they might say it derives from the profession's analysis of the concept of medicine. Some lay people may buy this argument, but it makes them very vulnerable to major life-and-death decisions for which they would be conceding no possibility of knowledge.

Alternatively, the profession may claim that lay people can turn to their own sources to determine what they think the proper duty of the physician is, but the profession is the ultimate standard of reference for its members.

That would be a truly relativistic or particularistic ethic akin to the two polytheists who would have to agree to disagree about ethics because there was more than one standard of reference.

It is hard to imagine why lay people would accept either of these understandings of the source of professional norms. Either the profession is the one definitive source, or it is the proper standard of reference for professionals, while some other standard (theological or philosophical analysis) would be relevant for the rest of the world. Lay people faced with either version of these claims would be subject to a set of moral norms that they would either have to take on faith (if the profession is the single definitive standard) or take with the knowledge of some other source that makes a different understanding of the duty of the professional appropriate.

Upon reflection, the idea that the profession is the definitive standard of reference for determining what is morally required of its members is terribly implausible. It makes the profession literally like a god—either the only god (for matters of determining professional norms), if the system is universalist, or one of the gods, if the system is relativist. It is hard to accept the notion that the profession actually determines the norms the way a god would or the way reason or natural law might. Surely it is possible, at least in theory, that the profession is wrong. The consensus of the profession about what is morally correct conduct for its members simply cannot be the ultimate reference point. Professionals and lay people alike must agree that the ultimate foundation of morality—even professional morality—must be outside professional agreement. Those who are members of religious traditions are likely to hold out that their religious framework provides the foundation for morality. Those who are more secular will turn to a basic philosophical system such as liberal political philosophy, with its use of reason as the grounding of moral norms.

PROFESSIONAL GROUPS AS ARTICULATORS OF MORAL NORMS

At this point professionals may retreat to a much less bold claim. When it is pointed out that it makes no sense to view a system of professional ethics as totally independent of more general moral systems, professionals may claim that, in fact, professional ethical duties do derive from more general systems. For example, many Western physicians are at least nominally within the Judeo-Christian tradition. Were they to claim that the profession is the ultimate standard of reference for professional norms, they would be committed to the view that professional ethics is in no way based on the morality of the Judeo-Christian tradition. This they should find discomforting.

This leaves the defender of a professional ethic in an awkward position. He wants to affirm a universal standard for morality and at the same time hold that the profession has some definitive role in determining the morality of the medical professional. One move at this point is to maintain that the duties of the physician are a set of role-specific duties derived from some more universal moral system, but that only the profession is capable of knowing what the implications of that system are for it. Only the profession can articulate what the role-specific duties are for its members.

The claim now shifts from an ontological one (that the profession generates the moral duty) to an epistemological one (that only the profession can know what the moral duty of professionals is). This may be based on claims about how moral norms for specific roles can be known. If, for example, experience in a role were a necessary condition for knowing how the general principles should be explicated to find the rules for acting in a specific role, then professionals could simultaneously hold that their ethic was universal and that only professionals could specify what the professional's duties were.

This still has the effect of leaving the lay person at the mercy of the professional definition of the professional's role. Some lay people may accept this conclusion, but it is far from plausible. Several problems arise.

First, there are cases where members of two professional groups must interact. For example, what should happen if a physician appearing before a judge in a judicial proceeding is faced with a dilemma about whether to reveal confidential information proving that a patient is not fit to be a pilot? The physician might hold that the problem is one of conflict between the principle of fidelity to the promise of confidentiality and the need to avoid harm to innocent third parties. The profession has traditionally resolved such a conflict in favor of fidelity to the promise of confidentiality.

The judge, however, may have a very different perspective. He may feel the responsibility to draw on his own profession to define the moral norms of conduct in the professional role. He may view the bar as the definitive source of knowledge about what is morally correct in resolving a conflict between fidelity to a promise of confidentiality and the duty to avoid harm to innocent third parties. Even if the two can agree that they are working with the same universal system of morality and that, in principle, there is a correct answer to the question of whether this confidence should be broken, they may not be able to agree on which principle should take priority. In fact, while the medical profession has tended to give priority to fidelity to promises, the legal profession has tended to give priority to avoiding harm to third parties in such cases. If each professional claims that the standard of his profession is definitive in applying the universal principles to the specific case, we are at an impasse.

The problem does not arise only between law and medicine. Imagine a conflict over whether physicians should perform abortions in a Catholic hospital. Even if the physician and the church hierarchy can agree on a system of ethics (such as Catholic moral theology), there is room for dispute over who has authority to determine what is morally appropriate conduct for the professional. The system of Catholic moral theology has, over the years, worked out a position on how moral truths are known. It appeals to the authority of tradition and reason as well as scripture and views the pope and other ecclesiastical professionals as being vested with interpretive authority.

Were this Catholic physician to claim that the medical profession had authoritative capacity to know what is moral for physicians, he would have to reject the theory of authority existing within his religious tradition. Likewise, Protestant and Jewish physicians will face a conflict between their religious traditions and the claim that only the medical profession can know what is moral for physicians.

An analogous problem arises for physicians who adhere to secular philosophical systems that include some theory of knowledge pertaining to how moral norms are known. One cannot simultaneously be in the Kantian tradition, with its emphasis on reason as a way of knowing, and hold that only members of a professional group can know the norms of conduct for that group, unless one were to hold that only the members of the group could be rational on such matters.

Medical lay people are in an even more precarious position when confronted with the claim that only professionals can know what is moral for professionals. For almost all actions of moral significance, professionals are interacting with lay people, or at least their actions have important impacts on lay people. The physician who insists that a treatment continue or that a confidence may not be revealed or that a placebo must be administered in a clinical trial is making a moral claim that has a substantial effect on those outside the profession. Even moral matters that appear to have direct impact only on intraprofessional relations can seriously affect lay people. For example, one element of traditional professional "ethics" that might appear to be a matter strictly among professionals is whether members of the profession or their families will receive professional services without fee. Yet a decision to treat other professionals without charge affects the availability of professional services and of scarce medical resources. To take another example, a moral decision about whether to report a colleague who is incompetent could be a life-and-death matter for some patient of that colleague. It is hard to imagine any matter of professional ethical conduct that does not have bearing on those outside the profession.

Is there any reason why lay people should accept the claim that only members of the profession have the capacity to know how to apply a universal ethical system to derive the norms of conduct for the professional role? It is hard to see what it would be.

The first defense of such a pattern might be that one has to know the relevant facts in order to make moral judgments. For medicine that could mean that one has to know the science of medicine in order to know what is morally appropriate conduct in the medical role. While knowledge of the relevant facts is a critical component of moral decisionmaking, that is really not the issue here. The question is whether knowledge of medical facts is in any way relevant to establishing moral norms.

Consider, for example, the question whether medical professionals ought to be governed by the rule that confidences may or must be broken when doing so will spare a third party from grave threat of bodily harm.

Certainly, professional knowledge may be necessary to know if there is actually a grave threat of harm, but that knowledge would appear to be irrelevant in making the actual moral decision whether information should be disclosed in such instances. Likewise, in considering whether physicians should be party to mercy killing in cases of intractable pain, considerable professional knowledge is surely required to determine whether pain is intractable, but that knowledge would seem to be irrelevant in determining the moral norm in regard to the acceptability of participation in mercy killing. It is just not plausible to hold that knowledge of the facts in a professional field is relevant to determining what the moral norms for the profession should be.

It may be, though, that experience in the professional role is what is needed in order to know the moral norms for that role. Here the claim is not based on knowledge of the facts, but derives more from long experience with the moral problems and the implications of alternative courses of action. It is conceivable that experience places one in a better position to assess moral norms for a professional role, but the implications of the argument are more radical than may be realized.

In military ethics this position has been widely rejected. We do not accept the notion that military generals (those with the relevant experience in war) should have authority to determine the moral norms for military conduct. To the contrary we take the view that that role may so distort one's perspective that military officers are actually poorer candidates for the task of determining moral norms. Those in the special professional role may have entered it because of unusual evaluative perspectives. Those inclined to think war is particularly evil, for example, would probably exclude themselves from the role. Having long experience in the role may further generate specialized moral and value perspectives that would be incorporated into moral norms articulated by the members of the profession. There is no reason to believe that the norms military officers would propose for themselves are superior to those that would be proposed by persons outside the military. It seems that a set of norms generated by a group with the richest, most diverse range of perspectives would be at least as good if not better.

Accepting the idea that members of a particular profession are specially suited to articulate the norms for that profession implies a willingness to accept the radical implications. Would physicians accept the proposition that lawyers are uniquely capable of articulating the moral norms for those in the legal profession—even when physicians are their clients? Would they accept the claim that only police can determine the norms of conduct for the police force? If the norms are derivative from a more general moral system (such as a religious or philosophical world view), then the question is, who can authoritatively interpret the implications of that world view for those acting in particular roles? The answer will depend on the ethical system involved. Those who hold to certain religious systems should be able to answer the question of who is authoritative in knowing moral norms from within those systems. Judaism has a richly developed theory of the role of rabbis, rab-binical councils, and Talmudic authorities in deriving moral norms. Like-wise, Catholicism has its theory of authority. Protestantism is known for its affirmation of the capacity of the lay person to know and understand. It has its secular analogue in democratic liberalism that affirms the capacity of the lay person to make judgments in this area. Anyone who stands in any of these traditions must reject the claim that professional groups have any special capacity to know and interpret the implications of a moral system for the professional role.

It is striking that even professionals themselves are increasingly accept-ing this conclusion. When the American Medical Association revised its code of ethics in 1980, it received a report from an ad hoc committee chaired by James S. Todd. That report acknowledged the increasing awareness that the professional role will be defined by society, saying, "The profession does not exist for itself, it exists for a purpose, and increasing that purpose will be defined by society."[7] This leads to the conclusion, not yet accepted by the AMA, that the lay person as well as the professional should be an active participant in defining the moral norms of the lay-professional relation. This will mean specifying norms not only for professional conduct, but also for the lay person who is an active participant in the relation. If a code of ethics is to be written for professional conduct, it should be written by lay people working along with professionals; it should be a public process, not one exclusively of a professional group.

PROFESSIONAL GROUPS AS ADJUDICATORS OF MORAL DISPUTES

There is one final claim that characterizes a professional ethic with particularistic tendencies. It is common for defenders of a professional ethic to hold that the profession should adjudicate disputes about its members' misconduct. This is presumably based on the belief that the profession either invents the norms or at least is most skilled in articulating what they are. If that were true, it would make sense for the profession to be responsible for deciding which of its members have violated the norms.

Often the question of violation of professional norms will raise subtle points of interpretation. If the norm requires disclosure of confidential information only when there is a threat of grave bodily harm, someone will have to decide how grave the harm has to be. If the norm justifies withhold-ing information from a patient in certain cases, the experts in the norms should determine whether such a case has arisen. It makes sense that those who are the source of the norm or those who are best at articulating it would be responsible for determining whether a violation has been committed.

If, however, the profession cannot justifiably claim to be the source of the norm or to be skilled in its articulation, then the presumption that the profession should adjudicate moral disputes is called into question. If, in fact, the members of a profession can be expected to have special moral perspec-tives (because that is what led them into the profession in the first place or that is what it socializes them into), then we would expect that if the profession adjudicates moral disputes, that special perspective will be reflected in their judgments.

Some criticize the use of professional mechanisms for dealing with charges that practitioners have acted unethically on sociological grounds that physicians are likely to protect their own. Convictions for professional misconduct, even for serious abuses of norms, were very infrequent until public pressures were brought to bear recently. It may well be that physicians have been lax on their colleagues, but that is not the real point. The real issue is that even if the professional group were impeccably conscientious in rigorously enforcing its own norms, it would still produce the wrong result if it had generated or articulated the wrong norms. Lay participation in the adjudication process not only will help ensure impartiality; it will also ensure that the interpretation of the norms reflects the full range of emphases and variations.

THE CONTRACT BASIS
FOR LAY-PROFESSIONAL MORALITY

If I am correct, it no longer makes sense for the moral norms of the lay-professional relation to be exclusively the province of professional groups. Physicians recognize the plausibility of this notion when they consider whether other professions (where the physician is a potential client) should have sole control over defining what the lay-professional relation should be. The alternative that makes the most sense is what in *A Theory of Medical Ethics* I called the *triple contract*.

The task is to define what the broad system of ethics ought to be for a society and then derive the proper norms for various lay-professional role relationships and the moral limits on individual interactions between individual lay persons and professionals. The theory ought to apply to all lay-professional relations. Thus, everyone should anticipate being the lay person in many such relations. A professional in one field will be in the lay role in many others. Arguing that the professional should be the sole determiner of moral norms for the relation will mean that all of us will be excluded from defining the norms for most professional relations.

The triple contract begins with the most fundamental task: formulating the basic ethical system—the general principles of right action that are perceived as applying to all human relations and from which more specific norms for more specific relations will be derived. Such a system will probably also include a theory of the virtues as well as a theory of how various principles and virtues are related to one another. Clearly the task is enormous, much more than can be attempted here. A summary of the method, developed more fully elsewhere, can be provided here, however.

In any moral community, the members have the task of agreeing on the basic principles. This implies that members of various religious and philosophical traditions will gather together to articulate their different ethical systems. Each will have its own presuppositions about who is authoritative and what the fundamental source (or sources) of norms may be. Members of various professions, who are also part of these traditions, would share with lay people in those traditions a common understanding not only of the right norms but of the theory of authority.

THE BASIC SOCIAL CONTRACT

Fortunately, members of modern society share a substantial consensus that no identifiable groups of experts exist in articulating what the basic principles are. Those who are committed to the universalist perspective and have a healthy skepticism about the capacity of individuals to make infallible judgments about moral norms often take the plausible view that the best ethical system will be the one that would be agreed to by people representing as many perspectives as possible.

The reason for this agreement is complex. Many people hold that there is a source of morality (a monotheistic god, reason, or natural law) such that the task is to discover as accurately as possible what the correct moral system is. Many Protestants, for example, hold that the moral order is defined or created by an all-powerful deity who has established a covenant with humans specifying proper moral conduct. They also hold, however, that humans are seriously flawed and fallible. The task is then one of knowing the content of that moral covenant.

Drawing on a long tradition dating back to the Old Testament, one attractive strategy is to gather the community together and ask it collectively to discern the content of that moral order. The Old Testament book of Nehemiah speaks of all members of the Israelite community—the gatekeepers and singers as well as the priests and Levites—entering into the covenant articulating its norms.[8] Insofar as the task is discovering the content of the ethical system that corresponds with the ultimate source of morality, those entering into the covenant will have to strive to make themselves as much like ideal observers as possible—eliminating imperfections in their relevant knowledge, their personal biases, and their lack of empathy with other points of view that could distort their perception of the moral order.[9] The result will be a goal of approximating ideal contractors similar to those described in hypothetical contract theories such as John Rawls's system.[10] It will differ, however, in that for those who are making use of a group of contractors to attempt to discover the moral system, the contract is simply an epistemological device—a strategy for knowing what that system is.

An important theoretical question is raised by those who believe that a moral system is simply invented by moral communities rather than discovered. They presumably would hold that the contractors can be much more arbitrary in articulating the basic moral system. While those holding that the system is discovered would have to concede that the contractors would be wrong, those who see the contractors inventing the system would presumably deny any such possibility. The practical significance of this difference is not obvious. There seems to be a real possibility that those who would discover the moral order and those who think they are inventing it can work together quite well. The result will be a system of ethics that is accepted by the contractors as a foundation for a moral society.

In *A Theory of Medical Ethics* I argued that the resulting system would include several fundamental principles, including beneficence and non-maleficence as well as autonomy, fidelity (or promise-keeping), veracity, avoiding killing, and justice. I further argued that the nonconsequentialist principles are coequal in their weight, but that taken together they take precedence over the consequentialist principles of beneficence and non-maleficence. This was, in effect, my reasoned speculation about what contractors would agree to under the conditions I specified. I, of course, cannot be certain that that would be the result without actually having the process take place. I think the evidence is overwhelming, however, that a system with these elements—that is, some nonconsequentialist principles such as autonomy and justice that take precedence over mere production of good consequences—is more plausible than the system of the traditional professional medical ethics that considers as right-making only the judgment of the clinician about what will benefit the patient. These principles will be summarized in chapter 6 of this volume.

Regardless of whether my own particular conclusions about fundamental principles would be sustained by such contractors, some basic set of principles, together with a theory of how they relate to one another, would emerge from the contract process. The result would be what I call the *basic social contract*. It specifies the norms of right action within the moral community.

THE LAY-PROFESSIONAL CONTRACT

Once this basic system is in place, with both parties contributing to its articulation, a second contract is possible: one defining the basic moral norms of the lay-professional relation. In medicine this would comprise the norms of conduct not only for physicians and other health professionals, but also for the other active participants in the relation, the lay participants. Since role-specific duties must be derived from the basic social norms, no formulation of professional or lay duties could violate the fundamental ethical system. On the other hand, special norms may be derived from the basic principles. Thus it may be agreed by lay people and professionals that the prima facie principle of avoiding killing should lead to a moral rule that those in the professional role of physician should never actively kill, even for mercy. Working from the prima facie principle of autonomy, it may be agreed that no physician has the authority to treat a patient without adequate consent. Deciding whether other ethical principles (such as beneficence) would support exceptions to this rule (such as in cases of "therapeutic privilege" where the clinician believed the patient would be better off if his autonomy were violated) will depend on the structure of the relation among principles in the basic system as identified by the social contract. The mere belief by professionals that beneficence justified a therapeutic deception would not be sufficient. A second contractual agreement would be needed to specify the norms of lay and professional role players within the framework of the basic social contract.

THE PERSONAL PATIENT-PHYSICIAN CONTRACT

Once the basic norms of the lay and professional roles are specified, there would presumably remain substantial room for discretion. For example, if the professional norm were specified that because of the principle of autonomy no physician would withhold potentially meaningful information from a patient without his consent, it would remain for the individual patient and physician to agree between themselves whether the patient might waive that right to consent. While the default rule would be that such information must be transmitted absent patient waiver of his or her right to it, in individual cases physicians and patients could agree to a therapeutic deception by having the patient authorize withholding diagnostic information of a certain type. The individual lay and professional actors would not be able to agree to any provisions that violated the basic social contract or the second contract between the lay population and the professional group. For example, if the basic social contract contained a norm that prohibited killing of the innocent, and because of that the second contract prohibited physician killing for mercy, then individual patients and physicians would not be able to agree to a mercy-killing contract. Barring such actions prohibited by the earlier contracts, however, the individual patient and physician pairs would be free to contract for whatever was mutually acceptable. An obstetrician and a woman patient could mutually agree that abortion would be outside the relationship and that the physician need not even raise the possibility in circumstances where most women would want to consider it. They could agree that birth control was out of bounds or was an essential part of the therapeutic relation.

The result is a triple or three-stage contract whereby the moral community comes together to articulate the basic ethical system, possibly constrained by what can be called the moral point of view, that is, the standards of ideal hypothetical contractors. Once that basic ethical system is in place, the social norms and rules for particular professional and lay roles could be defined. Finally, within the constraints of these two earlier agreements, the individual professional and lay person would be free to set personal moral limits on their relations. Both lay people and professionals are full, active participants entering into a partnership, first defining the moral limits and then selecting options within those limits.

The theory applies to all professional ethics, not just medicine. Lawyers would come together as a profession with lay people to define the moral limits of various legal roles within the constraints of the basic social contract.

Once those limits were defined, individual lawyers and lay people (including physicians in the role of lawyers' clients) would define the objectives of individual lay-professional relations. Some physicians would agree with their lawyer partners that their objective in responding to a malpractice claim would be to minimize the financial risk even if it meant accepting apparent guilt for an offense the physician knew he did not commit. Other lawyer/physician-clients would agree that even at the risk of financial loss, the goal of the relation would be to clear the client's name. The lawyer-professional would be constrained by the basic social contract as well as by the broad social agreement that defines the professional and lay roles for lawyer-client relations. That second contract would define such norms as lawyer-client privilege and its limits, as well as the extent of the moral duty of the lawyer to work for a client he knows is in the wrong.

We may not be able to agree on precisely what the foundation of professional ethics is, but we should be able to agree that it is something far different from whatever the profession says it is. We should be able to agree that both professionals and lay people have an active role in determining the moral norms of the relation and that individual contracts must function within the constraints of those earlier contractual arrangements.

CHAPTER THREE

The Physician as Stranger: The Ethics of the Anonymous Patient-Physician Relationship

In virtually everything that is written, said, or thought about the patient-physician relationship, the ideal of a close, long-term commitment is lurking. It is recognized that not all relationships between health professionals and lay people live up to that standard. In fact, physicians are often condemned for being distant, aloof, unconcerned about the life the patient leads in all its richness of beliefs, values, lifestyle, social involvements, and psychological problems. The "physician as friend," however, has been the ideal, and much of our medical ethical reflection has been oriented toward that ideal.

In contrast, a great deal of health care is delivered in a model in which the physician is a stranger. This is not because physicians are not warm, friendly, caring beings. Rather, the institutional structure of the health system available to increasing numbers of people today dictates that care will often be delivered between strangers, for example, in inner-city clinics, rural health centers, student health services, military and veterans' hospitals, tertiary care centers, and the offices of specialists seen for highly technical one-time referral consultations.

No one has explored what difference it makes in the medical sociology and the medical ethics of the patient-physician relationship whether the physician is assumed to be a friend, a long-term acquaintance knowledgeable about the beliefs, values, and lifestyles of the patient, or whether institutional constraints mandate that the physician will necessarily be a stranger. The nature of those medical ethical differences will be the focus of this chapter. The primary objective, therefore, is to explore the differences it should make in medical ethical theory whether the "stranger" or the "friend" model is operative, not to argue for the moral superiority of one or the other.

Only in the final section of the chapter will the normative dimension be broached, where it will be asked whether the traditional preference for the physician as friend is warranted, or if a case can be made for a morally normative distance between medical professional and lay person.

THE FRIEND/PHYSICIAN AS THE IDEAL

In labeling one model of the ideal patient-physician relationship as the "friend/physician," I have certain characteristics of friendship in mind. In the terms of Talcott Parsons,[1] the friendship relationship is functionally diffuse. It involves knowledge and even responsibility across a wide range of issues and many spheres of the individual's life. It contrasts with functional specificity, in which the physician and patient know each other and interact only in the narrower sphere of medicine. The character traits of the relationship are those of traditional friendship: compassion, kindness, sympathy, warmth, and fidelity. These stand in contrast to the character traits stereotypically attributed to the modern, more specialized, businesslike physician: efficiency, technical competence, impartiality, coldness, and distance.

THE FRIENDSHIP METAPHOR

I am using the imagery of friendship as a metaphor, recognizing that certain characteristics of friendship do not really apply. The ideal physician/patient relationship has more distance to it, more objectivity, than the more traditional friendship. The physician shows a concern that has been described as "detached."[2] While the physician is concerned about the plight of the patient, sufficient detachment ought to remain that emotional involvement cannot cloud the objectivity needed for good medical practice. Social interaction across a wide range of institutions outside medicine such as the church, schools, social clubs, and the like would be considered optional, but perhaps a desirable extra. Many essential characteristics of friendship, however, such as a long-term ongoing relationship, knowledge of family, and sensitivity to special interests, are included.

There is little doubt that the ideal physician is often considered a friend in this special, qualified sense in which I am using the term. Political scientist Richard Flathman, for example, says, "good physicians . . . have a close, perhaps even an intimate knowledge of their patients—knowledge extending well beyond their medical histories."[3] Physician Manfred Bleuler, writing in a journal with the remarkably unfriendly title *Diseases of the Nervous System,* makes explicit use of the friendship metaphor: "In the patient's pain, in his despair, in his misery, the patient called for a friend, a friend whom he can trust, a friend whose wisdom, whose willingness to help, whose integrity is beyond question, a man who understands his most secret and most personal problems, and the Doctor must be such a friend."[4] Physician Thomas P. Almy speaks of the need for the "personal touch" and for the patient-physician interaction to be "a more personal one."[5] The same longing for the model of the friend is expressed negatively in criticisms of the bureaucratization of medical care,[6] trends toward specialization, and "new intrusions" on the patient-physician relationship from institutionalizing medical care by moving into hospitals, groups, or teams, making the patient and the physician "units in a matrix."[7] There can be little doubt that this constellation of personal qualities that I have labeled "friendship" has been held widely to be an attractive, highly desirable way for patients and physicians to relate.

THE ETHICS OF THE FRIEND/PHYSICIAN MODEL

Assuming for the moment that the friend/physician is the model that should be normative for medical practice, one might inquire about its relationship to various theories of medical ethics. This analysis will require a few words about the notion of "theories" of medical ethics.[8] It is increasingly becoming apparent that medical ethics is not confined to ad hoc moral speculation about difficult cases and difficult topics such as abortion, experimentation, euthanasia, or genetic engineering. There is, and at least implicitly has been for centuries, a deeper, more coherent structure to moral reflection about medical decisions. Each major sociological or subcultural group has developed a more or less consistent *Weltanschauung*, a set of metaphysical and metaethical beliefs regardless of the topics that are at issue. Roman Catholic moral theology, for example, offers a rich tradition of ethics tracing back at least to Thomas Aquinas. Principles such as double effect and totality are derived from a teleological natural law doctrine that informs all work in medical ethics done from within this tradition.[9] Similarly, Jewish rabbinical scholarship offers a "theory" of medical ethics closely related to Jewish notions of the law, the sacredness of life, special obligations regarding the burial of the corpse, and the like.[10]

The mainstream of Western professional medical ethics, with self-conscious continuity from Hippocrates to the modern Western professional associations of physicians at least up to the middle of the twentieth century, also provides a theory of substantial consistency. The central principle, as stated in the Hippocratic Oath, is the physician's pledge to work "for the benefit of the sick according to my ability and judgment."[11] This paternalistic principle provides the moral foundation of the priestly model discussed in chapter 1. There is also a substantial emphasis on the ethics of virtue (although the specific virtues shift from the "purity and holiness" of the Hippocratic author to the "tenderness, steadiness, condescension, and authority" of Percival's code published in 1803,[12] and finally the modern AMA Principles emphasizing compassion and respect for dignity.[13]

Although it is not logically required, holders of the Hippocratic normative ethical principle that the physician should do what he thinks will benefit the patient normally make the kinds of metaethical claims we saw associated with professional ethics in chapter 2. In response to the question of how one knows that physicians should act on this principle, those working within what I am calling the Hippocratic tradition makes one of two claims. Sometimes members of the professional group maintain that they generate their own moral obligations as part of specifying what it is to be a member of the profession. Alternatively, they say that even though the moral norm is grounded in something more universal, only members of the professional group can know these principles. Thus, in either case, the professional group is the source or articulator of the moral norms.

The contract theory suggested in the last chapter is an alternative to this professional grounding of medical ethics that is attracting more attention. [14] While its characterization differs from author to author, its essential features include a broader base for the formulation of medical ethical principles, rules, and duties, including significant lay participation in medical ethical reflection; emphasis on deontological duties of fidelity, honesty, and respect for rights; and some notion of contractual or covenantal bond establishing the relationship between the profession and society and, on the individual level, between professional and patient.

What I am now suggesting is that the formulation of a model for the patient-physician relationship is influenced by the implicit medical ethical theory under which one is operating. In turn, within any given theory of medical ethics, whether the physician is viewed as a friend or a stranger may influence normative judgments bearing on the relationship. For example, if a theory included detailed rules of right conduct for lay-professional interactions, intimate, long-standing friendship between patient and physician might not be essential in determining right conduct on a whole range of issues such as sterilization, abortion, active mercy killing, etc. On the other hand, a hypothetical medical ethical theory operating on the principle that right conduct was determined by having the physician do what was most consistent with the patient's long-term subjective lifestyle preferences might require a substantial degree of long-term, intimate continuity of the sort I am characterizing by the metaphor "friendship."

The notion of theories of medical ethics gives us an analytical tool for exploring the ethical implications of the friend/physician and the stranger/ physician models of the lay-professional relationship. For purposes of simplicity I shall confine this initial exploration to the two major medical ethical theories competing in the ideological marketplace today: the Hippocratic and the contractual theories. We shall see that neither locks one in rigidly to the friend/physician or stranger/physician models. In fact, either can accommodate either of the models, but each requires considerable internal variation and modification to do so.

Hippocratic medical ethics and the friend/physician model

The Hippocratic ethic is often stated negatively as "First of all, do no harm," and even is rendered into Latin as *primum non nocere* (although it is possible that this is a late dignification of a modern folk ethic variant).[15] The priority of avoiding harm over helping does not exist in any ancient Greek or Latin texts of which I am aware. The Hippocratic tradition (whether stated in terms of positive or negative consequences) shows a particular affinity to the friend/physician model.

The Hippocratic ethic can be characterized as a form of individualistic, paternalistic consequentialism. It is an ethic in which consequences are what count. Furthermore, it limits the morally relevant consequences to those affecting the patient; it is individualistic. Finally, the standard of reference for judging what will benefit the patient is paternalistic: the benefits are assessed according to the physician's judgment.

In such a tradition, the friendship model is almost necessarily of crucial significance. If the physician's task is to use his or her judgment to benefit the patient, and one is at all enlightened about the significance of psychological, social, economic, religious, and cultural factors in the patient, then long-standing "friendship" in which the physician has knowledge of the broadest aspects of the patient's life is virtually essential. It is safe to say that Hippocratic medicine at its best must be holistic, must make the physician, if not a loving partner, at least a sibling or "best friend" in the medical sphere.

There is one way out of the friendship model for the Hippocratic physician—that is by retreating into an objectivist biological reductionism. This would require first of all that the patient's welfare be conceptualized as objective, that is, fixed in reality independent of subjective preferences. More than that is needed, however. If welfare were objective but still highly diffuse (dependent upon psychological, social, economic, and religious realities), the physician would still require intimate knowledge of the patient's objective situation. If, however, welfare were reduced to biological welfare (still conceptualized as objective), then quite possibly a physician could do what was in a patient's interest medically without any knowledge about the other spheres of the individual's life; in short, without the friendship. This is precisely what had happened in high-technology, bureaucratic, medicine by the mid-twentieth century. Physicians thought they could be a stranger in some tertiary care center and still do what was best for the kidney in room 374.

High-technology physicians are not the only ones who have made the biologically reductionistic move from within an essentially Hippocratic ethic. Ethicist Paul Ramsey, in his advocacy of a "medical indications policy" for establishing appropriate care for the incompetent terminally ill,[16] was committed to determining what was objectively in the patient's interest. He somehow accepted the strange, implausible assumption that such a determination could be made medically by a physician who was a total stranger to the patient, perhaps never having known that person while he or she was conscious, or anything about the patient's social system, family, psychology, or belief system. If the welfare of the patient is objective and can be reduced to biology, then one can be Hippocratic without the friendship. Otherwise it is hard to see how Hippocratic medicine could be practiced outside the friendship model.

Contract medical ethics and the friend/physician model

The relationship between contract or covenant medical ethics and the friendship model is more complex. Certainly the contract model, properly understood, can easily accommodate friendship between patient and physician.

One might think that the term *contract* implies a legalistic or businesslike relation between physician and patient and that the contract model is therefore inimical to friendship.[17] No one who takes this model seriously, however, has anything like that in mind. If there is to be a contractual ethic for medicine, all agree it must avoid those implications, emphasizing instead such notions as moral equality between the partners of the contract, fidelity to promises made, and a sense that the parties are autonomous agents capable of pledging and fulfilling pledges. The norms are trust, loyalty, respect, and faithfulness, not legalism and business bargaining. It will be along the lines of a "marriage contract," not the contract of the lawyer's office. That is why some now prefer the term *covenant*, which I take to be one special form of the more general notion of a contract.

The implications of this ethic for the friend/physician model depend somewhat on the exact working out of the contract theory. I shall illustrate this by using the triple theory of medical ethics, introduced in the last chapter and developed elsewhere.[18]

The contract or covenant theory of medical ethics accommodates the friend/physician model as easily as the more traditional Hippocratic ethic does. It does so, however, in a very different way. The Hippocratic ethic requires some degree of what we are calling friendship in order to fulfill the moral mandate to do what the physician thinks will benefit the patient (unless one retreats into the nasty world of an implausible objective biological reductionism). The contract or covenant ethic does not require friendship, but it can function effectively when the health professional and lay person know each other intimately over a long period, understanding each other's beliefs and values.

The contract ethic, when it functions within a friendship model, gives great prominence to the third contract. While fundamental principles for social interaction are established in the first contract, and the basic nature of the lay-professional relationship has limits set for it in the second, the third contract, the one between individual professional and lay person, will, when they have a long-term, trusting relationship, really be decisive. The physician and patient who know each other's beliefs, values, preferences, and tastes can incorporate them into their mutual understanding of the relationship. If they serve together on their church's "prolife" or hospice development committee, they may well already know each other's commitments so that the third contract can be an implicit, presumed agreement affecting many critical medical areas. If the physician sees his patient suffer when agony-prolonging extraordinary care is given to a dying patient, the foundation of spelling out a "third contract" regarding terminal care is already laid.

If the unique beliefs and values of the physician and the patient are to be respected and incorporated into the third contract, some degree of communication about them will have to take place. Over a period of time, patient and physician can determine whether there is a sufficient meeting of the minds that a mutually acceptable third contract can be established to provide a basis for the individualized friendship style of health care. It is the necessity for agreement at this third level of contract that will be explored in the final chapter of this volume.

Thus both the Hippocratic and the contract theories of medical ethics are compatible with the friend/physician model of health care. The Hippocratic almost necessarily requires it because the physician, charged with doing what he thinks will benefit the patient, must incorporate knowledge of the patient's life in order to make the judgments called for. The friendship is rather one-sided, to be sure. The patient need know relatively little about the physician's life. He is a rather passive partner in the friendship. An ongoing, trusting relationship is essential, however. The covenant or contract ethic can accommodate friendship in a truer, more reciprocal sense. Each needs to know the beliefs and values of the other to determine the content of the third contract, that is, to decide whether the commitments can be fine-tuned successfully to establish a unique relationship.

THE STRANGER/PHYSICIAN AS THE REALITY

The reality of the delivery of health care in most industrialized societies places severe constraints on the possibility of the development of the friend/physician model. A substantial portion of health care today is delivered in institutional settings where ongoing relationships are extremely difficult. The stranger/physician relationship is the norm in urban clinic and hospital outpatient services, student health services, military and veterans' hospitals, as well as tertiary care settings and specialist referrals. Some sense of the growing importance of anonymous contacts can be gleaned from the national and local data.

A 1978 National Health Interview Survey of the civilian, noninstitutionalized population revealed that, on an annual basis, for every 1,000 people, 642.7 physician visits took place in hospital outpatient departments and emergency rooms.[19] By contrast, 3,158.3 took place in doctors' offices or clinics or group practices. It is safe to assume that a substantial portion of the outpatient and virtually all the emergency room contacts were anonymous. Some smaller percentage of clinic and group practice contacts were also anonymous, and even some contacts in solo practice private offices were. Furthermore, these data exclude noncivilian care and care of "institutionalized patients" (in prisons, mental institutions, and other facilities where continuity of care is often minimal). Even among visits to office-based physicians, only 56.5 percent are to primary care physicians (GPs, internists, and pediatricians).[20] Even in a major university family practice center where continuity of care was a central commitment and patients were assigned to a specific physician, the average level of continuity of care was only 81 percent.[21] Given the mobility of the American population and the high incidence of "doctor-shopping" by dissatisfied patients (between 37 and 48 percent within a year depending on income level, in one study),[22] combined with the increasing incidence of institutionally based care, it is crucial to challenge the presumption that the ethics of the professional health care relation should be premised on the friend/physician model. It is critical to explore how the major theories of medical ethics can cope with the stranger/physician model.

HIPPOCRATIC MEDICAL ETHICS AND THE STRANGER/PHYSICIAN MODEL

It may not be an exaggeration to say that the Hippocratic ethical mandate cannot be fulfilled when the patient and physician are strangers. Aside from the move to biological reductionism, which is so implausible that it does not warrant further attention, there is no way for the stranger/physician to know what is really in the patient's welfare. There is simply no information upon which to base judgment.

When a misguided physician tries to continue in the Hippocratic mode even though the patient is a stranger, tragedy is likely to result. Dr. Robert Morse, the physician randomly assigned to Karen Quinlan, tried to guess what was in her interest in spite of the fact that he had never met her while she was conscious. His uninformed presumption about her welfare proved to be sadly out of line with the more informed judgments of her family, her friends, her priest—the unanimous judgment of all who knew her. The greatest danger of the Hippocratic ethic is that the friend/physician model may be assumed when the stranger/physician is the reality. If the physician must provide care for a stranger, it must be done on some basis other than Hippocratic paternalism, which requires knowledge of the patient.

CONTRACT MEDICAL ETHICS AND THE STRANGER/PHYSICIAN MODEL

It seems as though the stranger/physician relationship is also less than optimal under a contract or covenant ethic. In the language of the contract model developed here, when patient and physician are strangers, they cannot assume any content to the third covenant. There is no sharing of an understanding of unique belief and value.

In the case of the contract ethic, however, medical interaction between strangers is still possible. The moral structure is not limited to individualized judgments by physicians as to what counts as patient welfare given the subjective social-psychological, economic, religious, and other valuative dimensions of the patient's life. The care is delivered in the framework of the

two prior contracts. When the relationship is anonymous, the relative significance of the contracts simply shifts. The third contract decreases in importance. In the extreme case, when the patient is unconscious, for example, it
disappears altogether. The second contract (between the professional and the
society as a whole) remains to define the moral structure of the care to be
delivered.

In a world of anonymous health care, the second contract will have to
signal to all patterns of interaction that are to be presumed until the physician and patient (or agent for an incompetent patient) can reformulate them
by forming a limited third contract. For example, consider the doctrine of
the so-called therapeutic privilege, referred to in the previous chapter,[23]
under which physicians claim the "privilege" of withholding relevant information from patients such as the diagnosis of a terminal illness, the risk of a
therapeutic procedure, or even the entry of the patient into a research
protocol. The information is withheld on the grounds that disclosure would
be so upsetting that on balance it is in the patient's interest not to have it.

The therapeutic privilege is made for the Hippocratic ethic. Disclosure
and nondisclosure are dictated by the moral mandate to do what the physician, based on his or her judgment, thinks will benefit the patient. In the
ideal world of the friend/physician model, the physician, through long,
intimate contact, would know what information the patient would want to
know or have withheld on the grounds that it would be too upsetting. If the
goal of the therapeutic encounter is (paternalistic) patient benefit and the
model is friendship, the therapeutic privilege might be defensible.

In the contract ethic, a radically different approach is taken. If the
relation is one of friendship and the third contract dominates, patient and
physician can agree whether the physician (or anyone else) should have the
authority to withhold information on paternalistic grounds. If patient and
physician over the years have a clear understanding about what kinds of
information would be upsetting, and the patient has agreed that his physician
should treat him paternalistically regarding withholding information, then
the therapeutic privilege is probably tolerable. It is not a very dignified way
to treat one's friends, but in certain relationships paternalistic withholding
might be understandable. Likewise, patients might paternalistically withhold from their physicians information they think might upset them—that for
rational reasons a second opinion has been sought, that a medication has
been discontinued, or that some element of the physician's practice is
slightly offensive. The reciprocity of the therapeutic privilege will be explored further in chapter 17. The danger of such paternalistic agreements, of
course, is that one of the friends might guess incorrectly about what is really
in the other's interest. It is hard to argue, however, that limited agreements
authorizing mutual paternalism should be made illegal among consenting
adults.

Likewise, physicians and patients who know each other over a period of
time can negotiate a third contract excluding such paternalism. Most patients

today would not want information withheld on grounds of traditional therapeutic privilege. Many physicians are also finding that such a stance is uncomfortable or even offensive. If patients and physicians who share opposition to the therapeutic privilege wish to agree to such a lay/professional relationship, under the contract theory this is morally the appropriate way to handle the problem.

In the physician/stranger model, there is no basis for the therapeutic privilege in the Hippocratic ethic. There is no reason for the physician to know what information would upset the patient. The professional is reduced to the dangerous "golden rule" type of reasoning in which his or her own feelings, psychological set, and predicted reaction to bad news are substituted for those of the patient.

When patient and physician are strangers under a contract ethic, some pattern must be established at the level of the relationship between the society and the profession, that is, the level of the second contract. The two groups could agree that professionals would use their instincts to withhold information on therapeutic privilege grounds. It seems far more plausible, however, that the society and the profession would establish a fall-back position that stranger-patients should be told what reasonable people would want to know about their situations even if the physician believed this might upset them. This is precisely the position the society is adopting in the "reasonable person" court cases.[24]

Recently the question has arisen whether the reasonable person standard requires that patients be told what the typical "objective" reasonable person would want to know, or whether the information should be adjusted to take into account the special subjective desires, life plans, and values of the specific patient.[25] The emerging answer seems to be that, with certain qualifications, patients should be told what the typical "objective" reasonable person would want to know in order for a consent to be adequately informed, unless the one obtaining the consent has reason to believe that the specific patient would desire to know more or less in certain areas.

This recent development can be understood easily in the framework of the models of physician/friend and physician/stranger. In the pure case of the physician/stranger (where the physician knows nothing about the uniqueness of the patient), the "objective" reasonable person standard applies. The second contract in effect requires that patients be told what the objective reasonable person would want to know. As the physician gains knowledge of the patient's unique interests, the friendship model begins to become more appropriate. When the physician has reason to believe that the patient would reasonably require special kinds or amounts of information, the third contract requires that the more subjective reasonable person standard be substituted. The patient bears substantial responsibility for modifying the understanding of what a patient would want to know (although the physician may have the obligation to make reasonable deductions about the patient's uniqueness from the information available and to point out that those unique interests may be important in deciding what to disclose). The medical profession is increasingly accepting the wisdom of this position as well. In effect the second contract, the one between the profession and the society, establishes a fall-back position of the doctrine of the therapeutic privilege: it is unacceptable unless physician and patient concur on an individual basis for some authorization of it. The result is that the second contract establishes a societal, ethical pattern for all relationships between professionals and lay people that is publicly known and applicable to all unless modification is made between individuals who hold some other set of beliefs and values.

A wide range of problems in medical ethics can be handled in this way. Suppose, for example, a woman has been raped and seeks medical attention. Should the physician take the initiative to recommend diethylstilbestrol, which would function as a morning-after abortifacient? Some physicians may find even very early abortion following rape morally unacceptable. Furthermore, some may make the judgment that for particular patients, morning-after abortifacients may have serious psychological consequences. Given the wide range of beliefs and interpretations of potential consequences, some small percentage of physicians are likely to determine that it is morally unacceptable or contrary to the welfare of the patient even to initiate such conversation. Yet surely many such patients, especially those who are not aware of such a pharmacological option, would want to have that information.

Under the Hippocratic ethic of paternalistic patient benefit, the physician must use his or her judgment in deciding whether to initiate. If the patient and physician have a long-term friendship, perhaps knowing each other through a religious group as well as a medical relationship, the physician may well deduce correctly. In fact, some woman might be offended to have her physician suggest an abortifacient. If they are strangers, the physician can only guess.

Under the contract ethic, a community would mandate under the second contract a pattern of standard practice that both physician and patient could come to expect. The most obvious policy might be that physicians doing rape-crisis medical counseling should initiate such conversation until such time as the patient signaled that the discussion should cease. The physician who, for moral or other reasons, could not tolerate having to initiate such conversations would withdraw from rape-crisis medical services or limit such practice to patients with whom at least enough of a relationship had been established that a more individual (third contract) agreement was established that morning-after abortifacients following rape were excluded from the agenda. Once again the key is that with a contract ethic, some standard pattern of ethically acceptable behavior is established for stranger relationships. If the patient/physician relationship has evolved into a more personal one, special modifications can be negotiated to permit deviations from the standard, provided they do not violate more basic moral or legal obligations of the community.

The contract or covenant ethic is equipped to handle friendship relations when they exist. It is also appropriate, however, for structuring basic moral patterns for relationships between strangers that are increasingly the statistical norm.

THE STRANGER/PHYSICIAN AS IDEAL

The increasing frequency of the physician as stranger, of course, in no way implies that this relationship is morally normative. In fact, it is widely believed that the stranger/physician is at best an unfortunate necessity in a world of bureaucratic health care and a mobile society. Thus far the analysis of the implications of alternative medical ethical theories for the friendship and stranger relations has been descriptive. The goal has been to see how far each theory could take us in understanding the ethical dynamic of health care among those who are friends or strangers. It is interesting, however, to pursue a more normative assessment of the physician as stranger.

All of us would like to have a relationship with health professionals that takes into account our unique beliefs, values, ethical commitments, and lifestyles. Some degree of intimacy is required for this to happen, even if it is only assuring your oncologist that you would want to fight the cancer to the last gasp rather than be transferred to a hospice. I shall take the advantages of the friendship model as more or less obvious, the consensus wisdom of the community.

The interesting question is whether some people might actually prefer the physician as stranger, at least for certain kinds of medical encounters. Many patients seem to prefer the stranger in certain highly specialized, sensitive kinds of care. Patients seeking abortions, venereal disease treatment, and mental health therapy often seem to seek out strangers, wanting to avoid having to discuss such matters with long-term acquaintances. The anonymous patient-physician relationship offers privacy not available with more personal professional relations.

More generally, some personality types seem to favor maintenance of more compartmentalized lives. They simply prefer that those they know in one sphere are not deeply involved in other spheres, that those they see in church are not the same ones they deal with in business, in their children's school activities, in their entertainment, or in their health care. One type of contemporary personality seems not to require integration of the spheres of life. It is a pattern the psychiatrist Robert Lifton has labeled the "protean man."[26] Some people would rather not have to discuss their children with the grocery store clerk. Possibly these same personality types would prefer not to have to develop more sociologically diffuse relationships with physicians. Their reasons are numerous. Some, perhaps, would not want their "friends" to see them in weakness, which sometimes is the condition of patients seeking professional help. Others might simply prefer the sense of mystery that comes from being more private people or do not care to spend the time and energy necessary to build this particular set of friendships.

Another potential advantage of the stranger/physician model is that it avoids the danger of having the friend/physician attempt to estimate patient welfare or preferences based on what may be inadequate knowledge of the individual. Both Hippocratic and covenant medical ethics leave room for the physician to make judgments based on his or her perception of the patient's subjective position. The Hippocratic not only authorizes but actually encourages paternalism. The contract ethic leaves open the possibility that patients and physicians will gradually come to believe they have an understanding of a special set of normative relationships—of a unique third contract modifying the more general second contract. If one is concerned that there is a danger of misunderstanding in such presumed third contracts, then one might actually prefer the stranger relationship where no presumption could plausibly be warranted.

Upon reflection, it appears that one's preference for the stranger or friendship model of health care will depend on many variables, including personality type of patient and physician, the nature of the problem under consideration, and the specialty involved. It may also depend on how close one feels to what might be called the "core values" of the culture. Someone who is close to these values is likely to look approvingly on the general conditions of the second contract, so that his or her personal values will be reflected in the standard ethical presumptions that contract dictates for the stranger/physician. However, a patient whose personal values deviate greatly from the "core values" might make a special effort to find a physician who can accept the individual's uniqueness.

On the other hand, the patient whose values diverge from the core values may fear that a friend/physician will continue to act on the old Hippocratic ethic, doing what he or she thinks will serve the patient rather than what the patient might prefer. This individual may purposely seek out the stranger, knowing that such a physician ought to be less paternalistic and more confined by the second contract. The person with unique values would then carry the burden of informing the practitioner of that uniqueness, but would at least have the comfort of knowing that such a stranger/physician ought to behave in an ethically predictable manner and be open to patient-initiated discussions of variations.

One final argument in defense of the stranger relationship is quite subtle. It might be argued that patient dignity is often better preserved in this relationship than in the friendship model. For example, it might be felt that equal respect or dignity is best preserved between adults (age and other variables being equal) when each uses the same degree of familiarity in referring to the other—that both are on a first-name basis or refer to each other using surnames. In the friendship model, the physician will probably be referred to by title and surname, while the patient is often addressed on a first-name basis. In the stranger relationship, on the other hand, both parties may be inclined to use surnames. Increasing familiarity in a sociological context of substantial status differential may increase the gap in the degree of respect shown between the parties.

Certain types of medical practice may require the friendship or stranger relation more than others. For example, there is one type of practice where the stranger relationship is normative—actually preferred as the ideal. In psychiatry, establishing a therapeutic relationship with an old friend would be frowned upon. It is often considered especially important that the personal beliefs and values of the psychiatrist not be known to the patient. This is particularly strange, since if there is one sphere of medical practice in which the friendship model is especially important to patients, it would have to be psychiatry. Major therapeutic strategy choices and even the choice of underlying theory depend on the normative system of beliefs and values of the psychiatrist. If the patient, for example, exhibits a problem with a behavior that produces guilt, there is no way for the psychiatrist to know whether to treat the behavior or the guilt without deciding whether the behavior is appropriate, and there is no way of deciding that without a set of ethical and other normative commitments. One of the great differences between a psychiatrist and a minister/pastoral counsel is that the latter has stood before his or her potential client week after week, testifying to personally held theological, ethical, and philosophical beliefs that are certain to influence the counseling. In more ordinary kinds of medical care, however, some people may actually prefer to take their chances with the anonymous relationship, provided it is properly structured ethically by societal-level moral norms that we have been calling the second contract.

The implications for medical ethics of the identification of the unique ethical character of the anonymous patient/physician relationship are enormous. If the Hippocratic ethic is to be restored, the friendship model seems crucial. To the extent that more anonymous relationships are either inevitable or desirable, defenders of the Hippocratic ethic must look to the future with despair.

If the future includes medical practice by algorithm and eventually by computerized diagnosis and even mechanized storefront diagnostic centers (the grocery store coin-operated blood pressure machines being the precursors), then some other medical ethical theory will be a necessity. The contract or covenant theory is an alternative. It can accommodate the friendship model quite nicely, but also provides a foundation for health care relations among strangers. If it turns out that the stranger/physician is actually preferable, at least for certain people and certain kinds of care, then the contract ethic approach or some surrogate of it will be essential. It provides moral frameworks for both friendship and stranger relationships, although those frameworks are rather different.

CHAPTER FOUR

Values in Routine Medical Decisions

We have seen that there are alternatives to the Hippocratic conceptualization of the relation, that, in fact, the Hippocratic conception is probably dead. It rests on too many outmoded, implausible, and even unethical assumptions. We simply do not understand medicine, the physician's role, or the patient's, the way Hippocratic physicians did. While physicians were once thought to be members of a specially initiated elite possessing esoteric knowledge too dangerous for the lay person, now they are seen as mere human beings, people with special skills and knowledge who stand ready to help patients and their surrogates make choices that only patients are equipped to make. While patients were once thought of as helpless, infantile, passive recipients of the professional's largess, now they are increasingly seen as substantially autonomous agents capable of active participation in partnerships for the pursuit of their rights as well as their well-being. We are beginning to conceptualize medicine in a way that is radically different from medicine of the Hippocratic modern period.

This new conceptualization has implications for virtually every aspect of the professional-lay relation. Before we examine these implications for specific problems, though, something more general needs to be said about the basic conceptual shift that lies behind the adoption of the contractual approach to medical ethics and the partnership that this implies for the clinical relation. The new understanding sees values as being involved in literally every medical decision, not just in the ethically obvious cases.

The day is gone when medical decisions were seen as entirely value-free. Once we may have believed that good medicine was medicine grounded in good science in which physicians made technically correct choices. In that world compassionate, humane medicine was seen as important, but as fundamentally separate from technically competent medicine.

VALUES IN THE ETHICALLY EXOTIC CASE

The current generation of debate in medical ethics has changed all of that. Almost everyone recognizes that there are difficult choices in medicine that must incorporate value judgments. At the very least, most now recognize that so-called medical values underlie medical decisions. We choose a therapeutic regimen because it preserves life, relieves suffering, maintains health, or promotes well-being. These are values, albeit values thought of as inherent to medicine.

An increasing number of cases even pose ethical choices that cannot be made simply on the basis of values inherent in medicine. Karen Quinlan symbolizes the necessity of incorporating ethical and other value choices from outside medicine into therapeutic decisions. Medicine could tell us that this twenty-one-year-old patient was in a permanent vegetative state, that she could be maintained indefinitely, but that she could never be restored to consciousness. What it could not tell us was whether it was a good thing to maintain her in that state.

Sensitive clinicians now recognize that occasional decisions raise ethical issues that must be settled by appealing to beliefs and values from outside medicine. Different religious traditions hold different views about such matters. Catholics have a notion that some treatments are extraordinary because they do not offer benefits proportional to burdens. Orthodox Jews hold that life is sacred and should be maintained even if the patient will never recover from a coma. Secular philosophical systems offer analogous answers.

The need to incorporate ethical and other values arises not only in terminal illness but in many other cases as well: abortion and contraception, in vitro fertilization and the use of surrogate mothers, gene manipulation, organ transplant, resource allocation decisions when there are not enough ICU beds for the patients who could benefit from them. These are what could be called the exotic cases in contemporary medical ethics.

Most compassionate and sensitive physicians are now willing to consult with patients in such cases, explain the options, and permit patients to express their value preferences so that clinical decisions can be based, at least in part, on those values. The logic is that clinical choices in these cases involve both medical facts and nonmedical values. The clinician can supply the medical facts, and a set of nonmedical values as well, but patients can also supply those values. Since it is the patient who will be most affected, his or her values need to be recognized and incorporated into the clinical decision.

But clinicians may be tricked by these ethically exotic cases. As long as they believe that patient values are relevant to clinical choices only in relatively rare, special cases, most medicine can be practiced on the older model. Physicians can revert back to the idea that certain treatments are "medically indicated" and that most routine therapeutic decisions can be made based on their own clinical judgments without the necessity of using nonmedical values.

VALUES IN THE ROUTINE CASE

That assumption is now being called into question, however. A great deal of work has been done in the past decade on the nature and structure of clinical decisionmaking. The logic that has been developed for the ethically exotic case seems to apply to more routine medical decisions as well. Every routine problem involves a clinician's assessment of the medical facts of the case, an exploration of the treatment options, an assessment of the potential risks and benefits of those options, and finally, a choice based on some set of values among the plausible options. Consider a typical routine case.

CASE 1: THE ETHIC OF THE BROKEN ARM

A college student who had previously suffered a broken arm had pins placed by an orthopedic surgeon. He was now having day surgery to remove the pins. After the successful completion of the surgery, the surgeon placed a cast on the arm and, when the patient was comfortable and able to communicate, told him the following. "The standard practice would probably be to leave the cast on your arm for six weeks. I have found, however, that if you are careful, four weeks is enough. So I'll schedule an appointment for four weeks from now to remove the cast."

The surgeon and patient probably did not consider the possibility that evaluative judgments were involved in the selection of the four-week period. Yet some interesting choices were being made based on someone's values. First, it is striking that the surgeon reports the consensus of his colleagues and then announces he favors a different course. He may have believed that there was a scientific disagreement, that somehow it was a fact that either four or six weeks was the correct length of time to keep a cast on an arm for this purpose. Actually, what seems to be at stake is a values disagreement. To oversimplify, the shorter the time the cast is on the arm, the greater the risk of reinjuring the bone before the screw holes have mended. Shortening the length of time the cast is on the arm increases that risk. On the other hand, the cast is inconvenient and uncomfortable, and interferes with the student's schoolwork.

Deciding the correct length of time is really a trade-off between the risk of reinjury and the inconvenience of the cast. Moreover, if the cast can reasonably be taken off sooner if the patient is willing to be careful, that willingness and the impact on the patient's lifestyle become relevant. From this perspective, there can be no scientifically correct answer to the question of how long the cast should be on the arm. It could well be that this surgeon differs from his colleagues simply because his values differ.

If that is the case, what role ought the patient's values play in the decision about how long the cast is to be on the arm? There must be some period of time where reasonable people will disagree on exactly what the proper value trade-offs are. Conceivably, the patient is even more cast-averse than this surgeon. Or he may be even less cast-averse than the surgeon's colleagues.

When the patient who suggested this example was consulted, he introduced value dimensions that neither the surgeon nor his colleagues could have anticipated. The next time he would be home from school was in seven weeks. Coming home to have the cast removed before then would mean missing two days of classes, something he did not want to do. He was willing to wear the cast for a period of time even longer than the consensus would suggest because he placed high value on something unrelated to orthopedics.

If the patient's nonmedical values can play a central role in a decision as mundane as deciding when to remove a cast, they can, using the same logic, play a role in literally every move the clinician makes. Hundreds of other examples could be given. When a decision is made about having a patient leave the hospital, the economic and psychological costs of the hospital are traded off against the benefits of staying. Different physicians and different patients evaluate these choices differently. When salt is excluded from a diet, the blood pressure risks must be compared with the joy of salted food. When morphine is selected for pain control, the personal and social risks of addiction must be compared with the relief of suffering. When a decision is made to give routinely every patient a copy of his or her medical records or to keep them from patients, a trade-off is made between treating patients as autonomous agents and protecting them from the risk of possible harm from bad news or misunderstanding. Two very different sets of beliefs and values are at stake, incorporating, on the one hand, the Hippocratic notion that patients should be passive and, on the other, the more modern "Protestant" view that the lay person can be trusted with the text. Every prescription that is written, every lab test done, every recommendation of an office visit, every preventive strategy suggested has to incorporate what we now can call nonmedical values. To be sure, the stakes will not always be as high as in the ethically exotic cases. They will not be life-and-death value choices, but they will be value choices nonetheless.

Deciding to use any medication involves an assessment of the risks and benefits of alternatives and a decision that one set is superior. Those choices will involve economic alternatives, trade-offs among subtle psychological and social risks, as well as more obvious organic pharmacological risks. Clinicians with different value systems can and do routinely make different choices. There is every reason to assume that patients have value profiles that are relevant to these choices, and normally very little reason to assume that the patient's value profile is the same as that of the clinician. Even long-standing, ongoing physician-patient relationships normally have not been established on the basis of a value match at this level of subtlety.

CHANGING CLINICAL PRACTICE TO RESPECT PATIENT VALUES

The implications are radical. As long as the patient's values were important only for relatively rare "ethically exotic" cases, the clinician could easily call time out from the normal practice of technically competent medicine and consult with the patient or surrogate about which values should be used. If, however, values must be incorporated constantly in every move the clinician makes, it becomes impossible to stop and discuss every pertinent value with the patient. Yet it seems unfair to patients to have choices about their health and well-being made based on someone else's values, especially since we know that other clinicians would have drawn on other values. The values in routine medical decisions are going to pose pervasive problems for clinicians who want to respect patients' autonomy and dignity.

Several strategies are emerging to cope with these problems. One is to have patients and clinicians pair up purposely based on values. Hospice-oriented patients and clinicians come together in a special kind of value-oriented institution. Feminist patients and physicians cluster around feminist health care centers. Patients and physicians with similar views on abortion and contraception can cluster together. But will they be able to cluster around more mundane values? Does it make sense to make value-matching one of the appropriate elements in establishing patient-physician relationships?

One thing seems clear: the development of sensitivity to values that emerged around a few ethically difficult cases has now left us with a much different, much larger problem. Only when clinicians and patients begin to be aware of the value dimensions of even these routine medical choices will we begin to develop strategies for responding appropriately.

THE CONCEPT OF "DOCTOR'S ORDERS"

The active participation of patients (and patient surrogates) in medical decisionmaking is grounded on the notion that values from outside medicine must enter into such determinations. The patients in the partnership model are the primary persons with the skill to decide what is good medicine, because they are usually the ones who best know what will maximize their own well-being, and even in cases where a patient does not know best, he or she still bears certain rights of decisionmaking grounded in the principle of autonomy.

This partnership approach to decisionmaking poses serious problems for certain key concepts and terms used in traditional Hippocratic modern medicine. One of the most common and problematic is the notion of "doctor's orders." This term is pervasive in medical usage, accepted by lay person and clinician alike even though it implies authority and decisionmaking relations that no longer make sense.

One of the most common places where the term *orders* appears is in the "do not resuscitate order," to be discussed in more detail in chapter 25. The "do not resuscitate order" has become an important phenomenon in the evolution of more responsive and humane care of critically and terminally ill patients. Guidelines for decisions pertaining to resuscitation have been developed and are the source of much research,[1] therapeutic discussion,[2] and policy debate.[3]

What is going on when an institution as important as health care chooses the image of order-giver? At the same time, society and the health professions alike are moving toward a consensual or covenantal model in which the patient makes choices with the support of significant others including family, friends, clergy, and health care professionals.

As we have seen, we are at a point where we may have to choose among competing models for structuring the relation between the health professional and the lay person. One model, what I have called the priestly model, is a residuum from the day when medicine was viewed as the realm of experts with the authority that comes from possessing potent, secret wisdom, symbolized by the pledge in the Hippocratic Oath that the knowledge of the group was to be kept secret and that experts with that knowledge had authority to make decisions for patients. Another model, the partnership or contract model, emphasizes cooperation in which physicians work with patients toward the common goals of disease treatment, disease prevention, and health promotion.

It is hard to escape the conclusion that the language of order-giving had its origins in and fits best with the former model. The question then is whether it is meaningful or appropriate for the newer, more cooperative approach to decisionmaking. Part of the controversy stems from two quite different uses of the term. *Doctor's orders* in the first sense fits best with the more traditional model. The orders are authoritative instructions based on the physician's judgment about what, under the circumstances, is in the patient's best interest. It is assumed that the physician can determine what is most fitting for the patient. For matters such as ordering resuscitation or ordering its omission, where the choice is heavily contingent on the patient's own beliefs and values, we have seen that such decisions cannot be based on the practitioner's judgment. That is why most of the formal guidelines on resuscitation have insisted that the choice belongs to the patient.

Why, then, do the guidelines on resuscitation (and many other commentators) still speak of orders? It must be that the term is being used in a newer, more sophisticated way. Some say that *orders* is being used as the standard term for communication from physicians—including communications of the patient's judgment about whether care is accepted or refused. The physicians then are not ordering on their own; they are transmitting the patient's choice (the patient's orders).

But is that the right term for the newer, more cooperative era in which patients are viewed as more active decisionmakers? Many professions rely on authoritative transmission of instructions without giving orders. Business professionals do not speak of giving orders to their staffs; researchers do not talk of giving orders to their research teams. They ask, request, say "please," and adopt the other subtleties of respectful speech even when it is understood by all that such requests are to be carried out. Only physicians and military officers still speak of giving orders. Why is it, then, that physicians, even if they are only transmitting decisions patients have made about accepting or refusing care, are so firmly attached to the language of order-giving? It is just not appropriate to use such language in the newer, more cooperative model of the patient-physician partnership. The term *doctor's orders* is an offensive throwback to the more authoritarian days of Hippocratic paternalism when it was mistakenly believed that only physicians knew what was medically indicated for the patient. We now know that is not true.

CHAPTER FIVE

The Concept of "Medical Indications"

If the notion of doctor's orders is problematic in a partnership model of medical decision making, the concept of a *medical indication* is more so. Like doctor's orders, the notion of a treatment's being medically indicated is built on an understanding of medical decisionmaking that incorporates assumptions that are no longer tenable. The implication is that simply by knowing medical science well, a practitioner can determine the appropriate treatment for a patient independent of the patient's beliefs, values, and commitments. Central to the partnership model is the position that it is literally impossible to know what is good medicine without knowing whether an intervention furthers the rights and well-being of the patient, and it is impossible to know whether these are furthered without involving the patient actively in the decisionmaking process. The literature on the "do not resuscitate" order that so comfortably makes use of the notion of doctor's orders also frequently incorporates the notion of medically indicated treatment.

The Report of the 1985 National Conference on Standards and Guidelines for Cardiopulmonary Resuscitation and Emerging Cardiac Care states that "the physician has an obligation to initiate CPR when medically indicated. . . ."[1] In doing so, the report relies on the concept of a procedure's being "medically indicated." Federal regulations have been established in the United States to protect seriously afflicted newborns from unwarranted refusal of treatment. These so-called Baby Doe regulations require that states have in place programs to respond to reports of medical neglect "including instances of withholding of medically indicated treatment from disabled infants with life-threatening conditions."[2] Once again, major life-and-death judgments rely on the concept of a procedure being medically indicated.

The critical issue, of course, is what is meant by the term *medically indicated*. Pharmacology textbooks list medical indications. Package inserts list conditions for which various medications are "indicated." But neither the regulation writers nor their critics have ever really asked what it means for a treatment or procedure to be "medically indicated."

The dictionary defines *indicate* as "to demonstrate or suggest the necessity or advisability of." To say that a procedure is "medically" indicated apparently would mean that medical science or medical people have demonstrated or suggested its necessity or advisability. The nature of that demonstration, the kind of evidence that medical professionals would bring forth in the process, is not at all clear.

THE MEANING OF "MEDICALLY INDICATED"

"MEDICALLY INDICATED" AS A MATTER OF FACT

It is widely assumed among medical professionals that whether a treatment is indicated is a matter of medical fact. If a drug produces no imaginable benefits for a particular diagnosis, it seems to be a matter of medical fact that that medication is not indicated. On the other hand, medications or other treatment interventions that produce clearly desirable effects are said to be indicated. It seems to be a simple matter of fact.

Yet the judgment that a predicted result is desirable can never be a matter of fact, as we normally use the term. Such a conclusion is always a judgment involving values. Sometimes those value judgments are obvious and uncontroversial. But often they are not. For example, penicillin is said to be indicated for pneumonia (assuming that no "contraindications" are present, such as a history of anaphylaxis). But even in this apparently simple matter, it is not obvious that the result of overcoming a pneumococcal infection is always desirable. It is not only religious objectors to the use of drugs who might conclude that, on balance, killing the microorganisms through the use of a chemotherapeutic agent is not desirable. Some patients with painful terminal illnesses and short life expectancies might well conclude that taking penicillin for pneumonia might prolong their agony and delay the inevitable. In fact, it is even an evaluative judgment to conclude that it is a desirable result to prevent death from pneumonia when the survivor can live a long, healthy, happy life. It is an evaluative judgment about which there is a substantial consensus, but an evaluative judgment nevertheless.

What is the role of medical science and medical expertise in making these evaluative judgments? Modern science routinely relies on a fact/value dichotomy.[3] Science, it is held, can tell us the expected outcomes of alternative interventions and the probabilities of possible outcomes. It can tell us, for example, the probability of surviving a pneumococcal infection with and without penicillin of a particular dosage. It can predict the possibilities of various so-called side effects. What it cannot do is tell us whether the possible outcomes are good or bad.

Some people hold that the evaluation of outcomes is purely subjective, that "value judgments" imply that there is no objective basis for deciding whether an outcome is good or bad. One need not take the subjective position regarding all evaluations, however. It is sometimes held that certain evaluative judgments—such as ethical evaluative judgments—have some objective basis. They are grounded in natural law, in religious decree, or in reason that has an objective foundation.

It is not necessary to reach agreement on whether evaluative judgments are subjective or objective. Holders of either position ought to agree that the evaluations are not derivable directly from medical science. Regardless of whether it might be objectively good to preserve life of a particular form or only subjectively good, it cannot be determined from medical science alone that it is good to do so.

"Medically Indicated" as a Matter of Professional Evaluation

If deciding whether a treatment or procedure is good or bad is necessarily a matter of evaluation and cannot be determined directly from medical facts, then what is the role of medical professionals in making such judgments? A somewhat more sophisticated account of what it means for a drug, treatment, or procedure to be medically indicated concedes that evaluation must take place, but in relevant relation to medical professional competence.

The most important version of this position holds that medical professionals become experts not only on a set of facts and a scientific method, but also on a set of values, sometimes called medical values. These values, it is held, are inherent in a practice or profession.[4] They are inherent in what it means to be a physician. They are learned during the long process of socialization in medical school and the apprenticeship system to which young physicians are exposed. The values that are supposedly absorbed include the importance of prolonging life, relieving suffering, promoting health, and so forth.

Let us assume for purposes of discussion that physicians really do learn some such set of professional values and that they form the basis of clinical judgments about what interventions are medically indicated. If so, then a statement that a procedure is "medically indicated" means nothing more than that medical people have assessed the probable benefits and harms of its use in a particular circumstance and have found that, based on these special professional values, the net benefits are greater than those of any alternative course of action. If this is what it means for a chemotherapeutic agent or other medical procedure to be medically indicated, it creates two insurmountable problems.

Value Conflicts Internal to Medical Professionalism

First, assuming that medical professionals make assessments based on a set of "medical values," there will be evaluative conflicts internal to the set of those values we have identified. Any reasonable statement of the goals of medicine will contain multiple objectives—such as preserving life and relieving suffering. In order to determine that a drug is medically indicated for a particular condition, one must determine not only that it will preserve life or relieve suffering, but that it will offer the proper mix of these goals.

In recent medical history there was a deviant interpretation of the goal of medicine that gave a first and absolute priority to preserving life. That was never the position of classical Hippocratic medicine. It has been established that the duty to preserve life is, in fact, a duty without classical roots.[5] It has never been endorsed by an formal medical professional associations. To be sure, it is an accepted ethical position of some religious groups such as Orthodox Jews. It is, and should be, respected, but as a religious ethical conclusion, not a consensus of medical professionals about what is inherent in the practice of medicine.

The problem is that if judgments about when interventions are medically indicated are to be based on the values internal to the practice of medicine, then the medical profession as a whole must be able properly to balance these and other apparently competing values. We must be told not only that it is inherent in medicine to preserve life and relieve suffering, but also exactly when it is appropriate to sacrifice life preservation in order to prevent suffering and vice versa. There is absolutely no reason to assume that physicians as a professional group do or should agree on these value trade-offs. Health professionals, like all other persons, vary in their judgments about the balancing of competing values and goals. The task of reaching agreement about the proper balance seems both impossibly difficult and pointless.

Value Conflicts between Professional Medicine and Other Value Systems

Even if we could get the entire profession to agree that one particular mix of values internal to medicine is the correct one, there is no reason to accept the idea that that set of values is appropriate for persons who are not members of that professional community. Those persons would instead derive their own values from other sources—from religious, philosophical, and ethical traditions grounded outside professional medicine. Thus, even if we could get medical professionals to agree on a set of values as the basis for their judgments about what drugs and other medical procedures are "indicated," there is no reason to suppose that nonprofessionals would or should share those values. In fact, if special values about life preservation and relief of suffering lead people to choose medicine as a career in the first place, we should expect that the value consensus reached by such people would be atypical of the more general population. Medical lay people ought to hold different values, and therefore ought to get the wrong answer in deciding for patients when treatments are worth it.

This is especially true when we realize that a decision about an action will reasonably take into account a much wider range of value concerns than merely those on the medical professional's agenda. Reasonable lay people will want to consider not only life preservation, relief of suffering, promotion of health, and the like, but also economic costs, the impact on one's family, the long-term ecological concerns, and just plain matters of taste. In other words, even if some constellation of medical values would be served by an intervention, other concerns may rule it out.

One possible interpretation is that an intervention is "medically indicated" if it is in accord with the value consensus of medical professionals (even though it is unreasonable for lay people to share that value consensus). Another would be that an intervention is "medically indicated" if it corresponds with a lay person's medical agenda, while recognizing that any reasonable lay person has agendas well beyond the medical so that what is "medically" indicated may nevertheless not be the reasonable thing for the person to do. In either interpretation, claiming that a procedure is medically indicated says very little about what a reasonable person ought to do when all things are considered.

THE IMPLICATIONS: TWO EXAMPLES

The implications of this analysis are radical. It undercuts the widespread assumption that a decision that an intervention is medically indicated is a decision based on science or on the objective medical judgments of competent professionals. To see further the implications, let us examine two examples: the use of the concept "medically indicated" in pharmacology and related clinical sciences, and its use in public policy discourse.

"MEDICALLY INDICATED" IN PHARMACOLOGY

The idea that a chemotherapeutic agent is "medically indicated" is common in pharmacology. A similar notion is used in surgery, internal medicine, and other clinical sciences in referring to procedures and interventions that are thought to be beneficial on balance.

In pharmacology, an author of an article or a text often claims that a drug is medically indicated for certain conditions. Normally, this assertion is accompanied by a list of conditions under which the drug is "contraindicated." It appears that these are claims rooted only in good medical science, but that appearance is deceptive.

For an author to claim that a drug is indicated is to say that, according to someone's values, the medical or total benefits of the drug exceed the harms from the drug and the condition being discussed. Insofar as a pharmacologist is making claims about total benefits, she is clearly beyond her sphere of expertise. Such a judgment would require comparing the total benefits of the drug with the total negative consequences. This takes the pharmacologist into the realm of economic, religious, social, and aesthetic trade-offs, in which she clearly has no special competence.

Even if the judgment is limited to medical benefits, however, the claim is problematic. Consider, for example, the assertion that a particular nonnarcotic analgesic is indicated for the pain of headache. Underlying such a claim are some obvious evaluative judgments, such as that it is bad to have a headache, but also some more subtle judgments. For example, it might include the judgment that the benefit of eliminating the headache outweighs the potential harms of a one-in-ten-thousand or one-in-a-hundred-thousand risk of a particular blood dyscrasia that could result from the use of the drug. That is a judgment that is extremely difficult to make even for one limiting his attention to so-called medical values. It depends not only on how bad it is to risk the blood dyscrasia, but also on how bad it is to have a headache.

Closely related is the concept of a "drug of choice." Claiming that a particular drug is the drug of choice is simply to say that, according to the values of the one making the claim, its benefit/harm ratio is better than that of any alternative for the same condition. If deciding that a drug is indicated is a necessarily evaluative process, deciding that it is better than alternatives is an even more subtle evaluation about which pharmacologists have no particular authority.

"MEDICALLY INDICATED" IN PUBLIC POLICY

A similar problem emerges in public policy discourse. Often in debates over insurance, research procedures, the right of access to care, or the limits of treatment refusal by patients and their surrogates, policy makers make use of the concept of medical indication. Insurance will cover medically indicated treatments; community health clinics will provide indigents with the care that is medically indicated; parents will be permitted to refuse treatment only when it is not medically indicated.

These are all attempts to convert the evaluative judgment into a scientific judgment. They make it appear that medical science alone can determine when a treatment is appropriate and when it is not. A governor debating funding of medication for AIDS patients was quoted as saying he did not oppose care that was medically indicated. Controversy over drug funding in a catastrophic health insurance plan provided that generic medication should be dispensed except when trade names were medically indicated. In a DNR protocol, physicians were permitted to override familial treatment-refusal decisions when resuscitation was medically indicated.

Let us illustrate with a more extended analysis of one particular example, the Baby Doe regulations. Those regulations say that it is medical neglect to withhold medically indicated treatment from a disabled infant with a life-threatening condition,[6] to fail to provide "treatment (including appropriate nutrition, hydration, and medication) which, in the treatment physician's (or physicians') reasonable medical judgment, will be most likely to be effective in ameliorating or correcting all such conditions." "Medically indicated" is made to sound like a judgment based on medical science. However, it relies on the clinician's "reasonable medical judgment" that the intervention is likely to be effective in "ameliorating or correcting" the conditions. Both *ameliorating* and *correcting* are evaluative judgments with considerable ambiguity.

The criterion appears to be eliminating life-threatening conditions or lessening the probability that life will be threatened. If that is the case, the regulation writers are leaving to medical judgment only the determination of whether an intervention will increase the chances of survival. If so, they are, in fact, making a normative judgment—that treatment should always be rendered whenever it will preserve life. While that is a determination that policy makers might appropriately make, it is duplicitous to call all such treatments medically indicated. They are simply "morally appropriate interventions" if one believes that life should always be preserved. An ethical evaluation has been couched in language making it sound scientific.

This interpretation is further supported by the fact that three exceptions to the requirement of providing life-prolonging treatment are given: the term *medically indicated* does not include treatment that would merely prolong dying, treatment of the infant who is irreversibly comatose, or treatment that is virtually futile and inhumane. There is absolutely nothing aside from ethical judgments that makes treatment under these conditions not medically indicated; in all three instances it would prolong infants' lives. There may be good *moral* reasons why treatment ought not be provided in these circumstances: It is only temporarily life-prolonging in the case of the inevitably dying infant; it is deemed of no value in the case of the comatose infant; and it is inhumanely burdensome in the case of care that is virtually futile and inhumane. Many moral systems recognize that it is not morally required to offer treatment in such circumstances, but there is absolutely no reason to call treatment in these situations medically not indicated.

Likewise, there are instances where holders of many ethical values believe that treatment is morally expendable because it is useless or inhumanely burdensome even though none of these three conditions is met. For example, Catholic moral theology holds that treatment is morally expendable if it is gravely burdensome even though it is not virtually futile. An Orthodox Jew or a federal regulation writer who disagrees has every right to do so based on his or her religious or philosophical system of values, but it is meaningless to call treatment in such circumstances "medically indicated." That is simply an effort to buy an aura of scientific necessity for what is actually an ethical judgment.

The regulations provide one further example in their definition of "medically indicated" of an attempt to medicalize what are essentially evaluative judgments. The regulations specify that "appropriate" nutrition, hydration, and medication are medically indicated even in cases where no further treatment is necessary. The withholding of such nutrition, hydration, and medication is considered the withholding of a medically indicated treatment. But in what sense are these medically indicated?

Once again it is possible to adopt an ethical position that nutrition, hydration, and medication are morally required even for infants for whom a decision has been made that no other treatment should be provided. It adds nothing, however, to call such treatment medically indicated. It is simply morally required according to holders of this view.

To make matters more complicated, only "appropriate" nutrition, hydration, and medication are medically indicated. Presumably the authors had in mind excluding the feeding of an infant with a tracheoesophageal fistula when doing so would cause the infant's death. However, deciding that feeding other infants for whom other treatment is being withheld is appropriate is once again a moral judgment. There is an emerging consensus that any nutrition can be viewed as useless or burdensome when it merely prolongs the dying process of a comatose or semiconscious suffering patient.[7]

While there are also opinions and state laws to the contrary, the crucial point is that whether nutrition and hydration are ever expendable is a matter of ethical and other value judgment, not a matter of medical fact. That is why reasonable people might so understandably disagree on such issues.

To say that an intervention is indicated is to say that someone has assessed its probable benefits and harms and has found that, based on his or her values and beliefs, there are net benefits. If calling something medically indicated is really a subtle way of saying it is desired based on a particular set of values, then what is the implication for the relation of the medical profession, the government, and the general population in making such decisions? It appears to medicalize crucial ethical and policy determinations and to transfer decisionmaking from public officials and lay persons to those with medical expertise.

Since calling something medically indicated is really a matter of value judgment and not medical fact, it is understandable if reasonable people might disagree on at least some such assessments. It is for this reason that, at least in a liberal society, government regulation makes sense only in cases where the value judgments made are so powerful and so convincing that they can be imposed on a dissenting minority. That surely is sometimes the case, at least in decisions involving surrogates for incompetents. Parents are not permitted to abuse their children. The government has a legitimate role in preventing what is clearly child abuse. But, as I shall argue in chapter 24, it should permit some range of latitude in the judgments about what constitutes abuse. Determining what that latitude should be is necessarily a nonscientific question. Referring to treatments as "medically indicated" simply hides the true nature of the choices being made and transfers critical policy questions to medical professionals who may not share the broader public's ethical and policy framework.

Since what is being debated is the wisdom or correctness of a value judgment and not a matter of medical fact, it is odd that the standard of reference for deciding what would constitute an unacceptable result is, as the regulations specify, "the physician's reasonable medical judgment." It is not clear what is "medical" about the judgment that a particular kind of nutrition is required or expendable for a comatose infant. If the problem were one requiring medical knowledge, skill, or wisdom—the sort of question that at first appears at stake when one speaks of "medical indications"—then it would make sense for the physician's judgment to be the standard of reference. But if the issue of whether a treatment is indicated really reduces to a question of whether it is ethically appropriate, then it is hard to see why individual lay persons are not capable of making such choices.

Deciding that an intervention is indicated is really deciding that it fits some set of beliefs and values. As long as the lay person's beliefs and values do not lead to intolerable impacts on other persons, they ought to be the standard of reference for deciding what is appropriate. As long as that judgment is tolerable for the physician involved, he or she should be permitted to cooperate in the plan of care chosen. Government should intervene only where there is a strong possibility of harm to unconsenting parties. Calling treatments that are judged overwhelmingly beneficial "medically indicated treatments" adds very little except confusion.

CHAPTER SIX

The Principles for Medical Ethics

To build an ethic for the lay-professional relationship, we must go back to the basic principles of the first or social contract. In the professional ethics discussed and rejected in chapter 2, the professions themselves generated or at least articulated the ethical principles or norms for the professional role. They sometimes went so far as to define the moral requirements for the lay person in the professional relation as well.

NORMATIVE ETHICS: THE DEATH OF THE HIPPOCRATIC PRINCIPLE

Professional medicine at this point has provided a content for the second contract that is substantively different from that of other professions. Journalists, for example, have placed special emphasis on the ethics of protecting their sources. Scientists have stressed the value of knowledge. Each profession as it has articulated its code of ethics has emphasized certain normative principles. The task of those studying professional ethics is to identify what those unique norms are and how they relate to the norms of more general systems of religious and secular ethics.

The Hippocratic principle of benefiting the patient according to the physician's judgment[1] has been the moral norm of traditional, professionally articulated, medical ethics. That same idea was repeated in the ethical codes written by physicians and nurses throughout the centuries. It is in Florence Nightingale's Pledge taken by nurses over the past century. It is in the World Medical Association's Declaration of Geneva. Although at first it seems benign, it clearly is morally unacceptable on several counts. Fortunately, recent rewriting of professional codes has abandoned the Hippocratic principle in favor of much more sophisticated and more plausible ethical principles.

HIPPOCRATIC PATERNALISM

Of the many problems with the Hippocratic principle, three deserve special attention: its paternalism, its individualism, and its consequentialism. The problems can be illustrated by a case that, although it at first seems rather mundane, will, I believe, turn out to be the most important case in twentieth-century medical ethics.

CASE 2: CONFIDENTIALITY AND CONTRACEPTION

Dr. Brown practiced medicine in Birmingham, England.[2] In the early 1970s, when this case first received attention, he had been the family physician for a young woman and her family since her birth some sixteen years before. At the time the case became a problem, the young woman had decided she was in need of medical advice about contraception. She realized that Dr. Brown might not look kindly on such a request, so she went instead to the Birmingham Brook Advisory Center, the local equivalent of a Planned Parenthood clinic. After a physical exam and history, she was prescribed some birth control pills. During the course of the visit she was routinely asked the name of any family physician and whether it would be acceptable to communicate the prescriptions written to him in case of any need for follow-up. At this point the young woman made her mistake. Apparently without thinking, she disclosed Dr. Brown's name.

Soon thereafter Dr. Brown received in the mail information that his patient was on the pill. He was troubled by the pharmacological risks, but also the psychological and moral risks. After consulting with his colleagues, he finally decided his course of action. He disclosed to the young woman's father that she was on the pill.

In the proceedings that followed, Dr. Brown was charged with violating his patient's right of confidentiality. His defense, however, raised serious questions about the Hippocratic principle as a foundation for the ethical obligations of the physician. When charged with violating confidentiality, the physician could appeal both to the Hippocratic Oath and to the contemporary codes of the British and American Medical Associations. The Hippocratic Oath states that the physician should not disclose those things "which on no account one must spread abroad."[3] That, of course, leaves open the question of what ought to be spread abroad. That can be answered by the Hippocratic principle: the physician should use his judgment to try to benefit his patient and protect her from harm. Although Dr. Brown's judgment might not have been exactly what other people's would have been, that was precisely what he was doing. Should he really do what he believes will benefit his patient?

This ethical justification of breaking confidentiality to try to benefit the patient was repeated in the ethical codes of the British and American Medical Associations in effect at the time. Both permitted breaking confidence for the good of the patient.[4] The problems begin to become apparent. The Hippocratic principle is blatantly paternalistic. It justifies a physician's behavior whenever it is designed to try to benefit the patient regardless of whether the patient approves of it or believes it would really be beneficial. This paternalism also makes clear why the traditional physician might decide to withhold certain information from the consent process regardless of whether the patient would have wanted it. It reveals why physicians until very recently would often refuse to inform a patient of a diagnosis of a fatal illness.[5]

The historical evidence indicates that in its original context, the Hippocratic Oath was based on a philosophical system that saw physicians as possessors of information that could be too dangerous for lay people. The line that talks of protecting patients from harm has been interpreted as condoning paternalism. The physician was to protect the patient from harm that the patient might do to himself.[6]

What sort of underlying ethical principles for a society (i.e., those in the first contract) and beliefs about the facts would be necessary to justify this paternalism? It is the kind of ethical conclusion that might follow from a basic commitment to the position that a course of action is ethical if no other course would produce more good. If, for example, medical professionals began with the premise that the principle of beneficence should be the normative basis of the selection of more specific ethical principles for the professional, that would open the door to the Hippocratic formula. Beneficence is the principle that a right-making characteristic of actions is that they do good. Sometimes they also include the principle of nonmaleficence, that avoiding harming others is a right-making characteristic of actions. Sometimes beneficence is used as an inclusive term including both doing good and avoiding harm. The general principle of beneficence could lead professionals to conclude that in the professional role, the physician's duty is to do what he thinks will benefit the patient. Beneficence implies that even when doing good is paternalistic, that is, even when the good is done against the wishes of the one who is benefited, the action is morally justified. Any ethical system that includes no additional ethical principles such as autonomy is open to the possibility of paternalism.

A second, empirical assumption would be needed for the medical profession to accept the Hippocratic principle with its paternalistic implications. The profession would have to believe that the most reliable way for the physician to benefit the patient would be to do what he or she believed to be in the patient's best interest. On its face that seems a very implausible assumption when one considers the alternatives. Those in the liberal tradition often believe that individuals themselves are more likely than anyone else to know what will maximize their own welfare. If one accepted the empirical presupposition that patients themselves are the best judges of what will benefit them, then even for a system that included beneficence as its only principle, the role-specific duty of the professional would be to do what would benefit the patient according to the patient's judgment rather than according to the professional's judgment.

Upon reflection, there are many reasons why physicians ought not simply do whatever the patient says will be beneficial. Some of these have to do with the need to factor in benefits to others. That issue will be taken up momentarily. First, however, the case for paternalism should be examined more closely. Even the patient-affirming liberal should concede that in some cases the patient may not be the best judge of his own interests. At least for patients who are confused, and probably for those who are ignorant of the relevant facts or are suffering extreme anguish, it seems possible that some other parties may be better judges of their welfare.

That does not necessarily provide support for the Hippocratic form of paternalism, however. First, even if the patient is not always the best judge of his own welfare, it does not follow that his physician will be. Would it not make more sense, if one wants to be paternalistic, to let the consensus of professional medical opinion determine what is in the patient's interest rather than the possibly idiosyncratic judgments of the individual clinician? It seems odd to conclude that just because some minority of physicians, including the patient's physician, believes that laetrile or some other un-tested and potentially dangerous medication is best for the patient that it really is best. Even the paternalist who thought that the medical welfare of the patient should be decisive would appear more plausibly to use some more objective standard for medical welfare rather than the individual clinician's judgment.7

Those who consider the principle of beneficence to be the single and decisive principle at the level of the basic social contract face still another objection to medical paternalism even if a more objective standard were substituted. Is there any reason to believe that we would always maximize the welfare of an individual who was not the best judge of his own interests by going to the best, most objective judges of his *medical* welfare? The best interest of the patient as a whole presumably would require consideration of not only medical welfare, but also welfare in all other spheres, including psychological, social, educational, economic, aesthetic, and so forth. It seems unlikely that individual physicians are always the best judge of a patient's medical welfare, and it seems unlikely that the best judges of medical welfare are the best judges of welfare as a whole. The principle of beneficence, even in its paternalistic form, cannot support the Hippocratic interpretation of the physician's moral duty.

All of this discussion, of course, is built on the assumption that bene-ficence—the principle that an action is right that produces the most good—is the definitive principle for a moral community. In fact, even that assumption is widely rejected. If there are other principles that would be agreed to by our hypothetical contractors forming the list of basic principles to govern the moral community, then even if beneficence supports paternalism, it is not clear that other principles would as well. In particular, many would include a principle of autonomy as an additional right-making characteristic of actions.

This blatant paternalism of the Hippocratic tradition has been reassessed and found wanting. Not only is it rejected by virtually every lay medical ethical system grounded in religious and secular philosophical traditions. It is also rejected by the medical profession itself. The 1980 revision of the AMA's Principles of Medical Ethics deleted the patient-benefiting justification for breaking confidence. So did the most recent revision of the British principles.

HIPPOCRATIC INDIVIDUALISM

Paternalism is not the only problem with the Hippocratic principle. It is also individualistic. At least in its modern manifestations, the principle leads the physician to focus on the patient as an isolated individual. The Declaration of Geneva instructs that the health of the patient—in the singular—is the physician's first consideration.[8] It is widely recognized that medicine, at least until very recently, has been an ultra-individualistic profession. Considering the broader social, political, economic, and cultural dimensions of medical decisions was taboo. What is not widely appreciated is that this individualism is called for in the most sacred, respected ethical literature of the tradition.

The problems with limiting the physician's attention to the individual patient as an isolated entity are enormous. Some of the implications lead to absurdities. If the physician focuses exclusively on the individual, for example, research medicine designed to produce benefits for society as a whole is, by definition, immoral. It would also be unacceptable for a physician to choose public health as a specialty, since there the goal is the welfare of not the individual but the society. Cost containment, designed to save money for society rather than the individual, would also be prohibited from the physician's agenda.

It seems clear that the individualism of the Hippocratic principle must be modified. The difficulty is that the most obvious modification may lead to even more serious problems. For example, we could replace the Hippocratic principle with a more classical form of the beneficence principle, saying that the physician's moral obligation is to do the greatest good for the greatest number. That would surely justify research medicine, public health, and cost containment. But it might create even more problems than it solves. It would, in principle, justify the research that was done by the Nazis, if only they had been clever enough to design research that really produced substantial good for society.

The goal must be to modify the Hippocratic individualism without opening a flood gate of consequentialism so that the individual can be swamped in a sea of social welfare claims. There must be allowance for legitimate social considerations without abandoning entirely the rights and responsibilities of the individual.

Hippocratic Consequentialism:
The Case for a Deontological Medical Ethic

The only solution is to abandon the consequentialism of both the Hippocratic and utilitarian traditions. Professional medical ethics as we know it has taken for granted the notion that consequences are the sole determinant of right and wrong. The professional ethics of other professions may make a similar assumption. It might be found, for example, in the utilitarianism of most economists. By contrast, however, most major ethical systems of our world accept the idea that there is more to right and wrong than merely the production of good consequences. They hold that there are certain inherent right- and wrong-making characteristics of actions independent of consequences, or in addition to them, that determine rightness. This is the position of the Talmudic ethics of Judaism, of religious and secular natural law ethics in most of its forms, and of much Protestant thought. It is also the position of the ethics of such great thinkers as Kant, the natural rights tradition of our founding fathers, and the systems of such contemporary thinkers as W. D. Ross, John Rawls, and Robert Nozick.[9]

The patients' rights movement that has emerged in the past fifteen years has presented a significant counter to the Hippocratic tradition. It would have protected Dr. Brown's patient from having her confidences violated. It provides a check on the paternalism of the Hippocratic principle. But it still leaves us with problems. It focuses on the individual. Moreover, it seems to emphasize the individual as a center generating moral demands rather than as a locus of moral obligation. It has often been pointed out that there is a reciprocal relationship between rights and duties. If I have a right to information from you, then you have a duty to provide it. At least within limits, therefore, rights language and duties language are interchangeable. A good case can be made, however, for the priority of duties.[10] That is the perspective that should be taken by those operating within a religiously based ethic and by many defenders of more secular, philosophical ethics as well.

In such an ethic a set of principles, of prima facie duties, would become the starting point of a normative ethic for the lay-professional relationship. It would provide a framework for debating the principles at the level of the second contract, the one that defined the specific ethical duties of the lay and professional roles. It would provide a basis for overcoming the paternalism of the Hippocratic principle and give a limited mandate for consideration of impacts of actions on other parties, taking into account the justice of health professional actions. It would not, however, justify just any social utility consideration.

PRINCIPLES OF THE BASIC CONTRACT

If I am right, we need to know what reasonable people would choose in coming together to discover (or perhaps generate) a set of principles for governing a moral community. Assuming they would choose more than one principle as right-making, we also need to know what should happen when two or more principles come into conflict. Should the principles be rank-ordered into some priority, or should they be balanced against one another? Only when that basic ethical system is in place will we have a basis for assessing the Hippocratic principle and alternative sets of principles for the lay-professional relation.

THE BASIC PRINCIPLES

I discussed at length the principles that I thought would emerge from such a contractual meeting in *A Theory of Medical Ethics*. Only a summary can be provided here. There is a substantial consensus around the following principles.

Autonomy

First, reasonable people coming together to articulate the principles that should govern a moral community would include a principle of auton-omy, the principle that a right-making characteristic of actions or rules is that they respect the choices made by persons who are reasonably autonomous. Stated in this way, people have a right to formulate their own life plans and act according to those plans without interference from others.

This, of course, does not mean that people have the right to do anything they want. The ethical principle of autonomy is the source of a right that is often referred to as a negative right or a liberty right. It generates a right of noninterference. As such, it imposes some limits of its own. It does not permit actions that interfere with the autonomy of others. The autonomy of physicians to refuse to partake in actions they consider immoral may place limits on patients' efforts to pursue an abortion or a radical surgical pro-cedure.

Autonomy never provides entitlements; it does not give persons the right of access to resources to follow their life plans; it only restrains others from interfering with efforts of individuals to use what resources they have at their command to pursue those plans. It restrains others from interfering with voluntary agreements that are made ethically, that is, without violating other prior moral limits.

The ethical principle of autonomy has meaning only for persons who are, in fact, in some sense autonomous agents. It is vacuous for infants, the severely retarded, and the comatose who have not expressed wishes while competent, for example. For persons who are substantially autonomous, however, the principle of autonomy calls for noninterference, respect for the individual's plans, and granting of liberty to attempt to act on them insofar as they do not violate other moral limits.

Fidelity

Over and above the agreement that I predict would occur on the principle of autonomy, I see an agreement on the principle of fidelity, the principle that actions are right insofar as they express faithfulness to commit-ments previously made. The most obvious and important kind of commit-

ment a person might make is a promise. Thus promise-keeping is a
component of the principle of fidelity. Fidelity is broader, however. One
might be expected to be faithful to a set of relations—to long-standing
loyalties within a family, a friendship, or a partnership—even if no explicit
promises have been made. Perhaps one might describe such relations as
containing implicit promises. The precise language is not important. What is
important is the sense that fidelity to such previously established relations is
a right-making characteristic of actions over and above any benefits that may
come from such fidelity.

Some characteristics of the principle of fidelity are worth noting. In
order for a promise to be morally relevant, there must be some reciprocity. If
one person promises to provide a purported benefit to another, the promise
can never be cited as the reason why the benefit was offered if the one to
whom the promise was made did not accept it. Normally, there is some
reciprocal commitment by the other party, a promise in return to provide
something else. At minimum, however, the one to whom the promise is
made must acknowledge and accept it in order for the one who made it to be
bound by the duties of fidelity.

In some cases the paternalistic actions of physicians toward patients are
justified by the claim that the physician made a promise—took an oath—to
the profession that he would provide benefits to patients or preserve patients'
lives. Some patients, however, especially those hostile to paternalism, might
not want this purported benefit. If a promise is made to a third party, in this
case to the profession, no bond of fidelity is established with the patient. No
justification can be derived from such a promise for treating a patient against
his consent.

Even if a patient reciprocates by accepting the promise and endorsing
the desirability of the physician's benefit, it is generally the nature of the
ethics of fidelity that one can be released from a promise. If the physician
were to ask the patient to be released and the patient consented, no further
duty of fidelity would remain. Also, normally when a patient accepts a
promise from a professional, the acceptance should carry with it some limits.
For example, if a patient accepts a promise that the professional will do
everything possible to save the patient's life, the patient would reasonably
accept only with the proviso that the professional is authorized to make such
efforts only until such time as the patient declines further treatment.
Whether clauses prohibiting revocation can be incorporated into contracts or
promises is a matter of great debate. So-called Ulysses contracts in which one
party agrees (promises) that there will be no revocation may be possible
within certain limits. Regardless, it seems unlikely that such clauses would
make sense in many medical relations. For example, were a physician to
pledge to benefit a patient according to his judgment, no rational patient
would accept such an offer if it contained the clause that she could not
decline the help if she preferred. Exceptions might be made for special
circumstances where it might be rational to make limited irrevocable agree-

ments (such as in psychotherapies), but the promises and contracts governed by the principle of fidelity normally are revocable.

Veracity

Another right-making characteristic of actions is that communication be truthful. Insofar as a communication contains a falsehood, it tends to be wrong morally. Communications can be explicit or implied, direct or indirect. Those that are knowingly untruthful are wrong insofar as this dimension is concerned. Whether they can ever be justified on balance by other considerations will depend on one's theory relating conflicting principles. The untruthful aspect of a communication, however, will count toward making it wrong.

Some communications, especially in medicine, can be misleading by omission rather than commission. The physician may fail to disclose a serious risk of a piece of research or a malignancy that has a bleak prognosis. While sometimes efforts are made to defend such omissions on the grounds that one did not lie but only avoided telling the whole truth, it is often said that such omissions are as bad as lies. Sometimes they are even taken to be actual violations of the principle of veracity.

An omission may be morally as bad as a lie without being an actual lie. For example, if one had promised the patient (implicitly or explicitly) that a diagnosis would be disclosed, omission of the disclosure could be a serious violation not of the principle of veracity but of the principle of promise-keeping. On the other hand, it makes little sense to hold that veracity requires that everyone disclose every piece of information to anyone who could potentially find it meaningful. That is not only (or even primarily) because such disclosures might do harm. It is more because in some cases the one with the information is in no relationship with the interested party that requires or even calls for the disclosure. A consultant who is aware that a patient has not been told a diagnosis by the primary physician seems to be under no obligation to penetrate the primary physician-patient relation and disclose what he knows. He probably has not committed himself to such disclosures; he may even have promised to the primary physician that he would refrain from them. Were the consultant asked by the patient if he had cancer, it would be a violation of the principle of veracity to falsely deny it. It would not be a violation of the principle of veracity and perhaps not a violation of any other principle for the consultant to refrain from going out of his way to make the diagnosis known to the patient. It would, however, be a violation of an ethical principle—the principle of fidelity—for the primary caregiver to withhold the diagnosis assuming that such an explicit or implied promise had been made to the patient that such potentially meaningful information would be disclosed.

Avoiding Killing

There is debate about whether an additional fundamental ethical principle is that it is wrong to kill.[11] In the major religious traditions—not only Judeo-Christianity but also Eastern religions—it is considered wrong to kill, especially to kill the innocent. Of course, killing often is contrary to the welfare of the victim, so a general rule against it might simply be derivative from a principle of beneficence. The real test case comes when it is deemed to be in someone's interests to be killed, such as a person suffering intractable pain.

If the body were deemed to belong to someone else—to God, to the king, or to the community—then one might understand why killing would be wrong at least without the approval of the "owner." But even without the premise of external ownership, some view killing to be inherently wrong. In the Kantian tradition it violates the moral maxim that the person is to be treated as an end in himself. In other traditions it is seen as violating the natural law. The currently existing universal prohibition on active killing even for mercy is sometimes defended on rule-utilitarian grounds—on the grounds that legalization would lead to worse consequences on balance. However, the most reasonable way to make sense of the moral prohibition against active mercy killing is to acknowledge a fundamental principle that life is not to be taken.

That principle may, like the others mentioned, be only a prima facie principle. It may give way to other right-making considerations in case of conflict among principles, depending on one's theory of the relation among the principles. I approach medical ethics with the working conclusion that reasonable people coming together taking a moral point of view would conclude that killing is a wrong-making characteristic of actions.

Justice

Finally, a principle of justice may stand as an independent right-making principle according to such contractors. The key issue here is whether the pattern of distribution of good is morally important in addition to the amount of good that actions generate. Utilitarians since Mill have been interested in the pattern of distribution because of the notion of decreasing marginal utility. Increasing amounts of resources for individuals who are already reasonably well off will tend to produce less marginal good, so the argument goes, than if those same increments of resources went to persons who were less well off. To the extent that is true, the principle of beneficience by itself would support more equal distributions of resources.

Supporters of an independent principle of justice say there is more morally to the way goods are distributed than simply trying to maximize the aggregate amount of good. They may treat merit, effort, desert, birth, nobility, or some other consideration as relevant. The most powerful consideration independent of the aggregate amount of good produced is offered by the defenders of the egalitarian principle of justice. It holds that it is right-making to arrange resources so that people have an opportunity for equality of welfare. Especially in medicine, distributing resources to the least well off in order to give them an opportunity to be as well off as others may not lead to producing the greatest amount of good. While the notion of decreasing marginal utility suggests that giving resources to persons who are better off will tend to produce less good, in the case of medicine, giving resources to someone (or some group) who is relatively healthy may produce more good than concentrating resources on the sickest. In such cases holders of an egalitarian independent principle of justice will feel there is moral reason nevertheless to give some of the resources to the sickest. Whether that consideration is overridden by the fact that much more good in total might be done by concentrating resources on the healthier will depend on how competing principles of justice and beneficence are related.

Other Principles

The principles discussed thus far—autonomy, fidelity, veracity, avoiding killing, and justice, as well as those oriented to producing consequences (beneficence and nonmaleficence)—provide a rather complete list.[12] They appear in many contemporary documents dealing with medical ethics. This list is not necessarily meant to be complete, however. For example, W. D. Ross adds the duties of gratitude and reparation to his list. He holds that independent of consequences, one has a duty to show proper gratitude for kindnesses received and to make amends for damage done to others. There may well be a few other principles like these. Nevertheless, the list is quite short, and the principles listed here seem to cover the basic moral characteristics that most people feel need to be taken into account in assessing moral actions, rules, codes, or practices.

THE INTERACTION OF PRINCIPLES

The critical question remaining at this abstract level is what ought to be done when two or more of these principles are relevant to a particular action and their implications conflict. What should be done when responding to a patient's question truthfully will do great harm to the patient? Here the implications of the principles of veracity and nonmaleficence seem to pull in opposite directions.

THE SINGLE-PRINCIPLE SOLUTION

The simplest answer would be to hold that all of these principles are, in fact, derived from some single principle. For example, many utilitarians hold that all normative ethics reduces to maximizing of good consequences in some fashion. Some sophisticated utilitarians, often called rule utilitarians, claim that the goal of normative ethics is to opt for that rule or system of rules that will do more good than any other. They may actually develop a set of derivative rules that appear to be freestanding. These rules may even be called principles and may include autonomy, veracity, and the like. It is confusing to refer to these derivative formulas as principles if one is also going to call a foundational norm a principle. It would be better to call them rules. Otherwise we may hear of the principles of fidelity or justice being derived from the principle of utility or beneficence.

The chief problem with using a single foundational principle as the point of reference for adjudicating conflicts among the rules (derivative principles) is not this linguistic confusion. It is the implausibility of identifying a single foundational principle. Efforts to do so focusing on utility or respect for persons have been made, but they seem to fail to square with our moral sense of the complexity of what makes actions right. It just does not appear to be the case that the only reason it is right to speak the truth or keep a promise is that doing so means acting on the rule that has better consequences than any other set of rules.

Even if this single-principle solution is adopted, there is still the question of how to arbitrate conflicts among the derivative rules. It will not be enough to say that one would opt for the arrangement that maximizes the good, because we would still be left with the question of how much good truthful communication does in comparison with withholding the truth, and whether the various goods count on the same scale. Consequentialists face as questions of axiology (the theory of the good) the same questions they would otherwise face in attempting to rank claims when ethical principles conflict. In addition they must carry the added burden of the implausible claim that the only reason action can be right is that it produces good results.

LEXICAL ORDERING

Even if disputes among competing principles cannot be resolved by appealing to an overarching foundational principle, perhaps the principles can be rank-ordered so that those of higher priority take precedence. At first this strategy appears to offer no more promise than identifying a single foundational principle. It seems hard to argue why veracity should always take precedence over promise-keeping or even over beneficence. We can all think of cases where any one principle might have to give way to some other. A pure ranking of all the principles seems infeasible. Before returning to the lexical ranking approach for a possible resolution, let us look briefly at the other major option.

BALANCING STRATEGIES

If single-principle and lexical ordering do not appear feasible, what of the solution of claiming that all the principles are morally relevant, and that when they conflict an effort should be made to balance weightiness of the various considerations or to use some other nonlexical method of judging between conflicting appeals? Such an approach was used, to some extent, by W. D. Ross.[13] It has been favored more recently by Baruch Brody.[14] When two or more principles conflict, we take into account all relevant principles. Each contributes, prima facie, a dimension that is a right- or wrong-making characteristic. Only by seeing which dimension is weightier or more important can we decide what is our duty proper, the right action on balance.

While this approach can give a plausible account of virtually any moral conclusion, that may turn out to be its undoing. It can also give accounts in defense of terribly implausible conclusions, such as why it might be justifiable to experiment on patients without their consent, to abort women against their will, to lie to a patient to trick him into treatment, or to break confidences for personal gain. Each case can be described as a conflict between beneficence and some competing principle (autonomy, veracity, or fidelity). A defender of these morally unjustifiable actions can argue that it is a matter of balancing beneficence with the other principle and that, in his or her considered opinion, beneficence wins out. The critic is left quibbling about whether the benefit envisioned is really weighty enough to overpower the competing principle.

I am convinced that we are not this uncertain about the wrongness of the actions. It is not simply a matter of the beneficence not carrying enough weight to overcome the other principles. If that were so, the defenders could up the ante by envisioning another experiment or abortion or therapeutic lie or confidence breach where the consequences would be weighty enough. In theory balancing or intuitive judgment, strategies have to remain open to the possibility that any of these actions could be moral or that rules could be crafted defining circumstances where a consequentialistic exception to the moral prohibition would be justified. The argument against these actions is not that the consequences are not weighty enough. Rather, it is that no amount of consequences would count morally as a defense of these practices.

LEXICAL RANKING COMBINED WITH BALANCING

A more plausible approach combines the strategies of ranking and balancing. The consequentialist principles (beneficence and nonmaleficence) may reasonably be balanced. There is no absolute priority of avoiding harm over producing good. Likewise, the nonconsequentialist principles (autonomy, fidelity, veracity, avoiding killing, and justice) may have to be balanced or intuitively integrated by some judgmental method. However, between the two sets, the nonconsequentialist principles may take an absolute lexical priority over the consequentialist considerations.

For example, consider whether circumstances ever exist where beneficence should take precedence over autonomy. To make the comparison in a sophisticated way, consider first whether paternalistic beneficence should ever outweigh autonomy. Should a competent, substantially autonomous patient's refusal of treatment offered for his or her own good ever be overridden by the judgment that it is in the patient's interest to provide the treatment?

Certainly there are reasons why persons lacking substantial autonomy might have their wishes overridden, but by definition that is not a violation of autonomy. There are also possible reasons why benefit to others might justify overriding autonomy, but let us bracket that issue for a moment. At the level of law, the answer is clear: no competent patient ever has had autonomy overridden for reasons of strong paternalism. We may temporarily limit autonomy to determine competency, but once it is determined, the absolute priority of autonomy is clear. I believe it is also clear ethically. No matter how much we might view an autonomous agent's refusal as a tragedy, we will find it acceptable ethically.

What, however, of the case where the autonomy of a patient may be overridden for the benefit of others? At first it seems we justify that routinely. Yet even here there seem to be cases where we hold to the absolute priority of autonomy. In research involving human subjects, for example, we never let the argument that involuntary use of subjects is necessary to produce great good for society justify the use of autonomous human subjects without their consent. Here autonomy has an absolute priority over social (nonpaternalistic) beneficence.

What, however, of such practices as compulsory public health treatment of one patient for the good of others? We cannot be locked into an ethic so individualistic that autonomy always wins out over society's interests. Resolving such disputes requires careful description of the moral structure of the actions. It could be that here the aggregate amount of good overcomes autonomy. If that were true, however, it would seem that in principle when enough social good would come of it, patients could be used as research subjects against their will or could have the promise of confidentiality broken without their consent.

There may be another way of describing these cases where good to others justifies violating autonomy. It may be that in some such cases we are also allocating the good in a way that justice demands (because, for instance, the recipients of the good are particularly poorly off). If so, it is not simply that aggregate good is done by violating autonomy; rather, it is that another nonconsequentialist principle, justice, also demands the violation of autonomy. It may even be that the same amount of good done to other well-off people would not justify the infringement of autonomy. If so, it is not a case of aggregate good overpowering autonomy at all. It is a case of justice being in conflict with autonomy, requiring that the two principles be balanced against each other.

This strategy of a lexical ranking of nonconsequentialist over consequentialist principles and a balancing of each set of principles within its group leaves untouched our judgment that no amount of aggregate good from research justifies violation of consent, while at the same time it explains why some (but not all) benefits to others might be balanced against autonomy. It also explains why principles such as veracity, fidelity, and even avoiding killing are only prima facie principles when they conflict with other nonconsequentialist principles.

This complex interplay of principles with a mix of lexical ranking and balancing seems to me to be what reasonable people coming together from the moral point of view would pick as the basic social structure for a moral community. From this the more concrete rules can then be constructed as further negotiation takes place between lay and professional groups, giving rise to what I have called the second contract. It is to the content of duties for the lay-professional relation that we now must turn.

PART
II

The Individual Professional-Patient Relation

CHAPTER SEVEN

Informed Consent:
The Emerging Norms

Patients increasingly are insisting on their right to be informed about medications they are taking. Surveys indicate that they want to know a substantial amount about their medical treatment.[1] In one study comparing "acetylhydroxybenzoate" and a placebo,[2] hospital employees were given substantial details about the active drug, including the fact that it may cause fatal bleeding in ulcers, produce blood in the stool, prevent blood clotting, cause death on rare occasions with a large overdose, and lead to rare fatal allergic reactions, even in normal doses. In addition, the drug was presented as causing nausea, vomiting, heartburn, and allergic reactions, especially in asthma patients. Only at that point were the subjects told that "acetylhydroxybenzoate" was simply another name the researchers were using for common aspirin. The remarkable thing about the study was that after the subjects were told that the drug, with all of these potential side effects, was merely aspirin, only fourteen out of sixty-six felt the information should not be made available to the general public.

The idea of informed consent has emerged as a major doctrine in medical law and medical ethics in the last two decades. Prior to the twentieth century, there was virtually no recognition of the importance of informed consent, either for research subjects or for patients. The first formally negotiated consent on record was that signed by Alexis St. Martin. Soon-to-be-famous physician/researcher William Beaumont had treated an abdominal gunshot wound which St. Martin had received. The treatment had left an open gastric fistula. The consent gave Beaumont the authority to study the gastric physiology of St. Martin. That consent was really more of a contract for servitude, in which the patient pledged to be a research subject and travel with Beaumont as his "covenant servant," for the purpose of "exhibiting and showing of his said stomach . . . and the state of the contents thereof."[3] It only shows how far we have come in such a short period of time in developing the doctrine of informed consent.

THE FOUNDATIONS OF INFORMED CONSENT

There is real confusion about why health professionals are expected to obtain consent from their patients. I have examined the moral foundations of this issue previously in a study for the National Commission for the Protection of Human Subjects of Biomedical and Behavioral Research and in *The Patient as Partner*.[4] Here I shall only summarize the implications of the moral principles discussed in chapter 6 of this volume for the grounding of informed consent in the clinical therapeutic context.

PATIENT-CENTERED BENEFICENCE

Given their background in the Hippocratic tradition, some health care providers have assumed that the real purpose of obtaining consent is to benefit the patient. It cannot be denied that if patients know about the actions and side effects of the drugs they are taking, they are often likely to be better off. For example, in the above-mentioned aspirin study, a patient with an ulcer and another with eczema, both of which are contraindications for aspirin, were able to refuse to participate.

Often a patient may know of some peculiar medical problem that is a contraindication of a drug being prescribed. For example, a neurologist described amitriptyline for a patient with trigeminal neuralgia, an extremely painful inflammation of a facial nerve. Unknown to the neurologist, the patient also suffered from carcinoma of the prostate. The patient was not told of the drug's side effect of urinary retention. When this effect appeared, urinary catheterization was required to rule out the possibility of a recurrence of the tumor. It seems likely that the patient's interests would have been served had he been told about this side effect and the peculiar problems it would create for a man with prostate problems. In the partnership model, the patient and physician could explore together the potential advantages and disadvantages of alternative medications. Even if they jointly reached the conclusion to use the amitriptyline, at least the patient would have been relieved of the fears generated by the occurrrence of this side effect that was particularly threatening in his case.

Although informed consent will often be beneficial for patients, many have concluded that this is not the primary justification for informing them. If patient benefit were the basis, information could justifiably be withheld whenever a health professional believed that it might be harmful on balance.

TOTAL OR SOCIAL BENEFICENCE

Informed consent is occasionally justified on the basis of total benefits, including those to the broader society as well as to the patient. For example, in a research project in which hospital researchers wanted to obtain human placentas from the delivery room, a requirement to get consent of the women giving birth in that delivery room was defended, in part, on the grounds that if word got out into the general community that some research was being done in the hospital without getting consent, there might be a general hostility and suspicion against the hospital, thus doing more harm in the long run.

If the ethical foundation for getting consent is rooted in this general notion of social consequences, however, consent would not realistically be required often. In fact, research without consent would be justified whenever the greater good was served. This would justify potentially serious violations of individual rights and interests.

AUTONOMY

A third and more forceful reason for getting informed consent is rooted in the principal of autonomy. According to this theory, a patient has a right to the information necessary to make choices about his or her own behavior. The women in the delivery room should be told that their placentas may be used for research simply because it is their right. In 1914, Justice Cardozo articulated the patient's right to self-determination when he said, "Every human being of adult years and sound mind has a right to determine what shall be done with his own body."[5]

In 1960, the first important legal case dealing with informed consent in the modern period articulated that same principle. The patient was suffering from cancer of the breast and had had a radical left mastectomy performed. A radiologist had administered cobalt radiation that resulted in serious radiation injuries. The patient had consented to the treatment, but the physician had not informed her that it involved any danger. The court ruled that if the physician failed to point out the probable consequences, he had subjected her to unauthorized treatment. According to the court, "Anglo-American law starts with the premise of a thorough going self-determination. It follows that each man is considered to be master of his own body, and he may, if he be of sound mind, expressly prohibit the performance of life-saving surgery, or other medical treatment."[6]

THE ELEMENTS OF CONSENT

With that forceful commitment, the era of informed consent was launched in the United States. Soon thereafter, a Canadian case began to spell out exactly what kinds of information need to be transmitted for consent to be adequately informed.[7] In that case, a young college student had volunteered to be a research subject in order to earn money to put himself through school. He was administered an experimental general anesthetic, but was not told of the dangers of cardiac arrest that might be associated with it. The courts, in finding for the student, spelled out some of the basic elements that must be told in order for consent to be informed.

These elements have been expanded and qualified by the federal government's Department of Health and Human Services.[8] The regulations, written in the context of research medicine, require that patients or subjects must be given:

1. A statement that the study involves research, an explanation of the purposes of the research and the expected duration of the subject's participation, a description of the procedures to be followed, and identification of any procedures which are experimental;

2. A description of any reasonably foreseeable risks or discomforts to the subject;

3. A description of any benefits to the subject or to others which may reasonably be expected from the research;

4. A disclosure of appropriate alternative procedures or courses of treatment, if any, that might be advantageous to the subject;

5. A statement describing the extent, if any, to which confidentiality of records identifying the subject will be maintained;

6. For research involving more than minimal risk, an explanation as to whether any medical treatments are available if injury occurs and, if so, what they consist of, or where further information may be obtained;

7. An explanation of whom to contact for answers to pertinent questions about the research and research subjects' rights, and whom to contact in the event of a research-related injury to the subject; and

8. A statement that participation is voluntary, refusal to participate will involve no penalty or loss of benefits to which the subject is otherwise entitled, and the subject may discontinue participation at any time without penalty or loss of benefits to which the subject is otherwise entitled.

When appropriate, one or more of the following elements of information shall also be provided to each subject:

1. A statement that the particular treatment or procedure may involve risks to the subject (or to the embryo or fetus, if the subject is or may become pregnant) which are currently unforeseeable;

2. Anticipated circumstances under which the subject's participation may be terminated by the investigator without regard to the subject's consent;

3. Any additional costs to the subject that may result from participation in the research;

4. The consequences of a subject's decision to withdraw from the research and procedures for orderly termination of participation by the subject;

5. A statement that significant new findings developed during the course of the research which may relate to the subject's willingness to continue participation will be provided to the subject; and

6. The approximate number of subjects involved in the study.

It has sometimes been argued that the principles of informed consent for research are radically different from those that would apply to ordinary therapeutic relationships. If, however, the underlying moral principle is that principle of autonomy, then the same elements of information would appear to be necessary regardless of the purpose of the intervention. In research, there are normally more complex review mechanisms, including federal government requirements that all research involving human subjects be reviewed by an institutional board charged with ensuring, among other things, that adequate consent has been obtained. In the therapeutic situation, the burden for ensuring that consent is adequate is the same, but it falls on the health professionals dealing with the patient.

THE STANDARD OF CONSENT

In the last fifteen years, the theoretical development of the doctrine of informed consent has focused primarily on how much a patient must be told in order for the consent to be informed. Traditionally, it is held that the health professional must disclose the information that colleagues would disclose in a similar situation. Thus, in the case involving the mastectomy patient cited above, the court said, "the duty of the physician to disclose, however, is limited to those disclosures which a reasonable medical practitioner would make under the same or similar circumstances."[9]

The standard of the profession, as this is often called, has been challenged widely in court cases in a number of states[10] and in many articles in legal journals.[11] The courts have begun to conclude that if patients must have enough information to exercise self-determination, it should be logically irrelevant whether health professionals have traditionally disclosed certain information. It may be that practitioners have not customarily disclosed a piece of information, and yet that information would be significant in order for the reasonable person to make a judgment about the treatment. Alternatively, it may be that reasonable patients would find certain routinely transmitted pieces of information to be irrelevant.

CASE 3: CONSENT AND THE REASONABLE PERSON STANDARD

> In a 1969 case, a patient named Bernard Berkey had undergone a diagnostic procedure known as a myelogram. A needle was placed in the spinal column in order to remove fluid. The patient said that he felt a couple of mild sticks he did not mind at all, and then suddenly felt a terrific thrust as if someone were jamming an ice pick into his lower spine. He was left with diminished sensation in his leg, and weakness in his left foot.
>
> The physician admitted that he had not disclosed the possibility of such an occurrence, but when he was accused of not informing the patient, he brought forward testimony that his colleagues, similarly situated, would not have disclosed such a risk either. Should that have been an adequate defense?

The court rejected the physician's defense, saying, "we cannot agree that the matter of informed consent must be determined on the basis of medical testimony."[12] Other courts have found since then that the amount of information transmitted cannot be determined by the consensus of professionals, but must be measured by determining what a reasonable person in the patient's situation would want to have disclosed.[13]

This is what is now often called the objective reasonable person standard. It, of course, leaves open the possibility that the patient will not be able to be self-determining in cases where he or she would want to know information that differs from what the reasonable person would want to know. That suggests an alternative, sometimes referred to as the subjective standard: providing whatever information the actual patient would want, no more, no less.

There is one serious problem with the subjective standard. Virtually any information might be desired by some patients, yet it is impossible for the physician to disclose literally everything. The practitioner has an obligation to use reasonable prudence in deducing special interests. If the physician knows that the patient is a professional pianist, it is reasonable to conclude that he or she may have an unusual interest in potential risks to the hands. Furthermore, in the partnership model, the professional has an obligation to create an atmosphere in which the patient feels free to ask additional questions and to make special areas of interest known. Once the professional has fulfilled these obligations, however, the remaining burden rests with the patient to signal unusual concerns. To the extent that is done, the subjective standard must be met (or the physician should withdraw from the relation). If no such special interests are introduced, then the objective reasonable person standard is the only one that can be used.

IMPLICATIONS FOR HEALTH PROFESSIONALS

The implications are enormous. It means that, in principle, no professional can determine what to disclose to a patient by introspecting about what he or she would want to know in that circumstance. It also means that the question cannot be answered by turning to one's colleagues or examining what is normally disclosed in similar circumstances. If the principle of autonomy is the foundation of the informed consent doctrine, then patients will have to be told whatever they would reasonably want to know, even if it is not normal practice for that information to be disclosed.

It is unclear the extent to which health care professionals other than physicians bear responsibility for obtaining informed consent and ensuring that the patient has adequate knowledge of medications or treatments. It is also unclear whether the right to consent implies a right of access to written documents such as the *Physician Desk Reference* or patient package inserts prepared for the physician and pharmacist. It is clear, however, that we are entering a new era of informed consent, and the traditional answers will no longer apply. Some health professionals are beginning to take greater responsibility for ensuring that the patient has adequate information and education about medications being taken.

The principle of informed consent is built on the notion that the relationship between the health professional and the patient is a fiduciary one, that is, one of trust and confidence, rather than a mere business transaction conducted under the attitude of "let the buyer beware." If the foundation of the consent doctrine is the principle of autonomy and the notion that patients are to be treated as reasonable collaborators in the health care enterprise, then access of patients to documents such as drug package inserts and medical records may, in certain cases, be essential. Many jurisdictions have now recognized patients' right of access to their medical records, in part based on the same reasoning.[14]

It would appear that the various health care providers together have to take the responsibility for ensuring that patients are adequately informed, that is, that they are given information they would want to know in order to decide to participate in the treatment regimen. In some cases, especially when the physician has not fulfilled the responsibility and other health providers perceive that the patient is not adequately informed, it may be at least their ethical responsibility, if not their legal responsibility, to take a more active role in informing the patient.

CHAPTER EIGHT

Malpractice in the Contract Mode

Taking informed consent seriously in the contract or partnership mode may have unanticipated implications for areas of great difficulty in medicine. One example is the current medical malpractice crisis.

The clinician's attitude toward malpractice and legal involvement in medicine generally is summarized nicely in the title of an article in a medical magazine giving economics advice to physicians: "To Hell with All Those Laws: Let's Be Good Doctors." The implication is that physicians know what is ethical and that the law makes them do outrageous things if they want to be safe from lawsuits. They must practice defensive medicine and perform excessive tests that are both expensive and burdensome. Physicians must, according to this view, force life-prolonging aggressive treatment on inevitably dying octogenarians, order toxic tests, and generally violate their Hippocratic mandate. The mood seems to be that if physicians could just follow their codes of ethics and their consciences, the problem would go away. The law is the law and ethics is ethics . . . and ne'er the twain shall meet.

Many questions are raised by this approach to malpractice, including, what really is the source of the malpractice crisis, and what is the relation between codes, consciences, and the courts? The codes, as we have seen, differ significantly among themselves. That may turn out to be the first problem. The Hippocratic Oath is, at points, clearly incompatible with more modern codes—in its prohibition on surgery, its blatant paternalism, and its ambiguous commitment to confidentiality ("for those things that ought not to be spread abroad"). More modern codes are much more open to the physician's obligation to society (perhaps even at the expense of sacrificing the individual patient's interest). Some are opening to patient autonomy, a move never contemplated in the Hippocratic text. Some recent codes, such as the AMA principles as revised in 1980, even speak of the rights of the patient. Clearly, physicians who say malpractice would disappear if only they were allowed to follow their professional codes have a problem. Since the codes vary, someone or something must define which one would be followed. One function of the society—at least if we are working within a contract theory—is to facilitate ethical agreements between the profession and the lay public on precisely which codification provides a definitive ethical framework. To the extent that these codes are enforceable through state licensing boards or other public mechanisms, some court involvement seems inevitable.

As a way out, some physicians may say that since the codes differ, each physician should simply be permitted to follow his or her conscience. The AMA in 1980, for instance, said, "Ethics were never intended to be laws, but rather standards by which one may be measured. Ethics are broad and lofty ideals which permit individual discretion counterbalanced by individual accountability."[1] According to this view, ethics is a matter of following conscience, not of obeying the law. It is, of course, a long and respected tradition that ethics sometimes requires acting on conscience even when there is a law to the contrary. But physicians who adopt this approach should realize to what they are committing themselves. Ethics normally also includes a provision that, other things being equal, civil law should be obeyed. In our language, one of the basic principles of the moral community is fidelity to promises made. To the extent that one has accepted participation in the civil community and its laws, one has made some sort of promise to obey its laws.

Still, violation may be called for morally. The physician advising his colleagues to ignore the law is advocating civil disobedience. But he should realize the gravity of the stand he is taking. Civil disobedience requires a substantial moral commitment: that one's duty is so strong that it overcomes the underlying duty of keeping the promise of fidelity to the laws of one's land. Those who take this view ought to do so only after significant moral preparation—after the reading of Thoreau, Gandhi, Martin Luther King, and the draft-card burners of the 1960s. This is heady company. Civil disobedience requires commitment to some basic ethical criteria; an explicit defense by appeal to a higher law, a willingness to act publicly, and a willingness to take the consequences for one's actions including going to jail, if necessary.[2] Not many physicians are prepared to do all of this.

There are serious problems with this approach. First, just as with the codes, there are serious differences among us in the way our consciences guide us. Some sort of professional consensus could be used as a way of collectivizing the conscience of the medical profession, that is, as a way of producing a definitive code of ethics for professionals, but that leads to a second problem. Physicians as a group may differ from lay people regarding what is ethically acceptable in medicine. In the 1950s and 1960s, 88 percent of physicians would not disclose cancer diagnosis to a patient, while at about the same time 98 percent of patients said they would want to be told of the diagnosis.[3] Furthermore, by the end of the 1970s, most physicians had changed their views in favor of supporting disclosure.[4] If the earlier professional consensus had been used as a basis for determining whether the physician had done wrong by not disclosing, then patients' rights to adequate information would have been violated regularly.

If every physician simply followed his or her conscience or the collectively expressed conscience of the medical profession, patients would have their rights violated consistently. Laws are meant to shape behavior when individual consciences differ. We have learned that a better policy, a better *moral* as well as *legal* rule, is always to get consent before medical treatment even if you think you should not. Always resuscitate the patient when you can unless the patient or agent for the patient says not to. Always explain the risks that reasonable patients would want to know about unless individual patients have signaled explicitly that they differ from the objectively reasonable person in wanting to know more or less.

THE SOURCE OF THE PROBLEM

I suggest that the propensity of clinicians to follow the Hippocratic Oath and act paternalistically according to their own consciences or the collective conscience of the profession is the source of rather than the solution to the malpractice crisis. Under the old Hippocratic ethic, the physician's task was to do what he believed would benefit the patient according to the physician's ability and judgment. This meant withholding diagnoses if the clinician believed that would be better for the patient. It meant withholding information about drug side effects, about surgical risks, or about other possible unpleasant events.

The patient was viewed as an uninformed passive recipient of the physician's care. Often, when we were lucky, physicians guessed correctly. They told patients those things that benefited them—the side effects they needed to know about for practical reasons such as drowsiness or interactions with common food or drink. They avoided disclosing things that were not likely to be relevant to personal behavior and were not likely to occur in any case.

The result was that sometimes patients were quite happy—ignorantly blissful. In other cases they were surprised when some unexpected untoward event occurred. In both cases patients were treated as objects of the professional's paternalism. Regardless of whether the paternalism is found to be intrinsically offensive, I suggest that it is the cause of the current malpractice crisis. When patients are surprised with unexpected side effects, they are naturally distressed. Sometimes they sue—either out of anger at being treated paternalistically or simply because something happened that was not expected. One patient had not expected his spinal nerves to be pricked with a needle, leading to a permanent dysfunction of the foot.[5] It is only natural that he sued. Another had not expected the alopecia or the nausea. Others had not expected the mobility of a wrist to be affected by the orthopedic surgery, or the loss of a fetus from the amniocentesis. The patient naturally believes that the unexpected event resulted from physician negligence or incompetence.

INFORMED CONSENT: THE SOLUTION TO THE MALPRACTICE CRISIS

There is an alternative that I believe will largely put to rest the malpractice crisis, while incorporating superior ethical principles, those that result from the contract model. An ethic that incorporates the principle of patient autonomy and the derivative notion of the right of the patient to consent based on the reasonable person standard provides, as a fringe benefit, an easy solution to the malpractice glut. Even the codes of organized medicine have now largely bought into the model. The committee of the AMA that revised its code of ethics in 1980 says, "Paternalism by the profession is no longer appropriate."[6] The Judicial Council says that "the patient's right of self-determination can be effectively exercised only if the patient possesses enough information to enable an intelligent choice. The patient should make his own determination on treatment."[7] If a physician simply complies with that requirement, one that I am convinced reasonable people would agree to as part of the second-level contract between the profession and the public, the patient normally should not get surprised. The patient should be told all of the effects that a reasonable person similarly situated would want to know before deciding whether to agree to the proposed treatment. The only qualification is that with a patient who is in any way atypical in his or her preferences about information, the professional is obligated to meet the more subjective standard (or withdraw from the patient-physician relation).

A patient who is given accurate information about a known risk of a procedure and who nevertheless consents to it should thereby release the physician from responsibility for the untoward event. The patient is an active, substantially autonomous agent participating in a partnership and should be prepared to accept (or reject) the known, plausible risks of a treatment. Any risk that has been adequately explained by the clinician (or has been omitted on the grounds that the reasonable person would find it too infrequent or too trivial or too well known to want to be told about it) should, under the partnership model of medical ethics, become the patient's responsibility. (Of course, normally the patient's health insurance would cover any medical treatment necessitated by the reasonable acceptance of such risks.) Any risk that does not meet this standard would remain the responsibility of the physician who failed to obtain an adequately informed consent.

THE IMPLICATIONS

Under the contractual model in which the patient is viewed as an active partner in the clinical relation, the incentive to get an adequately informed consent would suddenly become enormous. I predict malpractice suits would diminish to almost nothing, as would complaints about being inadequately informed. Patients would have increased reason to trust their physicians and should, if the consent process is up to the reasonable person standard, assume responsibility for the outcome.

THE REMAINING GROUNDS FOR MALPRACTICE SUITS

Malpractice cases that would remain would be of two kinds. First, there would be some cases of what can be called "true negligence," the physician who is grossly incompetent and slips, cutting a nerve, when that would not have happened to a normally competent surgeon. Everyone should agree that cases involving true negligence deserve compensation, and the compensation should come from the physician or his insurer. The entire profession or the patient population should not be made to bear such costs. Certainly that patient's insurer should not. Presumably the malpractice insurance of the grossly incompetent physician would soon be priced at intolerable levels, and he or she would be driven from practice—an outcome about which no one can complain. While even normally competent physicians may occasionally make negligent errors, these should be covered by a low-level malpractice insurance premium. Patients should not object to having these minimal costs distributed over the patient population of the practitioner.

Second, there would in all likelihood continue to be nuisance suits by patients trying to take advantage of practitioners who have met the standards of an adequately effective consent. Here it will be key that by law or by judicial practice, the courts strenuously insist that patients who have consented to risks bear the responsibility for them. In addition, they should be informed as part of the consent process that there are always risks for which there is not yet adequate documentation and that they must consent to these as well. The physician should not bear these responsibilities either.

The defense of the physician against such a malpractice suit should simply be that an adequate level of information was provided based on the reasonable person standard and that the patient agreed to the risks. I believe it should not be difficult to establish whether this standard was met. In many cases pharmaceutical companies should be able to provide data on the desires of reasonable patients simply by testing sample groups of patients.[8]

Not all frivolous suits will be eliminated. That is asking too much of an ethic of medicine. The contractual ethic, however, does lead to the conclusion that there is an ethical obligation on the part of the patient to refrain from suits for events for which he or she has accepted responsibility. This is one of the duties of patients that will be discussed in chapter 17.

THE RESPONSIBILITY FOR BAD OUTCOMES

I have argued that the physician ought not to bear the responsibility for bad outcomes to which the patient had consented. Still, some patients will suffer even though they have rationally consented to some small risk of a serious untoward event. There should be, in effect, a no-fault insurance to cover such events. The easiest way to handle this would be to have the patient's own health insurance cover the costs of medical care resulting from such bad outcomes.

If there is a serious disagreement in society about the wisdom of taking a risk of a particular side effect, if the financial implications of the dispute were significant, separate risk pools could be created in the insurance system, one for those who chose to take the risk and another for those who did not. If the risk was small, the effect on the insurance would not be great anyway. This is, in effect, the way we presently handle ethically controversial choices by patients. Some insurance systems cover abortion and contraceptive services; others do not. Likewise, some insurance pools could cover the side effects of controversial procedures, while others would not. I will say more on the insurance modeling for coverage of the medical effects of voluntary choices in the contract model in chapter 20.

There is no reason why we should have a malpractice crisis today. The suits and defensive medical practices that are driving up insurance costs are easily amenable to a contract model of medical ethics and a consent solution. If patients are active participants who decline a marginal test because they think the risks and inconvenience of it are not justified, the clinician should be exempt from further responsibility for failing to perform the test. The practitioner cannot be held liable for failing to perform a test the patient refused to authorize. On the other hand, if the practitioner does perform a procedure and the unexpected but statistically predictable event occurs to which the patient has consented, the patient should bear that responsibility subject only to the provision that he or she should have the opportunity to have access to insurance that covers such effects. Treating the patient (or surrogate) as a substantially autonomous agent who is a full participant in the decisionmaking process will reduce malpractice to a modest mixture of cases of true negligence and nuisance suits.

Informed consent should provide a solution to one of the most serious problems in medicine today. It also provides a framework for many other controversial policy problems in health care, to some of which we now turn.

CHAPTER NINE

The Ethics of Generic Drug Use

Another of the current controversies in medicine that can be addressed by taking seriously the principle of autonomy and the informed consent doctrine that derives from it is the relation between generic and trade-name pharmaceuticals. Generic drug substitution laws have been passed in over forty state legislatures in the past decade. Antisubstitution laws, which were passed in the 1950s to prevent unscrupulous replacement of prescribed trade-name compounds with ineffective imitations, have been repealed because of pressure from consumer groups and government agencies seeking to reduce the cost of medications. They are supported by generic manufacturers claiming a right of free competition. In this rapidly evolving generic drug climate, health professionals are facing increasing pressures with often complex social, economic, and ethical implications.

The difficulties for the pharmacist, the physician, and the patient are illustrated by the following case:

CASE 4: WHEN IS IT RATIONAL TO USE A GENERIC DRUG?

A twenty-six-year-old woman employed as a file clerk was bothered by the pain of an earache and also was beginning to worry about possible damage to her hearing. About a week after noticing that the problem had not subsided, she sought the advice of a physician who, after an exam, wrote the patient a prescription. The woman asked her physician for "the cheapest thing that would do the job," requesting a generic drug, if possible, but the physician wrote a prescription for a trade-name antibiotic, saying, "You don't want to take any chances where an ear is concerned. Maybe that off-brand will be all right, but why take a chance with a company you've never heard of?"

The woman took the prescription to the local pharmacy and was upset to learn what a few days' supply of the medication would cost. She had a low salary, two children to support, and very little money available for discretionary spending, and so she decided to forgo the medication.[1]

This incident illustrates why people are concerned over the use of generics. It also illustrates how complicated the analysis of the issue can be. A physician motivated out of a concern to provide nothing but the best for the patient, quite possibly left her in a situation where no treatment was provided at all.

The generic drug laws raise social and ethical problems for the physician, the patient, and the pharmacist if they are to work in an active partnership. Three major issues must be confronted: the economics of generics, the structure of the decisionmaking, and the ethics of maintaining an incentive for research on new pharmaceuticals.

THE ETHICS OF THE ECONOMICS OF GENERICS

The economics of generics raise the most obvious problems. No one is denying that potentially a great deal of money is at stake: up to $400 million a year according to a federal government study. A 1979 policy shift that added seventy popular generic equivalents to the government's maximum allowable cost program was estimated to then-Secretary of HEW Califano to have the potential of saving $20 million just in Medicaid reimbursements.[2] The Federal Trade Commission has estimated that the savings will be 20 to 30 percent.

An actual study of prescription price changes under New York State's generic substitution law revealed savings of about 27 percent when brand and generic prescriptions were presented.[3] Moreover, the study, conducted both before and after the law was passed, found that the savings to consumers increased substantially after its passage. The prior average savings had been only 12 percent. Apparently the publicity of the law changed pharmacists' pricing policies. Pharmacists may be facing problems of professional ethics when they price prescriptions for generic drugs. Some have been known to fill a prescription with a generic product but price it at the level of the trade-name preparation. One study found that savings were not passed on to consumers in 29 percent of their comparisons.[4] According to some medical lawyers, many state laws require or imply that savings should be passed on to the consumer.[5]

Many have raised questions about the ethics of such pricing policies. The majority of pharmacists, who make appropriate reductions when dispensing generic compounds, resent the opportunism of their colleagues. Manufacturers of trade-name pharmaceuticals also have complained that such practices give pharmacists an unfair incentive to use generics, in effect charging patients for their version of the drug while dispensing the lower-priced substance. Pressures have been mounting to impose maximum price or maximum profit limitations on pharmacists as is currently done in Medicaid reimbursement formulas. Unless the profession comes to grips with this problem and develops a consensus on the ethics of such pricing, pressures for outside controls are likely to continue.

The economics of generic prescribing raises more subtle ethical issues, as is illustrated in the case of the woman with the ear infection. Not only did the pharmacist lose a sale and thus have loss of income as a result of the physician's insistence on the trade-name product, but the patient may have been harmed as well.

WHO SHOULD CHOOSE BETWEEN GENERIC AND TRADE-NAME DRUGS?

The insistence by the physician on the trade-name preparation at first seems to make sense. Many physicians' organizations are fighting vigorously for their right to retain discretion in the choice between trade and generic drug products. For example, one medical society is very much interested in the advantages of judicious use of generics, provided two conditions are met: that physicians not have increased liability and that no law curb the professional judgment of a physician in the treatment of the patient.[6]

In New York and most other states, the law provides just such protection. In New York State the physician is given a choice of two lines on the prescription over which to place a signature. In signing one of them, the physician is instructing the pharmacist to dispense as written. The other line indicates "substitution permissible." In one of the worst abuses of the English language on record and one that is surely confusing to pharmacists and patients, when the physician signs over the line indicating "substitution permissible," substitution of a generic is not merely permissible but, in fact, is required by law. The New York State attorney general has urged physicians to sign "substitution permissible" whenever possible, but the authority to choose a generic clearly remains with the physician, not the state, the patient, or the pharmacist.

Some have questioned, however, whether it is the physician who should have this authority. Two other candidates are also in a position to have knowledge relevant to the decision. Much of the technical pharmacological argument over the substitution of generics is based on the concern over whether they are truly biologically equivalent to the original trade-name compounds. Bioequivalence is questioned from many sources. Some studies have shown that, especially for certain compounds such as digoxin[7] and levothyroxine,[8] such problems have arisen. Thus, one of the demands of physicians before they prescribe generically is that controlled, scientifically valid studies establish conclusively equivalence is bioavailability and therapeutic effect.[9] Such studies are underway; in fact, they date back to the 1960s. An HEW task force, after twenty months of investigation, concluded that on the basis of available evidence, the lack of clinical equivalence among drug formulations meeting official standards had been grossly exaggerated.[10] Still, the problem is of concern to all involved. The physician, however, cannot realistically be expected to stay abreast of the pharmacological studies of equivalence. The pharmacist seems to be in a much better position to

make use of his or her expertise in evaluating the quality of generic manufacturers.

In virtually all states, legal substitution is limited to generics from
manufacturers whose preparation is contained in a formulary. This means
that substitution is permitted only of generics that have been demonstrated
to be equivalent.[11] (Some states have negative formularies specifying brands
deemed nonequivalent.) Thus the decision is really reduced to very subtle
choices about whether the generic manufacturer can be relied upon to
produce consistent, pure, properly labeled, and fresh pharmaceuticals.
Many would argue that the pharmacist is in a better position to compare
generic and trade-name manufacturers and to evaluate competing generic
producers.

Even if the physician retains control over the choice between trade and
generic preparations and signals that choice by authorizing generic substitution, the pharmacist still bears the responsibility for choosing among generic
manufacturers. Once again ethical as well as technical and legal responsibility exists. Several generic manufacturers may produce the "same" product. The pharmacist has a financial incentive to choose the cheapest, even if
he or she knows it may not come from the most reliable company, but legally
and ethically is bound to dispense the generic of high and consistent quality.
To the extent that professional skill is needed to make this kind of determination, the pharmacist seems to be in the best position to choose. He or she has
the skills, training, and sources of knowledge for that burden. Only in the
rarest of cases will the specific medical needs of a patient be relevant in the
selection. As long as the choice is made from a formulary of equivalent
compounds, it is hard to see why the physician's knowledge of the medical
condition of a particular patient would be critical. It is for these reasons that
many are advocating the increased role of the pharmacist in the decision.

Some are beginning to ask, however, whether the choice can be based
entirely on professional skill at all. Especially if choices are limited to a
formulary, the critical questions may turn out in the end to be nontechnical,
the kinds that lay people may be expected to answer based on their own
value systems. For example, the critical assumption made by the physician
in the case of the woman with the earache was that the trade-name manufacturer was more reliable, so "why take a chance?" Assuming the trade-name
product is more reliable, however, it is not clear whether all people in all
circumstances would agree that the chance is not worth it. For the woman
with the earache, for example, it might make sense to take some chance on
the generic manufacturer even if her physician, who is in a very different
financial situation, might think it foolish. The question becomes one of not
only whether the generic poses somewhat greater risk, but also how much it
is worth to avoid that risk. The answer will depend on the social and
economic position of the patient and also how he or she values the potential
benefits. It might make more sense to go with an unknown manufacturer
when buying medication for a headache (where the lack of bioavailability

probably means only that the headache will continue a little while) than in buying a drug for a crisis where failure could have dire consequences.

In short, many of the questions raised in choosing between generic and trade-name preparations are really value questions that can best be answered only by filtering them through the patient's own value system. If that is the case, then the patient should have an active role in deciding whether the "risk" of the generic is "worth it." The contract model of medical ethics, with its commitment to the principle of autonomy and the informed choice of the patient as an active participant in the partnership of decisionmaking, provides an obvious solution to the confusion over the generic substitution debate. This is a second major area of ethical concern for consumer and professional in the generic drug controversy.

The Research Incentive

A third area of debate involves the impact of the use of generics on the advancement of pharmacy. It cannot be denied that the United States has made a major contribution to the development of new pharmaceuticals. It is often claimed that patent law giving the original developer of a drug exclusive use (for a period of seventeen years) is crucial if the pharmaceutical industry is to continue making such a contribution. D. Craig Brater and William A. Pettinger, physicians and clinical pharmacologists at the University of Texas, Dallas, state the case for protection of research-intensive companies. Writing in the *Annals of Internal Medicine*, they say, "A tragic result from the reversal of the antisubstitution laws could be the curtailment of new drug development by the research-intensive firms of the pharmaceutical industry. Development of new drugs requires large quantities of high-risk capital. Revoking antisubstitution laws permits non research-intensive firms to benefit with essentially no risk and only modest investment."[12] They, in essence, state a moral claim of the developers of drugs to profit from them. The research-intensive drug manufacturers have generally supported this argument.[13]

The underlying moral issues are extremely deep. Should health care be a profit-making industry? What happens to the needs of those who do not have "profitable" diseases in such a world? If drug companies cannot retain a fair profit from their research investments, what incentive will there be to make the social commitments necessary for progress? The defenders of the generic substitution laws claim that research medicine can be preserved even if generic substitution is permitted. They argue that some critical basic research is already being supported by government and private philanthropic agencies. Brater and Pettinger point out that if the time needed to develop a new drug to the state of full FDA approval is too short to produce a fair profit, then as a matter of public policy, patent protection should be extended or should be begun only at the time of FDA approval.[14] (They cite the case of Minoxidil, which was approved on October 18, 1979, and had patent protection only until 1985.) Most people recognize that it would be foolish to cut off completely any incentive to conduct drug research. The broader society should, it would appear, decide if it wants to keep incentives by means of patent protection and, if so, give fair protection to provide a good incentive to develop new pharmaceuticals.

The generic substitution laws thus put both health professionals and society in the middle of a wide range of complicated ethical and social issues. We will have to cope with the ethics of pricing generics fairly; the ethics of relating the pharmacist's decisionmaking authority with that of the physician's and patient's must be addressed, as well as the ethics of fairly rewarding companies and individuals who serve the society by developing new drugs. A radical and controversial way of accomplishing this is to shorten the length of time between development and marketing by making new drugs available for use through what is being called a treatment IND. Patients are given a chance to decide that they want to receive the drug for therapeutic objectives even before the clinical trials are completed. This radical experiment in patient participation is the subject of the next chapter.

CHAPTER TEN

Treatment INDs: The Right of Access to Experimental Drugs

The emergence of AIDS has created a new controversy in clinical medical ethics. Some desperately ill patients are now asking why, when their cases appear hopeless, they cannot have immediate access to agents that offer some ray of hope, even if those substances have not completed clinical trials. They acknowledge that some of the agents they would like to try are potentially toxic, even lethal. They admit the chances of benefit are small. But they are increasingly claiming that they should have the freedom to take a long shot.

Two regulatory innovations respond to these developments. First, the FDA has developed an expedited process of treatment INDs (Investigational New Drug permits) by which patients suffering from serious or life-threatening conditions may gain access to certain drugs on a nonrandomized basis while clinical trials are being conducted.[1] Such drugs as the cardioselective beta-blocker metoprolol, certain cancer drugs including etoposide and streptozocin, and, most important, zidovudine (formerly azidothymidine or AZT) have been administered to thousands of patients under conditions that would now qualify for a treatment IND, and drugs, for example, teniposide (for treatment of certain patients with acute lymphoblastic leukemia), have been approved under the formal new regulations. Second, recently (October 1988) regulations were issued that will eliminate the need for Phase III trials in certain cases involving life-threatening and severely debilitating illnesses.[2]

All of this poses a serious threat to those committed to the importance of carefully designed random clinical trials prior to release of new drugs for therapeutic use. The ethics of research involving human subjects was the subject of *The Patient as Partner*. Those issues will not be discussed here. However, the proposals to rush new drugs such as zidovudine into clinical use based on decisions between physicians and patients prior to completion

of the standard experimental trials challenge the traditional distinction between research medicine and therapeutic medicine. A brief summary of a
few themes follows.

THE ETHICS OF RANDOMIZATION

By the 1980s it was clear that new pharmaceuticals could be potentially
dangerous. We have survived the thalidomide controversy. When a new
agent emerges, it is not only permitted but indeed morally imperative that
data be gathered about toxicity and efficacy. This should normally be done by
randomized clinical trials.

THE WINDOW OF OPPORTUNITY

It is morally important that such trials be conducted early with an
experimental pharmaceutical. Of course, only agents that offer real promise
are to be tested. There must be both theoretical and empirical reason (from
animal or in vitro analysis) to suspect that the agent is at least as good as
anything currently on the market. At the same time, until evidence is
gathered one cannot know for sure that the agent will be superior to or, on
balance, worse than the standard treatment.

It is at this point that investigators can plausibly hypothesize that there
is no significant difference on certain key variables between the experimental agent and traditional treatments. In the case of AIDS, a null hypothesis
might be that administering zidovudine (AZT) produces no significant differences in life expectancy, morbidity, and side effects when compared to
standard treatments. Of course, researchers hope that the null hypothesis
proves to be false, in particular that the experimental agent proves to offer
better life expectancy, less morbidity, and fewer side effects, but the question is always stated as a null hypothesis for purposes of statistical testing.

At the small window of opportunity when the null hypothesis is plausible, data must be gathered. Then we really do not have objective, impartial
reasons to believe that either the experimental or standard agent is superior.
For that reason, typical subjects cannot plausibly argue that they are at
serious risk from randomization (because no one really knows for sure which
treatment arm will prove better).

SUBJECTIVE VARIATION AMONG SUBJECTS

Even though they may be no confirmed differences in objective measures such as five-year survival rates, there may still be subjective differences
between the approved and investigational arms. Based on Phase I trials (the
first human trials, designed to measure toxicity), effects in such subjective
areas as feelings of well-being, sexual drive, vertigo, or nausea may be
expected to be different. The timing, place, or route of administration may
vary. While overall the differences in anticipated benefit/harm ratios may not
be significant to the typical, representative observer, they may legitimately

be so to an individual who has some atypical aversion to one of the side effects observed.

In a clinical trial of a potentially promising but toxic high dosage of a chemotherapeutic agent for cancer, a protocol called for hospitalizing patients in the experimental arm for seventy-two hours every three weeks so that the effects of the drug could be monitored. Those receiving the standard dosage could be seen on an outpatient basis. Investigators and the hospital's institutional review board were convinced that the risks of toxicity and the inconvenience of the hospitalization were justified by the potential increase in survival rates. A small group of potential subjects, however, was averse to spending so much time in the hospital. They concluded that they would be better off receiving the standard dosage and refused to participate in the study.[3]

Any competent scientist would argue that permitting subjects to opt out taints the quality of the sample. Moreover, it would take longer to recruit patients for the trial. If overall social benefits were the only consideration, quite possibly these atypical objectors to hospitalization, even considering the burden to them, should not be permitted to opt out. However, social benefit is not the only moral consideration. We recognize an autonomy-based right to refuse consent even if there are only personal, subjective reasons to refuse and even if it hurts the research. If the investigators are honestly in doubt about whether one treatment arm is superior to the other, then they ought to be able to find many patients willing to be randomized.

THE IMPLICATIONS FOR RIGHT OF ACCESS TO EXPERIMENTAL DRUGS

What should happen, however, if some other small group of atypical patients prefers the experimental arm? They may be so afraid of cancer that they are willing to take almost any risk. They should be told by investigators that there is no firm evidence of the extra benefit, that they will be exposed to serious, potentially lethal risks, and that they will suffer the inconvenience of hospitalization for one-seventh of the trial. They should be told that, on balance, the investigators consider that these risks approximately offset the possibility of longer survival. While most people presumably will be convinced (if the null hypothesis is plausible), some still may have an unusually high fear of death, great acceptance of the risks of toxicity, and low aversion to hospitalization. Should they be given the right of nonrandomized access? Should they be able to use the drug as a therapeutic agent, that is, as part of a routine physician-patient relation, while others are still not convinced that it has been demonstrated to be superior to the standard treatment?

Investigators are sometimes appalled at such proposals. They believe granting the right of access will destroy the research. However, they need to examine their arguments carefully. Some opponents argue that if nonrandomized access were granted, all potential subjects would insist on getting the experimental compound. These investigators are admitting that they believe they would be unable to convince a significant number of subjects of the plausibility of the null hypothesis.

Zidovudine is a good example. At one point in its development zidovudine was a promising agent for treating HIV-related thrombocytopenia and *Pneumocystis carnii* pneumonia. It had not been tested adequately in humans, however, and was known to pose serious risks. A clinical trial was ethically acceptable at the point at which the doubts about efficacy and fears of toxicity offset the expected benefit, at least for most people. At that point most subjects should have had no reason to object to being randomized.

It may be that with a disease as disastrous as AIDS, rational people would say that such a point never existed, that any risks of toxicity, even immediate death, would be better than going without the hope that the drug offered. In the earliest stages of development of most drugs, however, it is unlikely that the majority of people would be convinced that risking the untested agent is significantly better than going without the drug. If the doubts about the experimental compound are real, enough ambivalent people should be available who are willing to be randomized. However, does that small group who is atypical have a right of access?

As we shall see in the next chapter, if the agent is already on the market for other uses, there may be no legal basis for blocking access, provided, in the case of legend drugs, some physician can be found to write a prescription. That does not settle the ethical question, however. Defenders of a right of access should concede that granting it will taint the data and slow down the clinical trial. Those arguments were already faced, however, in granting persons the right to choose approved, noninvestigational therapy. Defenders of the right of access ask: If the principle of autonomy gives the right to the standard treatment, why should it not give a similar right to those who prefer the experimental agent? If we are working within the context of a partnership in which patients are viewed as substantially autonomous agents capable of making choices for or against medical interventions based on their own personally held subjective system of values, why should they not be permitted to opt for the experimental drug as well as the standard one in cases where investigators are convinced that there are not enough data to demonstrate that one or the other is superior?

There are additional relevant considerations. First, if we are dealing with an expensive agent or one available only in small quantities, society has an interest in making sure it is used efficiently to produce valid answers to the scientific questions posed. If the agent is scarce, certainly the investigators have a right to limit access to those willing to be randomized. Second, we should recognize that generally an investigator, clinician, or institution should not be forced to provide medications in ways that violate personal or corporate conscience. Thus investigators may be able to constrain access on a nonrandomized basis if they believe that supplying it would force them to participate in morally unacceptable risks with patients.

THE SEMI-RANDOMIZED CLINICAL TRIAL

Nevertheless, there might be scientific as well as ethical reasons for some people to be granted nonrandomized access. Any randomized clinical trial rests on an often unproved and controversial assumption: that those who will eventually receive the drug on a nonrandomized basis in routine clinical use will respond in a manner identical to randomized subjects. Randomized patients are quite different, however, from eventual clinical users. Randomized patients are told that what they are receiving is an experimental agent that has not been proved to be effective and may be toxic. Clinical users are told it is the therapeutic "drug of choice"; they use it believing it to be a safe and effective agent.

It is sometimes scientifically important to test the hypothesis that those who are believers in the drug will react in the same way as those who receive it as "nonbelievers." One way to do that is through what can be called a semi-randomized clinical trial. In such a trial, all are told that investigators believe there is no objective basis for preferring one treatment arm over the other. They are asked to consent to be randomized. Those who agree are randomized as usual. For those who retain a subjective preference for the standard or the experimental agent, instead of simply letting them drop out of the study, investigators could offer them a chance to receive treatment on a nonrandomized basis, following these subjects and recording data so as eventually to test the hypothesis that the randomized and nonrandomized subjects within each treatment group respond similarly.

In a fascinating study of ulcer treatment, patients were randomized to either medical or surgical treatment. Afterward, some of those randomized to surgery nevertheless refused it. They had to be treated medically. The investigators were wise enough to follow these postrandomization refusers and found, much to their surprise, that that group not only did better than the surgery patients, but they also did better than those randomized to medical treatment.[4] Hence, it seemed that the subject's preference for a particular treatment or the act of consciously choosing it improved the effectiveness of that treatment. Without following the group who had a strong preference for one treatment arm, this important finding would have been lost.

There may thus be scientific as well as ethical reasons why some atypical patients should be given access to treatment arms on a nonrandomized basis. On the other hand, if almost all patients who are presented the option of nonrandomized access have a strong preference for one arm, the investigators have evidence that the null hypothesis is not as plausible as they believed.

WHEN TO GRANT ACCESS ON A NONRANDOMIZED BASIS

Does this mean that investigators must always grant nonrandomized access when patients prefer the experimental drug? Probably not. We have already seen that the scarcity of the agent and the conscientious objection of the investigator provide bases for refusing access.

We have noted that the FDA policy making available treatment INDs and modifying Phase III trials is restricted to cases of life-threatening illness or serious and debilitating conditions. The moral justification of these limits is difficult to establish, however. Some people would argue that there are rational, if subjective, reasons why some atypical patients would want access to experimental agents even in cases where they are not suffering from life-threatening or serious illness. The most obvious response is that people ought not to have access to agents whose efficacy and safety have not been established. That, however, places the government in an overtly paternalistic role. In other aspects of medical ethics such as treatment refusal, we have now accepted the right of patients to make medical decisions even if those decisions appear to be contrary to their own interest. Moreover, if the null hypothesis is plausible, it is hard to argue against access on the grounds of the net risk to the subjects.

JUSTICE

If one rejects this general argument for a right of access to experimental treatments, there may still be a basis for granting an exception in life-threatening or serious illness as the FDA has done. I have suggested that contractors would adopt, in addition to beneficience and autonomy, justice as a relevant ethical principle. Many commentators have argued that this means societal resources should be arranged to give special consideration to those who are worst off.

This could provide a moral basis for differentiating between studies of relatively trivial conditions and extremely debilitating life-and-death conditions. Defenders of these theories of justice argue that the sickest patients should receive special consideration. This may be the moral insight in new FDA provisions granting patients nonrandomized access in life-and-death cases.

The arguments against granting nonrandomized access seem to rest solely on social utility. American society, however, has already reached the conclusion that social utility cannot dominate these ethical judgments. We grant patients the right to refuse randomization in order to get the standard treatment, so why should a similar right not be granted to those who have a strong preference for the experimental arm—at least in cases where scarcity is not a consideration? Assuming the null hypothesis is plausible, there is no basis for the claim that this will make it impossible to recruit subjects for the randomized trial or that patients will be harmed. In some cases there may even be good scientific reasons why we should gather data on nonrandomized patients receiving the experimental agent. At least in cases where justice also provides a basis for giving access because the patients are among the worst off in our society, some provision for access on a nonrandomized basis is morally defensible.

CHAPTER ELEVEN

Ethics of Drugs
for Nonapproved Uses

Another significant problem is closely related to the argument over treatment INDs. It also can be addressed using the contractual model of partnership. Physicians sometimes consider writing prescriptions for drugs currently on the market when they have in mind uses not covered in the Food and Drug Administration (FDA)–approved label. The examples run from uses widely accepted by the medical community (propranolol for hypertension before that use was added to the FDA-approved label) to controversial and highly deviant uses (thyroid for weight reduction or morphine for depression). On rare occasions these unlabeled uses may be based on nothing more than a physician's healthy imagination.

Important legal, social, and ethical questions confront the patients and health professionals involved with these prescriptions. Is it legal for the physician to prescribe such drugs or the pharmacist to dispense them? Are physicians aware they have opted for a so-called unapproved use? Should a pharmacist inform the physician or the patient that the use is not in the FDA's labeling? And if FDA-approved labeling is based on safety and efficacy, to what extent are these judgments questions of medical fact rather than value judgments?

A study by Erikson and colleagues at the University of Washington in Seattle reviewed the medical charts of five hundred drug uses in a three-month period in a family practice clinic. They found that forty-six (9.2 percent) were for uses not included in the FDA labeling.[1] An earlier study by G. R. Mundy and colleagues, of hospitalized patients using three drugs for which the FDA-approved labeling was particularly out of date found much higher rates of unapproved uses: 78 percent for cephalexin, 57.1 percent for allopurinol, and 65.7 percent for propranolol.[2] Erikson's study included some other disturbing findings. On no occasion did the medical chart show that the patient was informed that a drug was being used for an unlabeled purpose. Not only that, but in a related study of the beliefs of family practice residents and faculty, Erikson and colleagues found that unlabeled uses were frequently believed to be FDA-approved. For example, 63 percent thought dipyridamole was labeled for use as an antiplatelet agent, and 30 percent throught oral contraceptives were labeled for endometriosis when they were not.[3]

FDA regulations make clear that physicians are not prohibited from prescribing approved drugs for unlabeled uses.[4] Pursuant to the Federal Food, Drug, and Cosmetic Act, a drug approved for marketing may be labeled, promoted, and advertised by the manufacturer only for uses for which its safety and effectiveness have been established and which the FDA has approved. The law, however, does not limit the way in which a physician may use the drug, once approved. The physician may be constrained by state law. New York, New Jersey, and Wisconsin, for example, prohibit the prescribing of amphetamines for obesity. Moreover, physicians must follow rational medical practice or they may be subject to malpractice law. They are not, however, prohibited from prescribing for unapproved uses. In fact, there is no legal notion of an "unapproved" use. The FDA approves labeled indications, but it acknowledges that there may be acceptable uses beyond those included in its approved labeling. It recognizes that the FDA review process takes time and may not reflect the most recent scientific medical consensus. Some pharmaceutical manufacturers may simply not seek revision of labeling for new uses, especially if the market potential is negligible or if patent protections have expired. This policy has resulted in considerable confusion for physicians, pharmacists, and manufacturers.

Part of the confusion stems from the fact that several constituencies with differing agendas are being served simultaneously by the policies governing the use of drugs for unlabeled indications. Surely whatever moved Congress originally to require FDA determination of safety and then, in 1962 after the thalidomide scare, to add efficacy determinations had something to do with a desire to protect the public from unsafe and ineffective drugs. In fact, a drug that is not determined to be safe and effective for some use cannot be shipped in interstate commerce in the United States.

Both Congress and the FDA, however, have been eager to insist that whatever they do is not intended to infringe on the practice of medicine, by which they mean physician freedom. That concern, together with the fact that the legal hook on which the FDA law hangs is the right of the federal government to regulate interstate commerce, leads to repeated disclaimers on the part of the FDA that they have any intent to limit the medical judgment of the clinician. Clinicians are free to prescribe according to their best judgment. When other constituencies—manufacturers, pharmacists, and patients—are added to the agenda, it is easy to see why the current policies are complex and confusing.

SAFETY AND EFFICACY:
FACTS OR VALUE JUDGMENTS

The debate has much to do with whether safety and efficacy can be determined objectively without regard to particular uses in particular patients and the extent to which they are facts rather than value judgments. At first it might appear that both safety and efficacy are matters of medical fact. It would be for that reason that we leave such determination to scientific experts in the FDA, trained in medicine and the pharmacological sciences. Safety, at least it would appear, is a factual issue. That might provide the logic for authorizing physicians to use their own judgment regarding unapproved uses once the basic pharmacological and toxicological studies have been done and reviewed by the FDA. Many might think that once the drug is safe, it really does not matter how the physician uses it.

Those who are sensitive to more philosophical matters, however, both inside and outside the FDA, know that this is too simple an interpretation. Stuart L. Nightingale, FDA's associate commissioner for health affairs, says, "Safety is determined through a weighing of the potential risks and benefits of a drug for any given use."[5] Surely there are facts from pharmacology and toxicology that are critical in determining whether a drug is judged safe enough or not. Some of these are facts related to the basic pharmacology in normal subjects, the so-called Phase I clinical trial data done on normals. If a drug produced disastrous effects even on normals, we probably would never have the chance to test it for specific medical needs.

Increasingly, however, pharmacologists and philosophers of science are concluding that safety judgments are, as Nightingale says, essentially relative to the specific use envisioned. Consider a drug so toxic that it has produced serious side effects including ulcerative stomatitis, luekopenia, nausea, decreased resistance to infection, serious liver pathology, convulsions, and bone marrow depression. Some reactions can be fatal. One might at first be inclined to consider it so unsafe that it should not be on the market. That is a judgment that cannot really be made, however, until we know what the intended use is. If it were a cold remedy, then common sense would say it is much too dangerous. If, however, it were the chemotherapeutic agent that was the most successful treatment of some advanced, otherwise fatal cancers, then calling the drug safe enough to include in the hospital formulary makes sense. In fact, the adverse effects cited are from the FDA-approved labeling for methotrexate, an important antimetabolite cancer therapy.

There is rapidly developing controversy in the philosophy of science over the extent to which policy judgments, such as the decision to call a drug safe, can be made on a value-free basis. At this point it is fair to say that no one participating in that debate would hold that safety judgments can be made on the facts alone without the incorporation of some values. At least one must decide how bad some side effect is. The quantification of the harms for the harm/benefit calculus is essentially a value judgment.

Those participating is this fascinating new controversy over the role of values in government science policies are even quicker to point out that deciding the benefit side of the harm/benefit determination also is essentially an exercise in value judgment. The act of Congress giving the FDA its mandate to determine effectiveness does not define effectiveness well. When the FDA says a drug is effective, it probably means something like the following: based on *adequate* and *well-controlled* investigations by experts in the field, we believe the drug produces a *desirable* effect with *great enough* frequency to *justify* its use in the light of the *adverse* effects of the compound. If that is what is meant by effectiveness, it is clear that the FDA's procedure is to start with facts determined by recognized scientific methods and then make a series of value judgments. It would have to decide what effects are desirable and how desirable they are. Estrogen-progesterone combinations have the effect of preventing pregnancy. For a woman trying to avoid pregnancy, that is a good effect, although how good depends on many subtle considerations. For a female taking the combination drug to regulate the menstrual cycle who wants to get pregnant, that is a terribly adverse effect. The FDA also would have to decide how frequently the desirable effect needs to be produced. Forty or 50 percent success rates would be considered acceptable for some experimental cancer treatments, but would be an unsatisfactory rate for oral contraceptives. Finally, it would have to decide how the potential harms compare with the potential benefits.

This means there could not possibly be an all-purpose rationale for deciding whether a drug is safe or effective. It has to be done for the specific use and even for a specific patient. Erikson, for example, found physicians who prescribed indomethacin for dysmenorrhea even though it was not an indication in the FDA-approved labeling. For a woman who had not tried the standard treatments for dysmenorrhea, who had no objections to them, and who was not terribly troubled by her problem in the first place, indomethacin would seem wrong. However, for the woman who has tried the other commonly accepted treatments or who has principled objections to them (who refuses, for example, to take narcotics) and who is in agony from her problem, the indomethacin might be appropriate; that is, she might consent to using it if she were adequately informed and rational, given her values.

We are left with an intriguing set of policy issues raised by the problem of an FDA mandate to approve safety and effectiveness in order to justify marketing a drug that does not require physicians to limit drug uses to those included in the FDA labeling. It means, for example, that if two drugs existed each of which had been found safe by the FDA for some pharmacological use (perhaps prior to 1962 when only safety testing was required), but only one of them was found effective (and therefore only that one could now be marketed), physicians would have access to this one drug for totally unrelated uses while they would not have access to the other drug. They would have access to the one drug even though no scientific study had ever determined that it was either safe or effective for the use intended.

TWO POLICY OPTIONS

Those participating in the policy controversy over the use of approved drugs for unlabeled uses seem to be pressing for one of two policy options. They might be called the liberal option and the control option.

THE LIBERAL OPTION

One group, people such as Cincinnati physician Murray Weiner, emphasize the concern of the medical profession about retaining the physician's freedom of choice. They push the ethics of autonomy to its logical conclusion.[6] He would give the physician freedom to use not only those drugs which, by luck, have been approved for some unrelated use and are therefore on the market, but also, in special cases where the physician determines it is rational, even totally unapproved remedies. He cites as examples coumarin at the time it was found only "possibly effective" as an anticoagulant, and EDTA to reduce plutonium body burden, as well as laetrile for patients who have given up all hope for standard treatments and will go outside the system if they cannot get access from their physicians.

This solution, however, raises several problems. If harms and benefits are essentially subjective value judgments and people ought to be free to make such choices based on their own beliefs and values, it is not really the physician's freedom that has been violated if state or federal agencies restrict access; it is the patient's. Thus some proponents of the right of access to drugs for unapproved uses are arguing that somehow the freedom of choice would be the patient's. Lawyer Peter Barton Hutt, for example, suggests a model where consumers are free to obtain any drug regardless if it is proved safe or effective for a particular use.[7] Consumers would thereby be put on guard and would realize they need to be much more informed about their choices than they presently are. They would presumably rely on physicians to help inform them, but it would be a patient's own responsibility to decide whether to use a drug in an unproven or unconventional way. The FDA might continue with most of its present tasks. It would review the scientific quality of the safety and effectiveness data. It would not, however, serve as gatekeeper. Drugs could be marketed even if they had not been demonstrated to the FDA's satisfaction to be safe and effective.

In a story that emerged from the hearings before the House Intergovernmental Relations Subcommittee in 1971, an FDA dermatologist told of being approached by a patient inquiring about the use of methotrexate for the treatment of psoriasis. After pointing out that the FDA had not approved this use in the labeling of methotrexate and that it was a drug not without side effects, the practitioner indicated that dermatologists did believe it was a valuable agent in some recalcitrant cases of psoriasis. With advice that put the ultimate decisionmaking responsibility on the patient, he concluded that the patient "would have to weigh the potential advantages against the potential disadvantages in his particular case, and that this was not a decision that we could make here at the FDA."[8]

A similar conclusion was reached by the Department of Health, Education, and Welfare Review Panel on New Drug Regulation when it endorsed patient package inserts so that patients would be able to distinguish between what they called approved and unapproved uses.[9] They specifically recommended that if postmarketing surveillance revealed widespread use of a drug for unapproved uses, this should be a reason for requiring a patient package insert.

THE CONTROL OPTION

The second policy option, by contrast, sees the role of the government as protecting people from potential dangers to themselves that they may not know about. It would support controls, not only to protect third parties and incompetents, but even to protect competent patients making choices about their own drug use. That is the ethical stance that probably lies behind some of the original movement by Congress to require that a drug be demonstrated safe and effective before it can move in interstate commerce. The logic of the defenders of the control option, however, pushes them further than the FDA's mandate presently goes. They would argue that it makes no sense to protect citizens from a drug that has not been demonstrated to be safe and effective, but to permit unlimited access at the physician's discretion to approved drugs for uses for which safety and efficacy have not been demonstrated.

It should be clear how those working within the contractual framework of a partnership would handle this problem. There is in principle no way for either the practicing physician or the FDA to know whether any given drug is safe or effective enough to be used by a particular patient until it is evaluated based on that patient's system of beliefs and values. There is, of course, an important place for agencies such as the FDA in protecting third parties from the harm that might come from the use of medicinal agents. But it is remarkable how infrequently third-party risk is an issue. Certainly, the most dangerous drug in the world when assessed in terms of either consumer risks or third-party risks is alcohol. The state has a legitimate role in controlling the right of access to any drug that poses real danger to third parties, but not to those that simply pose some risk to the consumers themselves. Certainly, no drug on the market today should have more restrictive access than alcohol. There are a few others for which there are real third-party dangers, such as amphetamines and probably narcotics. Moreover, governments have a legitimate role in restricting parents and guardians from exposing their children to risks from drugs. Just as the government legitimately limits the right of parents to give their children alcohol, so it should limit their right to give other drugs; but that does not justify a total restriction on access even for adults themselves.

When a drug is on the market for one use, it does not follow that it is safe or effective for another. The belief by a physician that it would be good for the patient is irrelevant. If the patient is told of and makes an informed choice about the use of a drug for an unlabeled use, such use is appropriate. But then exactly the same should be said for drugs that are not approved for labeling for any use at all. If informed patients choose to take the risk in one case, the same logic could lead them to take the risk in the other. In the partnership model the physician will be critical in providing information for the patient about what uses have been considered for various drugs and what the findings are, if any, about safety and efficacy for the various uses. The physician certainly has the right to refuse to provide information and to end the partnership when he or she believes that a patient is acting foolishly, but the patient is the one who ought to make the choices about drug uses, whether those uses are condoned in FDA labeling or not.

CHAPTER TWELVE

When Should the Patient Know? The Death of the Therapeutic Privilege

CASE 5: LYING TO SERVE THE PATIENT

Mrs. Anna Domingues, a fifty-four-year-old woman, was born in Puerto Rico but lived most of her adult life in New York City. She came to the hospital with a complaint of severe abdominal pain and went to surgery on a Wednesday morning.

The medical student assigned to her case was unsure about what she should be told. He spoke to the resident responsible for the patient, telling him that Mrs. Domingues had stage-four cancer of the cervix, the most advanced stage. They had cleaned out all of the tumor they could see, but since it had spread to the pelvic wall, all they now could do was try chemotherapy and radiation. The five-year survival rate of stage-four cancer is 0–20 percent—bleak news for the woman.

The medical student was tempted to keep the information to himself, at least for the time being. He thought it could produce a severe depression, and maybe Mrs. Domingues would not cooperate as well in chemotherapy and radiation. On the other hand, he felt that it would not be fair to her to withhold the potent prognosis: somehow, she had a right to know her fate.

The student discussed the problem in turn with the resident, the attending physician, the staff psychiatrist, the hospital chaplain, and a social worker. An enormous dispute emerged. The attending physician was adamant that such bad news should not be disclosed, at least not with the full force of its meaning. The hospital chaplain was equally adamant in the other direction. The social worker seemed to side with the chaplain, stressing the need to prepare for the care Mrs. Domingues's three adolescent children were going to need. The resident was confused himself but reflected the consensus of the majority of his profession; he reluctantly concluded that it would be inhumane to let the woman know her poor prognosis.

Why are there disagreements about telling patients such as Mrs. Dominques about their medical conditions? When is it appropriate not to tell patients, and what are the ethical, legal, and clinical bases for making such decisions?

HAVING DIFFERING VIEWS OF THE SAME PATIENT

LOOKING AT DIFFERENT FACTS

Different ethical perspectives support the various stances taken by the student's advisors. First, his mentors were examining different data. The attending physician was afraid that there would be a bad medical outcome if the patient knew; he was afraid she would become uncooperative in the treatment regimen. The psychiatrist emphasized the psychological impact on the woman; to him the enemy was anxiety, fear, and depression, for which withholding the negative information was a powerful preventive.

The chaplain looked at very different facts. He knew that the woman was a devout Catholic and had an obligation to prepare spiritually for an impending death. For him, the religious or spiritual consequences dominated. The social worker, on the other hand, emphasized the social, economic, and familial consequences. She was concerned about the effect on the woman's family—the three children who needed care, and the enormous financial impact on this family of modest means.

Each of the consulting professionals, then, brought to bear very different information. Moreover, they seemed to be weighing the facts differently. The psychiatrist saw the psychological impact as very harmful. The chaplain was not at all convinced that disclosures need be so devastating. Physicians have a uniquely high fear of death, at least according to one study of the problem,[1] and that fear may cause them systematically to overemphasize the bad psychological impact of disclosures about terminal illness. Yet even if all consultants had agreed upon what kind of facts were relevant, they might have assessed the benefits and harms quite differently.

APPEALING TO DIFFERENT PRINCIPLES: THE THERAPEUTIC PRIVILEGE

There may well have been another, even more fundamental reason for the disagreement. The people involved in the dispute may have disagreed about the underlying moral principles that would influence the decision. The physicians probably applied the traditional Hippocratic principle of benefiting the patient when trying to decide whether to disclose a diagnosis to someone who is terminally ill. They were apparently working in the older, paternalistic, priestly model. The law calls the physician's argument "the therapeutic privilege." The idea has been with us since at least 1946, when Dr. Hubert Smith published an article in the *Tennessee Law Review* entitled

"Therapeutic Privilege to Withhold Specific Diagnosis from Patient Sick with Serious or Fatal Illness."[2] In spite of the fact that Smith recognized that there is no legal authority for such a privilege, there have been hints of its legitimacy in court cases ever since. According to this concept, the doctor is privileged to use his or her judgment to determine whether the patient would be hurt by disclosure, and if so, to withhold the information.

Cases Implying Support for a Therapeutic Privilege

The therapeutic privilege argument has arisen in both research and therapy settings. For example, it was used by Dr. Chester M. Southam of the Sloan-Kettering Cancer Research Institute in defense of his now-infamous study at the Brooklyn Jewish Chronic Disease Hospital in July 1963.[3]

CASE 6: THE BROOKLYN JEWISH CHRONIC DISEASE CASE

Dr. Southam injected cancer cells into terminally ill patients for experimental purposes. He admitted readily that no consent had been obtained, arguing that the physician has the right or even the obligation to withhold information that could be distressing to the patient, and pointing out that such information might indeed have been distressing to his research subjects.

He was charged by the New York State Board of Regents with a violation of his professional obligation to obtain consent from research subjects. The board concluded, "it is not uncommon for a doctor to refrain from telling his patient that he has cancer when the physician concludes in his professional judgment that such a disclosure would be harmful to the patient. The respondent overlooked the key fact that so far as this particular experiment was concerned, there was not the usual doctor-patient relationship and, therefore, no basis for the exercise of their usual professional judgment applicable to patient care."

The implication was clear: the Board of Regents thought that the therapeutic privilege argument is legitimate, but only in a therapeutic setting. One cannot argue that withholding the information would have been the most beneficial course to Dr. Southam's research subjects, because they simply could have been left out of the research entirely, thus avoiding the problem. Can we accept, however, the implication that it is morally permissible for a physician who is in a therapeutic relation to withhold information that he or she feels will be upsetting to the patient? May a physician ethically exercise the so-called therapeutic privilege?

In 1977, the same Board of Regents incorporated a limited therapeutic privilege argument in its policy on patient access to medical records. Acknowledging the general existence of such a right, the policy permits physicians to withhold access when they think the information would be seriously harmful to patients. While that policy has never been tested in the courts, it does represent the current thinking of an important state regulatory body, and apparently acknowledges the legitimacy of therapeutic privilege in cases where the physician believes disclosure to the patient would be harmful. In chapter 13, we shall see how the therapeutic privilege argument is applied in other state policies regarding the patient's right of access to medical records.

A case in Hawaii seems to accept the same idea. In *Nishi versus Hartwell* the court concluded, "the doctrine [of informed consent] recognizes that the primary duty of the physician is to do what is best for his patient. The physician may withhold disclosure of information regarding any untoward consequences of a treatment, where full disclosure would be detrimental to the patient's total care and best interest."[4]

According to the *Nishi* opinion, the law accepts the principle that physicians should use their judgment to do what they think will benefit their patients. Other early court cases defending the therapeutic privilege operate on the same principle.[5] I think that is a mistake. The model is one where medical therapy becomes the ultimate goal. The physician Bernard Meyer conveys this therapeutic metaphor when he argues, "What is imparted to the patient about his illness should be planned with the same care and executed with the same skill that are demanded by any potentially therapeutic measure. Like the transfusion of blood, the dispensing of certain information must be distinctly indicated, the amount given consonant with the needs of the recipient, and the type chosen with the view of avoiding untoward reactions."[6]

Cases Challenging the Therapeutic Privilege

A careful reading of some of the earlier court cases reveals that even then there were limits placed on professional judgment. The important 1960 case of *Natanson versus Kline*,[7] for example, often is cited as a justification for the use of professional judgment in placing limits on disclosure. The case, referred to in chapter 5, involved a woman who suffered injury from cobalt therapy and successfully claimed lack of informed consent. The court said that "the physician's choice of plausible courses should not be called into question if it appears, all circumstances considered, that the physician was motivated only by the patient's best therapeutic interests and he proceeded as competent medical men would have done in a similar situation."[8] That seems to be a blunt justification of therapeutic privilege based on professional consensus. However, an introductory clause in the opinion says that the physician's judgment is justifiable "so long as the disclosure is sufficient to assure an informed consent by the patient."[9] Thus even in earlier decisions, the information had to be full enough for the patient to exercise an informed judgment.

The therapeutic privilege argument recently has come upon hard times. Opinion in the last fifteen years has moved in the other direction. Challenges have increased among lawyers, philosophers, and even physicians.

There are two objections to therapeutic privilege. First, there is often a high error rate in assessing benefits and harm of disclosure. Physicians may give undue emphasis to medical or psychological consequences. They may incorporate their own uniquely high fear of death. They may overlook values dear to the patient. Predicting the psychological impact of bad news on someone whom the physician may not know very well is an enormously complicated task. The result is sometimes a rule or guideline at the level of the second contract that says that in order to do the most good in the long run, one should disclose all reasonable information to the patient, even if it appears the patient might be upset. The physician who decides that it would do more harm than good to disclose may be mistaken.

A second objection to the therapeutic privilege argument is far more fundamental. This view holds that all the arguments about benefit and harm miss the point: what is at stake is a basic right of the patient or a basic obligation on the part of the health care provider derived from what we referred to in chapter 6 as nonconsequentialist principles of the first social contract—principles of veracity, fidelity, and autonomy. If the patient is to be an active partner in the process of medical treatment working with the clinician insofar as the two can agree on mutually acceptable goals, then he or she has to know what would reasonably be relevant to any decisions.

Disclosure of a diagnosis and prognosis is at the very least a necessary part of any informed consent. Consent might be omitted only if the goal were merely maximum benefit to the patient. A physician may conclude that a prognosis should be withheld on this basis, but those who criticize the therapeutic privilege argument reject this logic in principle. They say that maximizing benefit is not the goal at all; rather, the objective is protecting the patient's autonomy. No exception is offered for withholding information necessary for an informed consent on the grounds that it would be disturbing to the patient. This excludes the therapeutic privilege argument.

While mere appeals to harm to the patient, psychological distress, or physical risks are not adequate morally or legally, an important legal case raises a problem that gives rise to what some are calling a therapeutic privilege "stringently formulated."[10] In *Canterbury* v. *Spence*,[11] one of the cases of the early 1970s that helped establish the reasonable person standard for consent discussed in chapter 7, the problem of therapeutic privilege was addressed. The case, involving a nineteen-year-old left paraplegic after an exploratory laminectomy, presented two exceptions to the consent requirement. The first was ethically obvious and consistent with the partnership model. It is often referred to as the emergency exception. When patients are unconscious or otherwise incapable of consenting, and harm from a failure to treat is imminent, we may presume the consent of the patient (unless previous objection has been recorded). In the language of the triple contract, reasonable patients and professionals would agree at the level of the second contract that clinicians are authorized to make such a presumption in these circumstances.

The second is the therapeutic privilege. It obtains "when risk-disclosure poses such a threat of detriment to the patient as to become unfeasible or contraindicated from a medical point of view."[12] The language is provocative and potentially offensive. It sounds as though the court was preparing to grant physicians the right to withhold information whenever they determined that it was potentially harmful to the patient. The court even uses the traditional medicalizing language of Bernard Meyer, suggesting that information can be "contraindicated from a medical point of view." That implies that it might be possible "based in pure medical science" to determine that it was medically wrong to disclose certain information. In chapter 5 I analyzed in greater detail the notion of "medical indications" and "contraindications." We saw that such expressions are usually simply jargon for the evaluative conclusion that based on the clinician's values, some action is appropriate or inappropriate. It should be clear that medical science alone can never disclose that an action is right or wrong; only value judgments about the outcome of the action can.

The *Canterbury* court backtracks somewhat from these implications when it spells out what it means by "unfeasible or contraindicated." It goes on to say:

> It is recognized that patients occasionally become so ill or emotionally distraught on disclosure as to foreclose a rational decision, or complicate or hinder the treatment, or perhaps even pose psychological damage to the patient. Where that is so, the cases have generally held that the physician is armed with a privilege to keep the information from the patient, and we think it clear that portents of that type may justify the physician in action he deems medically warranted. [13]

It is critical to distinguish those cases where disclosure will literally render the patient so ill or distraught as to foreclose a rational decision from those where it will simply hinder treatment or pose psychological damage. If information is withheld because it will hinder treatment or pose psychological damage without rendering the patient incapable of rational decisionmaking, it is withheld on purely paternalistic grounds. Especially when one realizes the enormous difficulty in predicting such harm and when the autonomy of the patient to participate fully in the decision is given proper priority, there seems to be no justifiable ground for authorizing withholding on this basis. The *Canterbury* court, in fact, makes clear that it "does not accept the paternalistic notion that the physician may remain silent simply because divulgence might prompt the patient to forgo therapy the physician feels the patient really needs." [14]

The cases in which disclosure would actually make the patient so ill as to foreclose a rational decision are •nother matter, however. In such a case a partnership with full sharing of decisionmaking is literally impossible. The patient will be rendered incompetent by the very action that is required to make him or her a partner in the decision. Appeals to autonomy to attack the therapeutic privilege become impossible. If the prediction of foreclosure of rationality is accurate, there can be no partnership. Such a patient is, de facto, incompetent to give an adequately informed consent.

This does not justify straightforward therapeutic privilege, however. If a clinician suspects the patient will be rendered incompetent by a disclosure, the proper course is to treat the patient as potentially incompetent. For incompetents, some surrogate must assume decisionmaking authority. If the patient refuses to yield this authority to a next of kin or other designated agent, the only avenue open is a competency determination. The clinician's argument that the patient is incompetent to offer a consent (because the informing process will render the patient irrational) should be presented to a court, which can determine whether the clinician's case is plausible.

If this sounds harsh or cumbersome, that is as it should be. The burden of proof needs to be on the one who claims that information alone will have such a devastating and unpredictable effect. Even if the case is made, the clinician is not hereby given license to treat without consent. Rather, the partnership is expanded. A full, active agreement will now have to be reached between the clinician and a surrogate acting on behalf of the patient. The surrogate will, as usual, be expected to act based on substituted judgment insofar as that is possible, that is, based on the patient's beliefs and values insofar as they can be determined. If they cannot be, then the surrogate will have to pursue the best interest of the patient. The surrogate judgment can be overturned only if the clinician can convince a court that it is beyond reason. (The full theory of the limits of reasonable surrogate judgment will be developed in chapter 24.)

If patients have the right of self-determination and the right of access to information so they can participate in decisions about their care, then the doctrine of therapeutic privilege is dead. This seems to be the conclusion one must reach from the law on informed consent and the principle of autonomy. It is even more clearly the ethical conclusion one must reach. Even so, sometimes the therapeutic privilege argument gets through the back door; other rationalizations that are really therapeutic privilege arguments in disguise are offered for withholding information.

RATIONALIZATIONS FOR
THE THERAPEUTIC PRIVILEGE

One such self-deception might be called the "you can't tell them everything" argument. Like the attending physician in Mrs. Domingues's case, some people justifiably point out that it really is impossible to tell patients everything about their conditions, and thus "fully informed" consent is impossible—adding, no one would be foolish enough to want full information even if it were somehow possible to define it. But that still leaves open the question whether the patient should be told reasonably significant or meaningful information regardless of a possibly negative psychological impact. While we cannot tell patients everything, we might still tell them the information that a reasonable person would find significant, meaningful, or interesting.

A second kind of self-deception is expressed in what might be called "truthful jargon." The patient had leiomyo-sarcoma with disseminated meta-static tissue growth. Dr. Charles C. Lund, who was then in Harvard Medical School's Department of Surgery, captured the technique's usefulness when he advised fellow physicians to proceed cautiously with blunt disclosure. He said, "certainly at the start of the interview [the physician] should avoid the words carcinoma or cancer. He should use cyst, nodule, tumor, lesion, or some loosely descriptive word that has not so many frightening con-notations." In other words, jargon may be truthful and still not communicate. Physicians using jargon such as this should not kid themselves into thinking they have fulfilled their moral obligation to convey to patients what reason-ably would be useful or meaningful in deciding about therapy.

Another type of self-deception might be called the "we'll never know for sure" argument. It begins with the profound clinical insight that medical prognosis is extremely subtle and complicated. At best, physicians are able to estimate the likely outcome with some degree of probability. But they can say truthfully, "we'll never know for sure." The deception comes when they use this as a rationalization for failure to disclose what they do know—that the prognosis is bleak and the likelihood of long-term survival is small.

Still another kind of self-deception occurs when the physician attempts to make a sharp separation between lying and withholding information. There may well be a moral difference between some omissions and commis-sions. For instance, in the related area of euthanasia, many believe that there is an enormous moral difference between actively killing a patient and simply letting him or her die. [15] The law seems to make a clear separation. [16]

The critical factor in omission, however, is whether the physician had an obligation to act. It seems clear that there is no obligation to act if the patient has withdrawn or withheld consent; in fact, continuing treatment on a terminally ill patient in such a case might be a battery. Withdrawal of consent for continued treatment is radically different from an instruction to actively kill a patient. Even the giving of consent does not necessarily justify any intervention that actively would hasten a patient's death.

With information disclosure, however, the physician is in a very dif-ferent situation. He or she has not been instructed by the patient to refrain from acting; in fact, the patient has not given a signal one way or another. In disclosure, the physician can be seen as in the process of negotiating consent for possible further treatment. Withholding information in a way that de-ceives the patient into thinking that he or she is going to recover is not lying, but it is a violation of the principle of fidelity, a failure to live up to the implied covenant with the patient to disclose what the patient would reason-ably want to know.

A final kind of self-deception is what might be called the "indirect communication" argument. Sometimes physicians and other health profes-sionals convince themselves that they are able to read signals from patients about their desire for further information or lack thereof. The patient in the midst of a cancer diagnosis workup may talk about long-term plans for building an addition to his home. Physicians have been known to take that as a signal that the patient does not want to discuss imminent death. It is conceivable that some communication between patient and physician may take place using such indirect signals or even body language, but there is great danger that the signals may be misread. It probably is safer to avoid the use of indirect communication arguments whenever possible.

In summary, all of these arguments are really self-deceptions. They do not justify withholding information or deceiving the patient. If that is justifiable at all, it will have to be established on some other grounds.

SOME SPECIAL CASES

There are a number of special cases requiring additional comment. These tend to be brought out in defense of therapeutic privilege. One special case occurs when the family requests that the patient not be told of the diagnosis. But how does the family know about the situation in the first place? Physicians have a well-recognized obligation to maintain confidentiality. In many jurisdictions, this is elevated to the level of law. If confidentiality is to be broken, it is the patient's right to authorize breaking it and not the family's. Whenever physicians disclose to family members first, without the patient's permission, they have violated confidence. Except in cases where the patient has specifically authorized a family member to advise the physician about the nature of the disclosure, the family seems to have no legitimate or justifiable role in deciding to withhold bad news. The partnership is between physician and patient, not physician and family.

That suggests a second special case in which the patient waives the right to information. Normally, patients should not make such requests. They have not only the right but the responsibility to be actively involved in decisions about their own care; but as we saw in the previous chapter, from the point of view of the law as well as of the medical professional, it really is not our business to force patients to have information against their wishes. If a request comes from a patient that such information be withheld, I see no problem ethically with honoring it. At the level of a special individual contract between physician and patient, an agreement for the patient to waive access to traumatic news is tolerable.

There is one final special case that may ease the burden on health professionals faced with the enormous task of telling patients about their medical conditions and futures. If patients have a right to all information that they would find meaningful in making a decision about the future of their care, might it still be possible that in some situations there is nothing a reasonable person would want to know?

In research medicine, this question arises when researchers want to make use of the waste products of routine clinical care, when a physician wants to use remainder blood, body waste, or the materials removed during surgery. Do such researchers have to get explicit consent from patients who would be unwittingly contributing to the research if they were not told, or would it suffice to obtain, upon hospital admission, a general consent statement that such waste may be used for research?

It seems that the proper test would be to ask whether reasonable patients would want to have information about a specific study. Normally, they probably would not, although if there were risks of confidentiality violation, or if the purpose of the study were unusually controversial, they might want more detail. Barring special circumstances, many have concluded that there is simply nothing the reasonable person would want to know. In that case, a general blanket consent statement might prove adequate.

Likewise, in therapeutic settings there may be some procedures so trivial or commonplace that patients would not want to know anything about them. Normally there is not a long explanation before routine blood samples are drawn in a laboratory, in spite of the fact that there is always a very small but real risk of infection and blood clots from the procedure. If reasonable people would not find such details meaningful in deciding to participate, then the current practice is reasonable and justified.

It seems unlikely, however, that people faced with serious illness—with a lump that looks suspiciously like a malignant tumor, for example—would be as indifferent to the information relevant to their case. The burden of proof is going to be on the medical professional to demonstrate that reasonable people would not want the information, unless a patient has explicitly waived the right to know. And the burden of proof ought to be very high.

It thus appears that the cases that seem to justify the therapeutic privilege may not make an exception to the general rule of telling patients what they would find meaningful. In some cases reasonable people would not want to know anything; in others patients are literally incapable of giving consent because of their condition or the traumatic nature of the information, and in still other cases patients explicitly waive their right to the information.

Our public policy is and should remain that competent individuals have the right to self-determination regarding participation in medical treatment, and that information necessary to make a decision about participation must be presented for a consent to be adequately informed. In cases where the patient is not competent to make such decisions, the legal agent for the patient must give permission for the medical treatment. The apparent exceptions to the requirement are really not therapeutic privilege arguments at all. Ethics and law both require that if patients are capable of understanding their conditions, they should be told about them. Many physicians have come to agree, but a consensus of professional opinion cannot be decisive. The ethical and legal mandate remains independent of professional medical opinion. The therapeutic privilege is dead if the patient is to be a true partner in the medical enterprise.

CHAPTER THIRTEEN

An Unexpected Chromosome: Disclosure of Genetic Information

In the previous chapter I traced the history of a radical change in physician willingness to disclose information to patients and outlined the moral and empirical presuppositions supporting more open disclosure. A patient who is to be an active participant in a partnership with a health care professional must have access to information that is potentially important or is meaningful in making decisions about care. Although the initial battles over truthful disclosure of such information were fought in the context of death-and-dying decisions, the logic of an active, informed patient jointly coming to an agreement with a physician about a plan of action applies to *all* health care. This chapter plays out the implications of the partnership model in the area of genetic counseling when a physician stumbles onto a piece of information of potential interest to a patient. It can be taken as the model for the moral conflict that might arise whenever the physician has potentially meaningful information regarding a patient's situation.

CASE 7: DISCLOSING POTENTIALLY DANGEROUS INFORMATION

Martha Lawrence was tense and nervous when she came to the Human Genetics Unit. She had been referred by her own physician because, unexpectedly pregnant at the age of forty-one, she was at risk for the birth of a mongoloid child. Mrs. Lawrence had given up her position as a high school teacher upon learning she was pregnant; she wanted the child, but wanted to consider abortion if there was an indication it was affected by Down's Syndrome. Since it was the eighteenth week of pregnancy, there was not much time to decide.

Mrs. Lawrence's first two pregnancies had been uncomplicated, and her sons (ages 16 and 13) were both in good health. The genetic counselor recommended amniocentesis, the withdrawal of a sample of the amniotic fluid surrounding the fetus, drawn from the abdomen with a needle. The fluid contains enough fetal cells for biochemical or chromosomal analysis.

The sample showed that the fetus had no extra twenty-first chromosome, and thus was free of translocational Down's Syndrome. But the sex chromosomes, rather than being "XX" (for female) or "XY" (for male), showed the abnormal "XYY" composition.

Some research has led to the hypothesis that XYY males might be "supermales," inclined to violent acts, including sexual offenses, while other recent studies do not confirm this.

Considering the inconclusive nature of such research, the possible danger to society and the Lawrence family, and the impact of the information on the way the Lawrences might treat the child, Dr. Gould faced a dilemma: What should he tell Mrs. Lawrence?

DISCUSSION

Dr. Gould's dilemma should dispel the common but naive assumption that the medical practitioner's role—even the genetic counselor's role—is to simply provide "the facts" to the patient. Dr. Gould has to decide not only which facts to communicate, but what the facts actually are. Which facts will fulfill his responsibilities as a counselor? Which will fulfill his moral obligation to the couple who have sought his advice?

The "Condition of Doubt" Problem

One fact that is clear, however, is that Dr. Gould has to decide something. There is no way out. This type of dilemma is becoming more common in the medical-scientific professions: some very human problem arises for which we have only a bit of scientific evidence, a promising theory, or perhaps only a wild hypothesis. Some day there may be more evidence, but the decision is demanded today. I call this a "condition of doubt" problem.

Whether patients who seek the professional's knowledge will get it depends, in part, on the physician's views about what to do when there is serious doubt. On the one hand the cautious person may say, "When there is real doubt, wait." He feels a moral imperative to wait until more evidence is in before acting positively. This view is firmly rooted in the Western scientific tradition, but it is clearly itself not based on scientific evidence. It is an expression of a judgment about the nature of the world.

At the other extreme is the position that when there is serious doubt, "proceed unless there is good reason not to." It makes sense to demand scientific evidence for confirming scientific propositions—for establishing "facts" as is done in the Western scientific tradition—but clinical medicine or counseling is a very different world. Some decision is demanded.

Do No Harm to the Patient

Mrs. Lawrence did not come to Dr. Gould worrying about an extra Y chromosome; she did not even ask him to tell her the child's sex (which he could have done). Her one concern was Down's Syndrome. Dr. Gould might decide he has fulfilled his professional responsibility by relieving Mrs. Lawrence of that anxiety, telling her that she is not carrying a fetus which would manifest Down's Syndrome. She would no doubt leave his office relieved, satisfied, and grateful. If the physician's moral duty is to do no harm to the patient (nonmaleficence), then he would have done his moral duty, avoiding the suffering and anxiety that could be generated by the revelation that the fetus's sex chromosomes were not normal.

If we were to assume that Dr. Gould was one of those enlightened physicians who considered his "patient" not just an isolated individual but the familial unit including the fetus, the case for not telling can be made, perhaps even more strongly. Anxiety and suffering might arise for the child as well as for his parents if the physician elected to "tell." To carry this argument a step further, when one considers that abortion is still possible at the eighteenth week of pregnancy, a strong case can be made that the most serious harm—death—could be done to a portion of the patient-family should the genetic status of the fetus be revealed.

THE HARM OF NOT TELLING

But the principle of protecting the patient from harm might also lead to argument in favor of telling Mrs. Lawrence about her baby's extra Y chromosome. If she later learns about it and hears or reads of the speculation about its implications, she may be subject to much greater suffering and anxiety than if she is told now. Her anxiety in this case would be compounded by her loss of confidence in her counselor.

BROADENING THE PRINCIPLE

Dr. Gould might broaden his ethical principle beyond the individual isolated case. The principle of doing no harm to the patient (or its positive counterpart of maximizing the good for the patient) is a variant of consequentialism. Limiting the consequences to just the isolated, individual patient makes the principle different from classical utilitarianism, in which the good of all is taken into consideration.

Dr. Gould may decide to abandon the individualism of the patient-physician relationship to broaden his ethical principle to include benefits and harms to all parties. This is dangerous to be sure, as it is the basis for the eugenic argument that an individual should be sterilized or a fetus aborted "for the good of society." From within the utilitarian framework, those arguments can be countered only by arguing that the harm done the individual—his loss of freedom or even loss of life—will always be greater than the good accomplished.

Yet even if Dr. Gould rejects the eugenic arguments, he may still look beyond the individual physician-patient relationship to the potential harm of the general practice of not telling when there is doubt or when there may be "bad news." The harm done in the long run—through breakdown in confidence in the professional group when it is learned that information may be routinely withheld—must be added into the calculation.

These long-term social considerations may lead to the conclusion that information should be disclosed even when the physician believes in the individual case that more harm than good will be done. Rule utilitarians will opt for the rule that produces more good than any other. Especially if one is concerned that physicians may tend to miscalculate the goods and harms that will come from a disclosure (because they have special value commitments, special psychological fears, or perspectives significantly different from the patient's), one might opt for the rule supporting disclosures in cases such as Mrs. Lawrence's where the physician believes that harm will result.

There are moral problems with this kind of support for a truth-telling rule, however. First, supporters of consequence-based ethics may be able to define special sets of circumstances where it can be predicted with great accuracy that more harm than good will actually come from the disclosure. For example, if an entire professional group were convinced that a particular class of disclosures would do harm on balance (such as disclosure of the extra Y chromosome), any idiosyncratic value biases would be overcome. If an interdisciplinary body (including patients as well as various kinds of professionals) reached that conclusion, even systematic evaluative and psychological distortions of a whole professional group such as physicians could be overcome. It is possible that in some cases, we really can conclude reasonably that more harm than good would come from a disclosure. A rule utilitarian would have to support nondisclosure in those cases if the class of disclosures could be described accurately and an exception incorporated into the rule. At this point, Mrs. Lawrence may make a moral appeal that moves beyond the consideration of consequences.

MOVING BEYOND THE CONSEQUENCES

The rightness of Dr. Gould's action may be determined not by consequences, but instead by certain right-making characteristics such as those identified in chapter 6, principles of autonomy, veracity, and the like. Were Mrs. Lawrence to ask explicitly if there were any other unexpected genetic anomalies, those who support a principle of veracity would hold that Dr. Gould is bound by it to answer truthfully. An outright lie destroys the trust of the contractual relation. More than that, it is simply the wrong thing to do. Perhaps the wrongness of the lie can be overcome in special circumstances by consideration of other moral principles, but insofar as veracity is a prima facie moral principle, it requires an honest response.

Of course, it is likely that Mrs. Lawrence will not think to ask if Dr. Lawrence has seen any other genetic anomalies. She may not understand that the amniocentesis is performed in such a way that other chromosomes including the XYY pattern can be seen. Is there any nonconsequentialist moral obligation for Dr. Gould to initiate the troublesome conversation, or can he simply rely on the claim that he did not tell a lie; he only failed to speak the whole truth?

If the relation between Dr. Gould and Mrs. Lawrence is a partnership built on a contractual moral commitment, that partnership generates moral expectations. The principle of fidelity to the contract requires that the implied understanding between the parties be honored. Is it a reasonable presumption—an implied commitment—that each party will disclose what the other would potentially find meaningful in carrying out the obligations of the relation? It is hard to imagine any other basis for a partnership.

We shall see in chapter 17 that this implies obligations for the patient as well as the physician to disclose potentially meaningful information. A patient in genetic counseling has a (moral) obligation to disclose, for example, exposure to potential teratogens, even illegal abusable drugs. That information is necessary for the professional to do his part of fulfilling the contract. Likewise, Dr. Gould has an obligation to disclose to Mrs. Lawrence information that she would reasonably find meaningful in deciding whether to carry her pregnancy to term. The working presumption is that fidelity to the partnership means giving her that information unless there has been an explicit agreement to the contrary. If Dr. Gould opposes abortion and does not want to be a party to one by providing the information, he has a duty to propose such limits on communication at the time the partnership is established. Since genetic counseling is an art developed up to the point that abortion is often the only option, Dr. Gould implies that he is willing to be a party to at least some abortions. In this case he is willing to be a party to abortions for Tri-somy 21 or he surely would not engage in this genetic counseling relation at all. If he is willing to provide information for Mrs. Lawrence to make a Tri-somy 21 abortion decision, but not for her to make other such decisions, he bears the responsibility to let her know his limits on the relation. Mrs. Lawrence can then decide whether she wants the counseling with the limits or prefers to establish some other patient-physician relation. Barring some "third-stage" contract, the principles of veracity and fidelity require the disclosure of the gratuitously discovered but potentially meaningful information.

Some analysts might conclude that the principle of autonomy also requires the disclosure, since Mrs. Lawrence cannot make an autonomous decision about her pregnancy without the information. Although that has become a common way of discussing such cases, I think it is a mistake. The principle of autonomy gives Mrs. Lawrence (and Dr. Gould) the right to be self-determining and to agree to enter the patient-physician partnership or refrain from doing so. It also gives them the right to withdraw from that partnership (barring special cases of irrevocable contracts). Autonomy, however, cannot generate an entitlement right, a right of one party to demand that another provide some good, service, or information. For instance, Mrs.

Lawrence cannot in the name of autonomy demand that Dr. Gould perform an abortion even if he has the required skill. To do so would violate his autonomy.

In fact, Dr. Gould does not generally have the duty to provide patients with potentially meaningful genetic information. A stranger who approached him demanding such information could justifiably be told to go away. What generates Dr. Gould's duty to disclose is the implied promises of the partnership contract. Physicians are expected to disclose what patients would reasonably find meaningful in deciding about their medical choices. Barring an explicit third-level contractual understanding to the contrary, fidelity requires Dr. Gould's disclosure to Mrs. Lawrence.

CHAPTER FOURTEEN

The Ethics of Dispensing Placebos

An active partnership between patient and professional requires fidelity to the commitment to disclose what the other party would reasonably expect to be told. This applies not only for terminally ill patients and to genetic counseling. It applies not only for revealing diagnostic information. It has important implications any time one of the parties knows something that reasonably would be of interest to the other. It has implications not only for physicians but also for other health professionals who may have potentially meaningful information for patients. The following case involves a pharmacist, but the same questions arise for the physician who prescribes, as well as for the pharmacist who dispenses.

CASE 8: DISPENSING PLACEBOS: THE PHARMACIST AS TRICKSTER

A pharmacist newly employed at a local pharmacy soon found himself in the middle of a case for which he had not been prepared during his professional education. It involved a prescription for an elderly woman who was a long-term client of the pharmacy. She had cancer of the colon that was managed medically. Some time earlier during her illness her physician had prescribed meperidine for pain and secobarbital for sleep. This barbiturate medication was continued long enough that she became addicted. After some months the physician was convinced that her tumor was under control and that his patient should be able to sleep without the medication. He had arranged with the pharmacist to dilute the secobarbital capsules gradually in order to detoxify his patient. The owner of the pharmacy began by opening the stock capsules and replacing some active medication with inert lactose. Gradually the percentage of lactose was increased to the point where the patient had for some time received completely inert placebos. The new pharmacist found himself with a prescription for secobarbital placebo.

He was disturbed by the prescription. Somehow he had a vague feeling that it was unfair to the patient, and he did not like to be a party to the deception. He was concerned about the expense involved. He learned that the pharmacist charged four dollars for the placebo prescription—far less than the real cost in time and material to compound the capsules. The physician had reduced his fee to a dollar for writing the prescriptions. Both fees seemed reasonable to him, but still this patient of modest means was having to pay sixty dollars a year for some lactose and gelatin capsules. What really bothered the pharmacist, however, was a vague sense that there was something unethical about the use of placebos. He suddenly found himself a part of something like a conspiracy to deceive a patient, to trick her into thinking she was getting real pharmacological help.

THE NOTION OF PLACEBOS

Placebos are an ancient medical tool. Not specific active therapy, they are used for their psychological effect. Some commentators point out that much of the history of medicine is really the history of placebo effects. It is true that many medical treatments—magical incantations, botanical extracts, leeches, a laying on of hands—probably have been effective, if at all, only through their nonspecific psychological effects, but in many of these cases those administering the therapy as well as those receiving it believed there was a specific, organic therapeutic action. The ethical problem of placebos arises when the prescriber is deliberately deceptive or misleading, knowing the compound is inactive but keeping this information from the patient.

Health care providers select placebos because they feel the substances will help patients and help them more than any of the alternatives. There is little doubt now that the placebo effect is real. A study by a New York psychiatrist points out that placebos can have an impact in virtually every therapeutic area.[1] They can reverse the action of potent active drugs, affect organic illnesses, even incurable malignancies, and mimic the effects of active drugs. A physician with a Ph.D. in philosophy who has written extensively on the placebo effect summarizes the literature showing that placebos have an effect not only on pain but also on cough, mood change, angina pectoris, headache, seasickness, anxiety, hypertension, status asthmaticus, depression, and the common cold.[2] Placebos can lower blood sugar levels in diabetics, control nausea, and even produce toxic side effects. In one study these included somnolence, palpitations, irritability and insomnia, weakness, temporal headache, diarrhea, collapse, and itching. Studies consistently find that 30 to 40 percent of patients report placebo responses, some of which are quite dramatic.[3]

The reason placebos work is not so obvious. The fact that they do is often used by commentators to prove that older notions that attempt to make a radical separation between the psychological and the organic are outmoded. Those intrigued by the wholistic health movement find support in the consistent presence of placebo effects. Norman Cousins, for instance, in a fascinating book devotes an entire chapter to the placebo effect as support for his thesis that the patient's mental state can have profound impact on the body's ability to heal itself.[4] One theory coming from a group at the University of California Medical Center in San Francisco headed by Jon D. Levine and his colleagues suggests that placebos may activate endorphins, stimulating natural pain-relieving and healing mechanisms.[5]

Although placebos are now known to have some toxic side effects, it is clear that these are normally much less than the side effects of other, more traditional pharmacological agents. This low pharmacological risk combined with their demonstrated effectiveness has provided the implicit moral justification for the use of placebos. If a little deception can help a patient, so the argument goes, what harm does it do? Even Thomas Jefferson, one of the Western world's most articulate defenders of rights and liberty, seems to have fallen for this appeal to good consequences. Writing to a physician friend, "If the appearance of doing something be necessary to keep alive the hope & spirits of the patient, it should be of the most innocent character. One of the most successful physicians I have ever known, has assured me, that he used more bread pills, drops of colored water, & powders of hickory ashes, than of all other medicines put together."[6]

MORAL PROBLEMS

Bread pills, colored water, and hickory ashes seem innocent enough, at least if the moral goal is to produce good effects for the patient. But those more skeptical of the morality of placebos raise two kinds of objections.

HARMFUL EFFECTS

First, there is the firm belief that the goal of the health care provider should be to do what he or she thinks is for the benefit of the patient. This, after all, is good Hippocratic medicine. Critics from within this framework, however, can easily point to problems that might occur with the use of a placebo. The young pharmacist noticed that there are economic costs to the benevolent ruse. There are more serious problems, as well.

Sissela Bok, the Harvard philosopher, summarizes some of the other harms that placebos can cause.[7] She mentions the pharmacological effects mentioned above—the nausea, headaches, and other side effects. She cites a case of dependency where a psychotic patient was given placebo pills and told they were a "new major tranquilizer without any side effects." The patient after four years was taking twelve tablets a day and complaining of insomnia and anxiety.

Even more serious is the damage that can be done to a patient by relying on a placebo when more active therapy would have provided even more help. Brody points out that many of the suggested uses really just substitute the placebo for some other therapy, perhaps more difficult to administer, but also more effective. He cites temporary anxiety states and situations where placebos might be used initially to placate a patient until a doctor-patient relationship can be established for more direct use of psycho-therapy or emotional support. He points out that there are more effective, pharmacologically active antianxiety agents readily available that are known to be effective in a larger percentage of patients than the placebos. He also suggests that it is hard to buy time in order to build a solid, trusting physician-patient relationship by beginning the relationship with a decep-tion.[8]

This suggests a more serious set of bad consequences that may come from the use of placebos. Even if there are no pharmacological harms done, there may be psychological harms. Some patients are going to discover that there has been a deception, that the physician has purposely maneuvered them for their own good. Eventually the health care profession could gain the reputation of a group prone to deception, thus breaking the lay popula-tion's confidence in the professional and defeating the intention of the deception.

NONCONSEQUENTIALISTIC CONSIDERATIONS

For defenders of the deontological view of ethics, deception is simply wrong independent of its consequences. It violates the basic moral duty to be respectful of others in human relationships. Insofar as there is a con-tractual commitment requiring fidelity among the partners in the relation, that fidelity is violated when one party is deceived by the other. Patients have been known to mislead their physicians by withholding potentially important information from them. For example, they may fail to disclose exposure to some environmental factor that would explain an illness and change a course of therapy. They may fail to reveal that they are not taking medication as prescribed. This can be done from the most benevolent of motives. The patient may want to avoid hurting the physician's feelings. It makes no difference that such benevolent deceptions are shortsighted, that such nondisclosures actually jeopardize the patient's interests. The *moral* wrong is that the physician is deceived; he is treated without the respect that the relation requires. Likewise, patients who are given placebos are treated without respect. There is a violation of the trust required of the relation. This is a second, quite different, basis for opposing placebos.

In the partnership model, lay people have a duty, a responsibility, to be actively involved in their own care. Because of the very nature of placebo therapy, it is almost impossible for a patient to give an informed consent to such treatment. If one is told the basis on which the placebo works, its effectiveness will be destroyed. There is one study that found, paradoxically, that some patients still experienced placebo effects even after they were told the medication they were given was inert,[9] but generally the placebo effect is incompatible with the moral and legal requirements of informed consent. It is impossible for the patient to be an active partner in the therapeutic process and simultaneously be deceived about the very nature of the therapeutic strategy.

There is only one other situation where placebos can be used effectively without deception. In the double-blind clinical trials in which an active compound is compared to a placebo, the validity of the research is preserved if subjects are told there is a placebo in the design. Of course, neither the subjects nor the investigator knows who gets the inert substance, but subjects can consent to having the placebo in the design and thus having a chance of receiving it.

Barring these special situations, however, the placebo necessarily involves a deception. For those who believe there are moral obligations to be honest and faithful to a relation independent of the consequences, placebos will be morally impossible. One suspects that the new pharmacist given the prescription for a placebo had a twinge of moral conscience because he felt there was just something wrong with treating the patient this way, that it was violating her rights or her dignity, that it was violating his obligation to treat her as a respected person even if it did not produce bad consequences in her case.

The patient, the physician, and the pharmacist are morally in quite different positions when it comes to deciding the ethics of placebo use. Patients probably differ on whether they would approve of having their physician prescribe placebos. Some certainly would object; others probably would approve. Yet in principle there is normally no way that either the physician or the pharmacist can inquire about the patient's views. To do so would destroy the effectiveness of the therapy. In regular, ongoing relationships between a patient and a physician, the professional might take the initiative and ask the general question whether the patient would approve of placebo use if ever it was thought valuable. A blanket "uninformed consent" at the level of the third contract in which the patient and the physician agree that such deceptions are acceptable provides the only possibility for an ethically justifiable use of placebos.

CHAPTER FIFTEEN

The Patient's Right of Access to Medical Records

Compared to the ethical controversy surrounding heart transplants, psychosurgery for behavior modification, manipulation of the human genetic code, and in vitro fertilization of human egg cells, a patient's right of access to his medical records and control over his medical treatment may seem mundane. As a result, this issue tends to be overlooked. But because of growing pressure from patients who want to know what their records contain, physicians may soon be forced to deal with regular requests for such information. They may then find that this issue has a more fundamental effect on current medical practice than any of the more exotic forms of medical care.

The inherent inequality of the physician-patient relationship is probably the major reason why the contents of medical records have not traditionally been made available to patients. In the old Hippocratic model of health care, patients went to doctors for their highly specialized knowledge and skills, and in most cases simply trusted physicians to act in their best interest. Physicians have moved dramatically in the past generation toward more open disclosure. At least with regard to critical pieces of information such as diagnosis of a terminal illness, they are more willing to inform patients. Yet patients are still expressing an interest in more information than physicians disclose. As the partnership model replaces the more paternalistic model, shielding patients from their own medical information makes less and less sense. Some patients are pressing for the most complete sharing of information possible, including direct access to their medical records.

THE NEED FOR RECORDS

In the past, patients rarely challenged physicians' handling of their medical affairs. But in any system where the contents of personal files are kept from the person concerned, abuses can occur. Furthermore, since medical treatment can affect an individual's life dramatically, patients often need access to their medical records to make more informed decisions about that treatment, or about their future.

In addition to the ethical questions that surround the issue of access to medical records, there are legal considerations.[1] Many patients consider their records their property—a part of the "service" they have purchased from the physician rendering care. According to this view, access to records is a basic civil right. Statutes dealing with confidentiality of medical records appear to support this right. Confidentiality belongs to the patient; with some special exceptions, such as conditions requiring compulsory reporting of venereal disease, it is the patient whose permission is needed in order for physicians to be released from the bounds of confidentiality.[2]

Patients with the most urgent need for access to their medical records are probably the terminally ill. Although the right of dying patients to refuse treatment is now well established, these patients sometimes lack the information necessary to make a responsible choice. While many physicians routinely consult a patient before or during extraordinary and heroic life-saving and dying-prolonging treatment, this practice is by no means universal. Even physicians who are concerned about whether to begin or cease heroic treatment on a terminal patient often discuss the question with their colleagues, but not with the patient. In other words, even from the perspective of concern, many physicians see their responsibility as deciding what procedure to "perform on" a human being and, as a result, deny the patient the fundamental right to control his or her own treatment.

What kinds of cases have led patients to insist on access to their records? The need may be more common than most physicians think. For example, a woman with a nineteen-year-old daughter was given a fertility drug 20 years ago. She had been trying—unsuccessfully—to find out whether the drug her physician gave her was diethylstilbestrol. The following case provides another example.

CASE 9: WHAT IS IN MY COMPUTERIZED MEDICAL RECORD?

> A middle-aged man with a history of inactive diabetes was excluded from his company's group medical insurance coverage. His fellow employees agreed to change companies if another would agree to take him. They found a willing company and made the switch. However, the man was informed by the company's agent that he should say nothing about the diabetes, because the information was not yet in the central computer where the insurance industry stores patient medical records. Alarmed that the insurance industry was keeping a file on him, the man has been trying to find out what his record contains and how the information stored in the computer is used. So far, his efforts have been unsuccessful.

Growing concern over the contents of medical records has also been voiced by those who have participated in research studies. One family consented to take part in a longitudinal study by a major medical center on the relationship of prenatal factors and child health and development. The mother and her son were examined at regular intervals for seven years, until the parents became concerned over the large amount of psychological and neurological data that was being gathered about their apparently normal child. They said they would continue to participate in the study only if they could examine their son's records. Their request was denied. The reason given was that the study was funded by the government, and while records were sent to the child's pediatrician, there was no budget provision for copies to give to the parents. The parents became even more concerned when they learned that the government received copies of test results, and they asked to see the contents of the files the government had on their son. So far, they have been allowed to see the medical center records from some of the early tests, but have not yet seen any recent records or the contents of the government files.

THE ARGUMENT AGAINST ACCESS

The main argument against access to medical records is the traditional Hippocratic one: truthful information about their conditions can be upsetting to patients. From the paternalistic point of view, the health professional has a duty to protect patients from themselves. If patients would become upset at the truth or if their misunderstanding of it would lead them to harmful behavior—to irrationally refuse surgery or withdraw from a professional relation—then the physician, according to this Hippocratic stance, has a duty to protect them by withholding information.

The problem arises most frequently in the case of psychiatric records. Particularly with paranoid patients, it is argued that disclosure of the diagnosis and other notes made by the clinician in the record could undermine the therapeutic strategy. For this reason many state laws granting patients a legal right of access to their medical records, such as those of Maine, Massachusetts, Nebraska, Nevada, New Jersey, Oklahoma, Pennsylvania, and Texas, exempt psychiatric records.[3]

The argument is essentially a manifestation of the therapeutic privilege argument examined in chapter 12. There we saw that clinicians may not be good at predicting the harm that can come from the disclosure of information. Physicians who have made it a routine practice to give patients copies of their records do not report serious harmful effects. To the contrary, their experience has been overwhelmingly positive.[4]

Even if it is true that patients will occasionally be upset or even hurt by disclosure, it still does not follow that withholding is justified. If patients are to be treated as partners in the health care relation, then access to the information and documents necessary to participate fully in that partnership seems essential. A partnership in which the patient would like to have access that is not provided will be deficient regardless of whether there is anything in the record that the clinician wants to keep from the patient. Such access can become an important symbol of partnership even when it is not substantively important.

Access to the medical record becomes one element of the right of access to information. In the partnership model, both parties have to have the access needed to fulfill their responsibilities as well as to feel fully and actively responsible. The clinician thus has a right of access, and the patient has a duty to disclose information that is reasonably necessary for the clinician to fulfill his or her responsibilities. The patient who withheld critical information from a psychiatrist, such as sensitive thoughts and feelings, not only would risk jeopardizing the clinician's ability to help but also would be reneging on the implied promise of open disclosure. If the sensitive thoughts and feelings happened to be in written letters or other documents, the psychiatrist would be justified in wanting to see the actual documents rather than have the patient present a mere oral summary of them.

Likewise, if the physician possesses information that is reasonably likely to be meaningful to the patient in making key decisions about the therapeutic relation (including the decision to remain in the relation), then the patient has the right to that information. If it is in writing, he or she has the right to the written form. If it contains information embarrassing to or incriminating the clinician, it is that much more likely to be meaningful to the patient. If patients are to be taken seriously, they have to have such access.

Of course, there are limits to that right of access when the patient is incompetent. If the patient is a minor or is severely retarded, for example, there must be a surrogate medical decisionmaker—a parent or guardian or other person with legal authority to make medical decisions for the patient. In that case, the surrogate has to be brought into the partnership with a right of access to the record. That surrogate will have to decide how much, if any, of the record should be in the hands of the incompetent one. Some parents might routinely want their older children to have such access. Provided mechanisms are available to explain potentially confusing or misleading information, that would seem to be a wise practice.

In chapter 12, I concluded that if information is merely disturbing to a patient, that fact does not preclude disclosure, but if the information is so disturbing that it renders the patient incompetent, then procedures must be undertaken to assure that a suitable legal surrogate is appointed to function as the patient's decisionmaker. The same conclusions seem to apply to written medical records as to oral information about diagnosis and prognosis. If there is a patient, say a psychiatric patient, for whom the clinician believes the disclosure of the record will be so debilitating as to render that person incompetent to consent or refuse consent to further therapy, then it is literally impossible to get an adequately informed consent to treatment. The very process of giving the information makes the patient incompetent to process it. While I believe this degree of trauma from medical records is extremely unlikely, we should concede that it can occur.

The only recourse is to seek to have such a patient declared incompetent and have a guardian appointed who can process the information and offer a proxy consent on the patient's behalf. The incompetent patient, like the child or the retarded incompetent, does not have an automatic right of access to the record. That guardian may still reach the conclusion that some or all of the record should be disclosed to the patient now, not for the purposes of obtaining a consent but to bring the patient as fully as possible into the partnership relation. I remain convinced that there are very few disclosures of written or oral information that would really make their patients incompetent. It is extremely rare to see competency hearings on these grounds. If the clinician is not prepared to follow through to the point of seeking a guardian, then he or she should not argue that the information itself would render the patient incompetent.

A good case can be made on both consequentialistic and nonconsequentialistic grounds that offering a copy of the record should be routine practice. On pragmatic grounds alone, the number of cases involving patients traveling to other towns or receiving emergency medical care when their own physicians cannot be reached suggests that great good could come from routine patient retention of a copy of the record. We are increasingly a mobile society. The ability of the clinician to get a copy of the record to the patient's bedside when it is needed is increasingly problematic.

This moral and legal right of access does not necessarily imply that all records must be disclosed. There may still be special cases where the clinician believes that access to the record would be harmful or where the patient does not want to be bothered. In the partnership model, there is room at the level of the third contract for the individual clinician and patient to agree to an exception to the normal rule in favor of disclosure. The clinician might in these exceptional cases propose a waiver on the part of the patient to the right of access to the medical record. Should the patient agree, that special arrangement could become a part of the terms of that particular partnership. Should the patient disagree, he or she at least retains the right to break the relation knowing that the record is being withheld.

It is a difficult question whether the clinician should be able to make such a special third-level contractual limit on right of access a necessary part of a lay-professional relation. If there were an ample supply of clinicians willing to disclose medical records and other critical information, I would have no strong objection to such a contingent contract. In the present world, however, the patient who insisted on his or her right of access might not be able to find any clinician willing to establish a relation on that basis. As long as the power of the clinician is so strong, there are some rights of the patient that shold be unsurrenderable, at least at the clinician's behest. Should the patient refuse to exercise his right of access, no one can seriously complain, but for clinicians to make a physician-patient relation contingent on the patient's waiver of a right of access to medical records seems to be a coercively limiting stipulation. Of course, legally guaranteeing patients the right of access to their records would not necessarily solve the problem once and for all. Some physicians, for example, say that if they were forced to show patients their records, they would simply start keeping a duplicate set. Not only would this be a violation of the spirit of these guarantees, but once the patient's right of access to his records is established, physicians could be sued for engaging in duplicity.

A better solution would be to reeducate both physicians and patients concerning the necessities of the partnership model of the lay-professional relation. If the patient and the professional are each to be viewed as full, active, and responsible partners in a common enterprise, then each has to have full access to the data necessary to make the relation work. Each has to treat the other as a partner in the full sense of the word. The lingering doubt on the part of the professional that patients can handle the truth makes such a relation impossible. Unless the patient consents in special circumstances to waiving the right of access, medical records should routinely be in the hands of patients.

CHAPTER SIXTEEN

The Limits of Confidentiality: The Case of the Homosexual Husband

David, the oldest of three children, was the son of a well-to-do manufacturer. David's father valued physical prowess and athletic accomplishments, areas in which the boy showed little interest. When David was twelve or thirteen years old, conflicts with his father resulted in almost nightly arguments. It was evident that David's father had become concerned about his son's mannerisms and considered them to be effeminate.

David's schoolwork deteriorated considerably, and he became withdrawn. His father decided to send him to a military school, but he remained there for only six months. By this time, David had told his parents that he was a homosexual, that he had engaged in and was engaging in homosexual practices. He came home and completed his high school studies but he did not go to college and continued to live at home.

He was treated for gonorrhea, asthma, and infectious hepatitis. At the age of twenty-one, to gain exemption from the draft, his physician attested to the fact that he was a homosexual.

Five years later, Joan visited her family physician for a premarital serological exam. The physician was the same practitioner who had treated David. Joan was twenty-four years old and had been under his care since the age of fourteen. A close and warm relationship had developed between the physician and Joan's family, so it was normal for him to ask about her fiancé. When he did, he learned that she was about to marry David. She had known him only briefly, but well enough, she felt, to be certain about her choice. Nothing more was said at the time.

David and Joan were married shortly thereafter and lived together for six months. The marriage was annulled on the basis of nonconsummation. David told Joan that he was homosexually oriented, and she learned as well that not only did they share a physician but also the physician was aware of

138

David's homosexuality. She subsequently suffered a depression as a result of this experience and was angry that her physician had remained silent about David. She felt that she could have been spared this horrible episode in her life—that it was his duty to inform her. His failure to do so was an act of negligence resulting in deep emotional scars.

To whom did the physician owe primary allegiance? Do the interests of one patient prevail over the requirements of confidentiality surrounding another's case?

At least in uncomplicated cases, the practitioner should convey to the patient any medically relevant information that would be potentially meaningful or useful in medical decisionmaking. The physician's Hippocratic ethic instructs him to do what he thinks will benefit his patient. Lay people form similar conclusions from other systems of ethics focusing on principles of autonomy and honesty.

The tradition of physician ethics on confidentiality is not at all clear. The Hippocratic Oath, marvelous in its ambiguity, says that the physician should keep secret things he learns in his practice that ought not to be "spread abroad."[1] Which things those are is not specified. The World Medical Association's (WMA) twentieth-century version of the Hippocratic Oath states simplistically that the physician will keep confidences entrusted in him.[2]

On the other hand, the 1957 version of the American Medical Association takes a quite different approach. Its principle of ethics says that the physician ought not to disclose things learned in confidence except in three cases: when disclosure is required by law, when it is in the patient's interest, or when it is in the interests of other people.[3] The AMA during that period insisted on the physician's duty to disclose to persons other than the patient from whom the relevant information has been learned, thus taking a much more social course. But it opens the door for a wide range of disclosures.

Nowhere does traditional physician ethics say anything about resolving conflicts between duties to two patients whose interests may diverge and may differ from the practitioner's. By the time the physician has reached a dilemma such as that cited above, there may simply be no morally acceptable resolution. If the problem of potential conflict had been faced earlier, several solutions might have been acceptable. The problem is one of clarifying the ethical covenant between the profession and the society, i.e., the second-level contract. The grounding of the ethic of confidentiality is not as clear as it might appear. Some hold that there is something intrinsic to the professional role in medicine that requires confidentiality. There are obvious advantages in creating an environment in which professional and patient trust each other. I think it makes the most sense to view confidentiality as a promise made by the profession to the lay population as part of the second-level contract. Fidelity to the promise is then the moral grounding of the confidentiality rule.

This provides a basis for resolving what appears to be the intractable conflict in the case of the homosexual husband. The promise of confidentiality has to be made in such a way that it will not conflict with the promise to serve another patient's welfare (or at least so that there is a clear priority rule covering cases where the welfare of others requires breaking confidence). The AMA rule during the period of 1957 to 1980 provided that a confidence may be broken if necessary "to protect the welfare of the individual or the community." That would clearly arrange priorities for the physician in our case. Assuming the woman has a real interest in knowing about her future husband's inclination, confidentiality would give way.

Upon reflection, however, it is doubtful that reasonable lay people and professionals would agree to the provisions endorsed by the AMA. It suggests that whenever third parties stood to gain even in the smallest amount, confidences could be broken apparently at the discretion of the physician. Taken literally, it condones breaking confidence to serve other people's trivial interest even if doing so hurts the patient seriously. Surely that is not a rule to which rational lay people and professionals would agree. It violates not only traditional professional standards but also what reasonable lay people would want of their health professionals.

On the other hand, reasonable people probably would not shift as far in the other direction as the WMA's total prohibition on disclosure. I believe they would insist on a promise of confidentiality with a compulsory exception clause to be exercised only when there was a grave threat of bodily harm to other persons. That is the kind of standard that emerged in the Tarasoff case, the most well known legal case requiring a professional as a duty (not merely a right) to warn third parties of serious risks of harm.[4] Although in a contract approach to medical ethics it is not definitively important what the professional group adopts, it is encouraging that the AMA has adopted this view in its interpretation of its recent revision of its principles of ethics. Although the principles themselves unrealistically eliminate all exceptions to the confidentiality requirement except in cases where disclosure is required by law,[5] the Council on Ethical and Judicial Affairs interprets this to mean that "where a patient threatens to inflict serious bodily harm to another person and there is a reasonable probability that the patient may carry out the threat, the physician should take reasonable precautions for the protection of the intended victim. . . ."[6] If such a proposal were agreed to by reasonable lay people and professionals meeting together taking the moral point of view (and I am convinced that it would be), then the only question in our case is whether the physician believes that David poses a serious threat of bodily harm and exactly who should be warned.

Although the drafters of this proposal probably had in mind threatened assaults, certainly the exposure to a continued risk of veneral disease would count as a grave threat of bodily harm, as would those who purposely plan to continue sexual activity after testing positive for HIV infection. Whether the history of homosexual preference itself constitutes a threat of *bodily* harm to a young woman planning marriage is somewhat more difficult to assess. Those of us advocating requirements to break confidentiality in cases of threat of harm to others have insisted on the reference to bodily harm as a way of avoiding disclosures justified on the basis of vague psychological threats. Certainly there is no reason in principle why serious threats of grave psychological harm that can be accurately predicted should not also justify disclosure. This woman's risk seems quite predictable and severe. When it is combined with the physical risks of infection, I would have no difficulty concluding that the promise of confidentiality must give way.

If that is the nature of the appropriate promise, however, all patients need to understand the limits on such a commitment. To the contrary, David most certainly was not told and did not understand that confidences he conveyed to his physician would be disclosed in cases of grave threat of bodily harm. The working understanding of many health care professionals and patients is a promise of confidentiality without exception. If that is David's understanding, and at the same time Joan had good reason to believe that the physician had promised always to treat her by acting in her interest, then the physician has made two incompatible promises. Is there anything he can do to make the best of this impossible situation? I think there is.

Assuming that the physician is convinced that the information would be important to the woman, he could explain his perception of the situation to her future spouse, determine whether she does know about the homosexuality, and try to convince him of the importance of telling her. If he agrees, the physician's problem disappears. If he does not, the physician has three options.

First, he could continue in both physician-patient relationships without disclosing. This seems to me to be the least acceptable option, a basic violation of the implicit promise of trust and confidence. Second, he could disclose anyway, after explaining to the man that he has a moral obligation to do so. (Although I am convinced that such a case might arise, I am not convinced that this situation fits the description.)

Third, he could withdraw from one or both relationships. He might claim that his practice was so busy that he had to transfer one or both to a colleague—a blatantly deceitful explanation. He could say openly that he had to break the relationship because of information received in confidence, but that would provoke so much curiosity that it might lead to violation of the confidence. He could say vaguely that conditions in his practice were such that he had to transfer one or both to colleagues. As unsatisfactory as this solution is, I believe that it may be the best moral compromise available.

In transferring the woman to another physician, he no longer has a duty to do what would benefit her as his patient. That satisfies the Hippocratic rules, but somehow to me it is still morally very unsatisfying. In fact, from my standpoint as a nonphysician, the duty to disclose is strong even if the person who may benefit from the disclosure is no longer the physician's patient. Nevertheless, breaking the relationship is preferable to continuing in a relationship that must be based on trust without disclosure.

This case shows how important it is to know clearly what the ethical ground rules are at the beginning of a relationship. I prefer openness and disclosure, even if privacies must occasionally be violated. If patients know in advance that the physician may be forced by conscience to break confidences in certain limited situations, I do not think they have grounds for objecting to such disclosures.

CHAPTER SEVENTEEN

Patients' Duties
and Physicians' Rights

Traditional Hippocratic medical ethics has tended to view the patient as a passive participant in the physician-patient relation. This passivity is exacerbated by those who continue to insist that patients seeing physicians are so ill that they normally cannot function as rational agents in a partnership of decisionmaking. The Parsonian sick role casts the patient as dependent and exempt from the normal social duties of adulthood.[1] Some establishment sociologists of medicine insist that the appropriate analogy of the relationship between physician and patient is that of parent to child.[2] Even practitioners who try to be enlightened about the relationship speak of the physician's goal as "restoring autonomy." Physician Eric Cassell often expresses the traditional image of the patient as infantile, out of control, and helpless:

> If I had to pick the aspect of illness that is most destructive to the sick, I would choose the loss of control. Maintaining control over oneself is so vital to all of us that one might see all the other phenomena of illness as doing harm not only in their own right but doubly so as they reinforce the sick person's perception that he is no longer in control. . . . The sick have much in common with the infant. . . . It is perfectly apparent that the sick person is dependent. . . . Therefore, when we say that the sick are dependent, we say they are takers of what others give. . . . In the contract between doctor and patient, the dependent sick person's willingness to receive is part of the currency of the bargain.[3]

The typical patient-physician relationship is actually far from this image of infantilism. Especially in the era of health maintenance, immunizations, and chronic illness, most patients interacting with physicians are relatively healthy. They are there to obtain physical exams or routine health screening, to take infants to well-baby clinics, or for counseling. Those who are ill often have conditions that are far from all-consuming. Some have colds, influenza, or other rather minor problems. In addition, many of those with more serious problems can hardly be said to have regressed to infancy. They have broken arms, heart arrhythmias, diabetes, hypertension, or other conditions that hardly leave one incoherent. A large number of physician-patient interactions involve follow-up visits, say from surgery, in which the patient is ambulatory, reflective, and lucid. Even with prototypical chronic serious illness such as cancer, heart disease, or renal failure, the typical patient is not so debilitated that he or she should be analogized to an infant.

Some patients, of course, really are seriously incapacitated. They are unconscious or compromised with Alzheimer's disease. They are in such pain that they cannot think clearly. Even they, however, are not really like infants. Adults or adolescents will have developed a system of beliefs and values. They may have left living wills instructing others about their wishes for medical care. They may have views so clear that their wishes can be constructed. Even for those who do not, other members of the lay health care team—the family, friends, and relatives who stand with the patient—will normally be reasonably autonomous, thinking agents capable of stepping into the surrogacy role and acting as substantially autonomous decision-makers.

If the old image of passivity is inappropriate for most patients today, there are important implications for the ethics of the lay-professional relation. In the partnership I am describing, both parties have duties and, reciprocally, both have rights, derived from the basic contracts that I have outlined. Both patients and physicians will be bound by the ethical constraints of the first social contract just as all other members of the basic social community are. The basic principles of respecting autonomy, fidelity, veracity, avoiding killing, and justice will provide the framework within which the second contract, governing the roles of health professional and lay actor in the medical role, will be defined. While medical ethics historically has tended to articulate the duties of the health professional as the more obviously active, responsible party in the relationship, recently we have begun to see scholars and reformers writing aggressively about the rights of the patient—the corollary to duties of the physician. But relatively little is written about the converse duties and rights, the duties of the patient and the rights of the physician. Before we turn to a more detailed analysis of the implications of the individual principles of medical ethics, something should be said about this less obvious dimension to the patient-physician relation. Only if we view the dynamic as one involving duties for patients and rights for physicians as well as the other way around will a true partnership model with a convergence of interests and mutual responsibility be possible.

HISTORICAL PRECURSORS

There is nothing in the Hippocratic Oath about the duties of patients. Thomas Percival's classical medical ethics written at the end of the eighteenth century goes into enormous detail about the duties of professionals, both to each other and to their patients, but has nothing on the duties of patients.[4] Percival, writing in the context of a local intraprofessional dispute among physicians, surgeons, and apothecaries, thus provides a framework whereby one might establish correlative rights of professionals vis-à-vis one another. He never uses the term *rights* in referring to rights either of professionals or of patients, but were a set of rights to be derived, the rights of professionals that one might find in Percival are claims only against other professionals, not against patients.

When the American Medical Association wrote its first code of ethics in 1847, it included a set of eight "obligations of patients to their physicians."[5] Their tone is conveyed by the introductory paragraph:

> The members of the medical profession, upon whom are enjoined the performance of so many important and arduous duties towards the community, and who are required to make so many sacrifices of comfort, ease, and health, for the welfare of those who avail themselves of their services, certainly have a right to expect and require, that their patients should entertain a just sense of the duties which they owe to their medical attendants.

The obligations that are then spelled out seem rather archaic today. They are set in the context of the intraprofessional controversies of the day when orthodox medicine was emerging from alternative, sometimes dubious medical systems. Thus one of the duties of the patient is to "prefer a physician whose habits of life are regular, and who is not devoted to company, pleasure, or to any pursuit incompatible with his professional obligations." Others focus on showing proper deference and respect: patients should "faithfully and unreservedly communicate to their physician." They should, however, simultaneously "never weary the physician with a tedious detail of events or matters not appertaining to [the] disease." Patients should obey the physician's prescriptions promptly and implicitly, without being influenced by their own crude opinions about their fitness. And a patient should avoid even friendly visits of a physician who is not attending him. He should declare his reasons for dismissing the physician. Justice and common courtesy require this, we are told.

THE DUTIES OF PATIENTS

The AMA's nineteenth-century list may have excluded some duties that patients should bear within the context of the contracts I have outlined. The duties of patients are as broad and as specific as the implications of all the principles of ethics derived from the basic social contract and the secondary obligations of the contract between the medical profession and the lay population. Thus all the moral obligations of being a member of a moral community apply.

FIDELITY

Paying Bills and Keeping Appointments

Perhaps the most fundamental ethical obligation of each party in a contract system of ethics is the duty of fidelity to the commitments made or implied in the contract. In a multilevel contract theory with basic social contracts as well as contracts among individuals, this does not reduce ethics to agreements among individuals. It also means keeping commitments to the basic ethical principles and the socially articulated understandings of the various professional and lay roles. It will include, however, individual commitments made at the third stage of the contract process. Some of the promises may be as mundane as the commitment to pay bills and keep appointments. It is odd that in medicine, services appear to be authorized without any discussion of prices. In other contractual relations, we would not think of signing up for services without knowing the monetary terms. Even among lawyers there is normally an agreement stipulating what the hourly rate will be. It might even be argued that the establishment of a convenantal relation between physician and patient is not complete if there is no mutual understanding about financial terms.

The same is true regarding the keeping of appointments. A professional's time is important. Normally a physician will have made promises to other patients that will be compromised by a late arrival. Certainly it is well within a physician's rights—other things being equal—to charge for appointments missed.

This, of course, is a mutual promising. Each party agrees to see the other at a specified time. A physician who misses an appointment or is late is just as much in violation of the covenant, is just as much breaking the fidelity. It would seem reasonable that a physician who follows a practice of charging patients who miss appointments should suitably compensate patients who are kept waiting when he or she is late. Something like waiving a quarter of the fee for each fifteen minutes a patient is kept waiting seems reasonable to me. The point here is not to work out the details of fair compensation when the promise of the appointment is violated, but rather to suggest that each party has a moral obligation grounded in fidelity to assure that—other things being equal—the appointment is kept.

I say "other things being equal" because, as was outlined in chapter 16, sometimes the requirements of fidelity conflict with other ethical principles. Regardless of which theory is used for resolving conflict among principles, sometimes the promise of the appointment may have to give way. Either party may have weightier promises that have been made—to care for one's children, for example.

When we examine the medical implications of the principle of justice, I shall argue that it requires that resources (including time) be arranged so as to benefit the least well off. If another who is not a patient has a desperate need for immediate medical attention, justice might require a physician temporarily to abandon a patient (say, one who has been promised a physical exam). In later chapters I shall suggest that there is a general provision of the second contract that normally exempts physicians from what might appear to be a duty of justice to abandon patients when a nonpatient may have marginally greater medical need. Nevertheless, in some cases the duty of justice may so overwhelm promises made, including the promise to keep an appointment, that on balance appointments ought to be missed. Even more obviously, the conflict may arise when another patient to whom the physician has promised loyalty has an immediate medical need. Then two promises are in direct conflict; one must be broken. In such cases, however, physicians owe something to the patient; they have what is sometimes called a duty of reparation to make amends for the violation of the patient's trust.

Likewise, a patient may have some conflicting obligation that justifies breaking the promise of the appointment. If we accept the argument that beneficence alone can never override nonconsequentialist duties, the patient's reason for missing an appointment can never be based simply on consequences. It may, however, involve conflicting nonconsequentialist duties, such as the need of a child to whom one has made a promise of fidelity or the need of someone who is worse off and therefore has a conflicting claim grounded in justice. If the patient does respond to these conflicting duties by violating the promise of the appointment, there is once again a duty of reparation, of paying for the missed appointment as well as phoning to apologize and minimize the harm done.

This same logic of conflicting duties may even justify failure to pay the bill. Justice would seem to require using scarce resources so as to keep fundamental commitments (such as to one's children) or to benefit the least well off. On these grounds, if a patient is unexpectedly strapped for resources, it seems reasonable to pay bills according to the principle of justice—to benefit the least well off first. The key here, however, is the term *unexpectedly*. Promises, including the promises of the physician-patient relationship, should not normally be made if there is any likelihood they cannot be kept. In the normal relationship, the duties of fidelity require things such as paying bills on time and keeping appointments.

Confidentiality

Another aspect of fidelity is confidentiality. In chapter 16 I suggested that the normal duty of the health professional to keep confidences should be understood as derived from a promise made at the level of the second contract. There is a reciprocal promise that information disclosed within the lay-professional relationship will not be disclosed to third parties. If the parties negotiating that second-stage contract are at all reasonable, they will include some limits on that promise, probably including an exception clause in those cases where failure to disclose will do serious bodily harm to third parties.

They might also include what is called the therapeutic privilege exception, a provision discussed in detail in chapter 12. It would permit violating confidences whenever the clinician has reason to believe it would be in the interest of the patient to do so. In that chapter I argued that it would be irrational of patients to include the therapeutic privilege exception in the general promise of confidentiality between the professional and the lay population. Nevertheless, within the constraints of exceptions agreed to, the duty of confidentiality rests on a set of promises and thus within the context of the principle of fidelity.

Like physicians, patients bear the responsibility to keep the promise of confidentiality. Both parties ought to be under the constraints of the second-level contract, in which each promises not to disclose private information learned about the other in the course of the relationship (unless there is a serious threat of bodily harm to third parties).

Of course, much of the information a patient might want to disclose could be of great interest to third parties. If a patient believed that a physician was intoxicated, that a surgeon was grossly negligent, or that sexual indiscretion had taken place, disclosure would be called for, in fact morally required, if it could protect third parties from serious harm. In other cases, however, patients may learn things in the professional relation which they have a duty to keep confidential. The most obvious example would be information they learn about other patients by observation, accidental disclosure, or even careless indiscretion of the physician.

Were the physician to disclose personal information about himself during the course of patient education and counseling, the duty of confidentiality might apply. The patient being comforted following disclosure of a stigmatizing diagnosis (alcoholism or mental depression, for example) who is told by her physician that he also has suffered from the condition owes to that physician the same duty of confidentiality that the physician owes to the patient. If both are significantly responsible moral agents, they both bear the duties of confidentiality. The second-level contract would contain a promise of mutual respect for the private information of the other.

VERACITY

Another basic ethical principle is veracity. In chapter 12 I explored the implications of physician disclosure of information to patients. It is increasingly clear that there is also an ethic of patient disclosure to physicians. Physicians, like patients, have a right to be informed about anything they reasonably would want to know from the patient before agreeing to the third-level contract. This could be information about the patient's plan to make use of the diagnostic information from the relation. If a geneticist is asked prior to amniocentesis about the sex of a fetus, he has the right to know what use will be made of the information. Just as patients have the right to know of any objections to abortion on the part of the clinician that could cloud the communication, so the physician has the right to know if the patient is contemplating an abortion, especially for problematic reasons such as sex selection.

Regarding the therapeutic privilege exception to the physician's duty to disclose, I have suggested that there are good reasons why reasonable lay people and professionals agreeing on the terms of the second-level contract would not include a clause giving the professional the right to withhold information he or she believes would be harmful to the patient. If that argument is rejected and a therapeutic privilege is included, there are implications for the duty of the patient to disclose truthfully. Often patients are heard offering what amounts to a therapeutic privilege argument to explain why they have not related potentially important information to their physicians. Out of fear of upsetting the practitioner, they decide not to reveal that they have not been taking their medication or that they have seen a second physician or that they are consulting unorthodox therapists.

It would appear that if clinicians are going to insist on a therapeutic privilege as part of the general understanding between the profession and the society, then lay people are entitled to reciprocity. Patients also would insist that they have the right to withhold information they believe would be harmful to the clinician. It is the nature of the therapeutic privilege argument that it may not matter if the assessment of harm is accurate or plausible. The Hippocratic therapeutic privilege exception permits nondisclosure whenever, in the physician's judgment, harm would result. The decision is based on the clinician's subjective judgment of harm. Likewise, some patients may make inappropriate assessments of harm, but if the exception is based on subjective assessments rather than justifiable expectations of harm, then patients, like physicians, would be authorized (perhaps required) to withhold.

Even if the therapeutic privilege exception were revised to justify withholding information only when there is a reasonable expectation of harm, the exception is still paternalistic. It still involves a subordination of the principle of veracity to beneficence, a subordination that I cannot accept. Patients then have a duty to speak truthfully to their physicians just as physicians do to their patients. A faithful, trusting relation is impossible without such a foundation.

JUSTICE

Malpractice

The principle of justice also implies duties on the part of the patient. In chapter 8 I suggested that in the partnership model, malpractice should be less of a problem if patients take responsibility for predictable undesirable effects of medical procedures to which they have consented. This would leave only cases of real negligence to be handled through the malpractice tort system. I acknowledged that some unscrupulous patients may nevertheless try to sue physicians for untoward consequences. Even though they ought to lose such suits if a contract model is fully in place, there is nevertheless serious harm to the physician so sued. The principle of justice requires, among other things, that people be treated fairly. This means that such abuses of the malpractice system on the part of patients are clearly unethical, even if they occur. Justice requires that equals be treated equally. Physicians who faithfully inform patients of anticipated and justifiable risks would not be held accountable for those effects when they occur. Most physicians would, thereby, avoid such suits. Fairness requires that no physician be sued for consequences about which the patient was informed and consented.

The Duty to Step Aside

There is another implication for patients of the principle of justice. We have already seen that this principle may permit physicians in certain exceptional cases to temporarily abandon patients in order to serve others who are in greater need. The justice claim of the one in great need will have to be so strong that it overcomes the moral claim of the patient to have the physician keep his or her promise. That ought to happen only rarely, so rarely that in the next section I shall suggest that clinicians should, as a matter of the second-level contract, generally be exempt from the duties of justice in order for them to be able to keep their commitments to their patients. Nevertheless, patients should ask what their duty is if such a circumstance should occur. Even though they have a right to insist on fidelity from the physician, they also have a duty to promote justice. This may mean stepping aside in order to benefit someone who is in desperate need.

It is crucial that this argument not be generalized to the point that the patient has a duty to step aside whenever someone else could benefit more from the physician's attention. This is one of the most convincing cases supporting the lexical priority of nonconsequentialistic duties (including justice) over consequentialistic ones (such as beneficence). The lexical ordering of promise-keeping over beneficence explains why physicians should remain loyal to patients even when abandoning them may do a bit more good.

THE RIGHTS OF PHYSICIANS

For the most part, the rights of physicians are simply correlative to the duties of patients. Subject to the exceptions already discussed, physicians have a right to expect fidelity of patients to the commitments they make, including keeping appointments, paying bills, and maintaining confidences. They have a right to expect truthful disclosures and to be treated justly.

There is one additional right they may claim with respect to their patients, related to the duty to respect the autonomy of others. While physicians must respect the autonomy of patients in the consent process and in recognizing patients' rights of refusal, patients must also respect the autonomy of their physicians.

One of the most crucial elements of the second-level contract is that parties to lay-professional relations should generally reserve the right to withdraw from the relation if they discover that the limited convergence of objectives no longer applies. If patients realize that their goals of medical treatment are no longer compatible with those of their physician, they should be able to withdraw. Likewise, physicians should normally be permitted to sever the partnership when they no longer can accept the patient's goals and objectives.

There are some complications, however, when the professional exercises this right. It seems fair to say that the common understanding of the second-level contract is that professionals can normally withdraw only after providing suitable competent medical referral. To hold otherwise could leave the patient stranded with no access to life-saving medical support. Two problems arise, however: when no referral is possible, and when the physician perceives referral to be grossly immoral.

When Referral Is Impossible

In some special cases, there may be no one to whom the physician can refer the patient even though the patient is pursuing some legal course of action that he or she perceives to be moral. In some isolated communities, there were times when no physician was willing to perform a legal sterilization on a young woman who had few or no living children. Some women believed the sterilization to be not only their right but their moral duty.

It is not obvious how such conflicts should be resolved. The real problem seems to be mismatching of supply and demand. In the long run in cases where the controversial practice is legal, the solution seems to be to make sure enough physicians are trained to do it who consider the practice ethical that patients insisting on the service can receive it.

In the short run, this will not be possible. In some cases, society may perceive the service to be so fundamentally important that practitioners will be required to deliver it as a condition of their licensure. In other cases, society may perceive the service not so fundamental and will support the clinician's right to withdraw without referral. The case of Elizabeth Bouvia can be understood as such a dispute.

Case 11: Elizabeth Bouvia and Physician Right of Refusal

Elizabeth Bouvia wanted to receive medical care in a hospital—including a continuous narcotic drip for pain relief for severe arthritis while she exercised her right to refuse medically supplied nutrition and hydration.[6] The court recognized her right to refuse, but the dispute centered on whether she had the right to insist on staying in the hospital to receive the pain relief while refusing nutrition and hydration. Physicians objected to having to provide medical care to a patient who was, in effect, starving herself to death. Assuming no physician was available to provide the care on Ms. Bouvia's terms, should the physicians providing her care have been required to continue without the right to feed her, or should they have gotten court authorization to feed her as long as she stayed in their institution?

A lower court first sided with the physicians (while confirming her right to refuse nutrition if she left the hospital).[7] The California Court of Appeal later found that her position was sufficiently plausible that she had the right to refuse nutrition even while in the hospital.[8]

I suggest that cases such as this present a head-on conflict between the right of the physician autonomously to withdraw from the case and the right of the patient to a decent level of medical care. In those situations where what is demanded by the patient seems to be beyond a decent minimum, physicians are going to retain the right to withdraw, but in cases where the service seems fundamental to the decent minimum, society will necessarily make agreement to deliver the care a condition of continued licensure. Of course, the physician will still retain the right to act as an autonomous agent and withdraw, but only at the price of withdrawing from the terms of the second contract, the contract under which he or she is licensed to practice medicine and receive the privileges thereof. Normally, there should be someone available willing to provide a legal service that patients believe to be ethically necessary. In those rare cases when temporarily there is not, society will have to mediate the ethical conflict. One hopes that only in the rarest of circumstances will physicians be required to deliver care in conflict with their consciences.

WHEN REFERRAL IS IMMORAL

A more intriguing case arises when the physician perceives that even referral to another physician would be immoral. Some of those cases may involve relatively minor moral compromises on the part of the physician such that he or she is willing to respect the autonomy of the patient and make a referral nevertheless. A physician practicing medicine in a state such as Minnesota without a brain death statute may have some moral doubts about the legitimacy of pronouncing death on a patient who has suffered irreversible destruction of the entire brain. If the family were to ask to have the case transferred to someone willing to use brain criteria even though that had never been authorized, the physician, though finding the transfer morally objectionable, might nevertheless cooperate.

What, however, of an obstetrician who receives a request for a late-term abortion from a woman who argues that her health will be jeopardized by the pregnancy? She has the legal right to the abortion, according to the Supreme Court,[9] but, especially if the health risk is admittedly minor, the physician nevertheless has strong moral objections to murder. A referral to another physician would be, in his eyes, a referral for murder. That normally is not morally acceptable.

I consider this problem to be absolutely intractable. Surely the physician should have the right not to refer for what he considers to be murder. Surely the woman should have the right to speak with a physician who may condone the legal abortion. Here again we need a better matching of physicians and patients. In this case, however, it is not a matter of training physicians with the needed views. Some such practitioners already exist. It is a matter of figuring out how patients and physicians can be properly matched up.

Eventually a purposeful exploration of such basic moral positions will have to figure into the establishment of every patient-physician partnership. Until then there must be a presumption that clinicians are operating on some core, consensus morality unless they inform patients to the contrary. The Orthodox Jewish physician who believes that stopping life support is unethical and that referring to another physician who would do so is likewise ethically unacceptable has a duty to inform a patient of this special ethical position prior to the establishment of the relation. If he does not, he must be bound either to accept the patient's terms or to refer. In the case of the obstetrician who objects to a legal abortion desired by the patient but considered unethical by the physician, the practitioner's ethical objection to abortion must be stated as part of the initial agreement establishing the lay-professional relation; otherwise he or she must accept the obligation to refer the patient. The long-term solution is to make sure that everyone understands that such basic moral commitments must shape the patient-physician relation and to ensure that patients and physicians establish their covenantal relations only after exploring these commitments.

Regardless of the details of the duties of patients and the rights of physicians, a partnership or contractual theory of medical ethics will insist that there is a mutuality of obligations, that if the partners in the relation are given the autonomy and respect they are due, then patients will have duties and physicians will have rights, as well as the other way around. In addition to the duties and rights resting on the more traditional medical ethical principles focusing on the individual dyadic relation, this will include those based in the principle of justice and other social obligations. It is those social obligations to which we now turn.

PART
III

The Social Professional-Patient Relation

CHAPTER EIGHTEEN

Autonomy's Temporary Triumph: On the Alleged Conflict between Autonomy and Justice

In Part II the partnership between the health care professional and the patient was viewed as a relation between two isolated agents. The rise of the understanding of the patient as an active decisionmaker led to concern about informed consent, truthful disclosure, and access to medical records and nonstandard therapies. These were the problems that emerged in the early years of the current generation of medical ethics, dating from about 1970.

On all fronts patients were seeking freedom from what was becoming a tyranny of technology. Now that amniocentesis could determine genotype prenatally, pregnant women were demanding to know the condition of their fetuses even if clinicians believed they would be better off not knowing. Patients and their civil-rights lobbying groups were demanding the right to refuse electroshock and psychosurgery even when psychiatrists were convinced these treatments would make their patients better. Teenagers were demanding the right to have their contraceptive use kept confidential, even if their physicians thought the teenagers would be better off if their parents knew. Terminally ill patients lying in agony were pleading desperately for the right to be left alone—to be allowed to die—even if caregivers believed it was in their interest to be treated.

It was these cases that led us in the 1970s to see medical ethics as a conflict between the old Hippocratic paternalism and the nonconsequentialist principles of veracity, fidelity, and especially autonomy. We discovered that never in the history of professionally articulated ethics had there ever been any acknowledgment of the patient as a dignified agent free to participate in and exercise self-determination over medical decisions. As we have seen, it does not exist in the Hippocratic Oath, in the prayer of Maimonides, in Percival's ethics, or in the codes of the AMA or the World Medical Association prior to this period. The cultural roots of autonomy lie elsewhere. Some trace them all the way back, at least proleptically, to Adam. Certainly they are in the right tradition—with the Judeo-Christian notions of covenant, commitment, and conversion. By the sixteenth century, especially in the left wing of the Reformation, the concept of the individual as a free, choosing person was emerging full-blown.

It is in this context that autonomy has won the day, even if John Stuart Mill and modern utilitarians tarnish the victory somewhat by insisting that liberty is only a means to maximizing benefit. Respect does not mean simply doing what one thinks will benefit a person, *even if* others really can determine what is in that person's best interest. It is not that benefiting the patient is morally irrelevant—of course not, and hard work is in order to determine what will benefit—but rather, respecting the free choices of autonomous human beings must take precedence.

The case is overwhelming that autonomy takes moral priority—a full lexical priority—over the paternalistic implications of the principle of beneficence. I have made this argument elsewhere and summarized it in chapter 6.[1] That conclusion has led people such as Paul Ramsey to label me and others who place strong emphasis on the autonomy of individual patients in such situations as "extreme libertarians".[2] In that very special situation he was right, but he failed to realize how limited the implications of the principle of autonomy are. It is a principle that responded to an extreme paternalism. The result was a temporary triumph of autonomy.

SOCIAL ETHICS

By 1975, those of us involved in medical ethics were waging an internecine fight between two ethics of individualism: should the physician's Hippocratic paternalism or the liberty lover's respect for the autonomy of the individual win out? In that year Karen Quinlan left us the legacy that established firmly and finally that there are limits on the physician's authority to do what he thinks will benefit the patient. We discovered that to deal with an increasingly important group of cases—cases of research medicine and health resource allocation, of national health planning and the planning of hospital budgets, of cost containment and Diagnosis-Related Groups (DRGs)—we needed a social ethic. The goal became recovering our sense of a moral community and discovering the claims that its members have on our health and other social resources.

If the lay-professional relation is to be viewed as a partnership, we will need to deal not only with conflicts between paternalism and nonconsequentialistic principles such as autonomy at the individual level. We will also have to confront the fact that clinicians are in partnership relations with more than one patient at a time. As we saw in the case of the homosexual husband, fulfilling the duties of one relation may necessarily mean sacrificing some interests of another patient to whom the clinician also has obligations. It may mean having to deal with the claims of nonpatients who could be benefited substantially if the clinician would only make marginal compromises with his or her patient. It may mean having to deal with cost containment, public health, decisions about reporting carriers of AIDs, and willful exposures of patients to small risks for the benefit of research. The partnership about which we have been speaking can never truly be limited to the individual level of two isolated actors pursuing mutually acceptable goals. It must always be embedded in a social ethic. We need to turn now to the contractual limits imposed on the partnership by the various social contracts.

In the process we may learn from the earlier debate over ethical principles at the individual level. Just as there is a tension between merely benefiting persons and showing respect for their autonomy at the individual level, so also at the social level we must choose between merely producing benefits and producing benefits within the constraints of moral principles not committed solely to maximizing aggregate benefits. In individual medical ethics we have learned that respect for autonomy takes precedence over producing patient benefit, and in social ethics we must realize that respect for justice takes precedence over producing social benefit.

MAXIMIZING AGGREGATE BENEFITS

One possibility in a social medical ethics is simply to opt for the policies—the physician and nurse behavior, cost containment strategies, and health promotion budgets—that produce the greatest net benefit overall. This strategy is used by those seeking health policies that will do the most to lower overall mortality and morbidity rates or maximize average life expectancy. This ethic of cost-benefit and cost-effectiveness analysis poses serious ethical problems, however. The most critical is that maximizing aggregate net benefits ignores the possibility that some people may be harmed a great deal while others are being helped. It treats certain people unfairly while producing the greatest good.

The shift to cost-effectiveness analysis is an attempt to finesse the problem of justice. Let policy makers pick the policy objective, so the defenders of this type of analysis say. Simply use cost-effectiveness as a tool for choosing the most efficient means to a predetermined end. As long as means are different, however, benefits may be distributed differently. In subsequent chapters I shall explore the implications of this conflict between efficiently maximizing aggregate benefits and distributing resources more fairly, but possibly inefficiently. One example will help illustrate the difference between these goals.

CASE 12: EFFICIENCY VS. EQUITY IN PUBLIC HEALTH

British researchers were interested in studying the cost-effectiveness of two methods of screening schoolgirls for asymptomatic bacteriuria—a condition for which early detection and treatment may prevent kidney damage.[3]

The first method involved sending the girls home with a kit containing a dipslide. The accompanying letter of instruction directed parents to ensure that the child placed a urine sample on the dipslide in the manner specified. They were to exercise certain precautions in storing the sample and return it to the classroom the next day. This method of screening was compared to a method that involved sending a mobile laboratory to the school, where samples were collected under the supervision of trained personnel.

The first method cost considerably less per case screened: 0.26 pounds per case for the home dipslide method as compared with 0.77 pounds per case for the supervised mobile laboratory method. A cost-effectiveness analysis might therefore lead a policy maker quickly to conclude that the home dipslide method was more efficient and therefore preferred.

Closer analysis of the data, however, revealed two additional pieces of information. First, the mobile laboratory method was successful in getting usable specimens in a higher percentage of cases (96 percent vs. 70 percent). Since it is often more expensive to achieve success in more marginal cases, a cost-effectiveness analysis that strives to minimize the cost per case will often push policy makers toward more conservative, more minimalist programs. In this case it could lead them to exclude 26 percent of the schoolgirls who would benefit from the less efficient screening.

Second, when the social class effects were analyzed, it became clear that the failures were not randomly distributed. The home dipslide method was successful in 84 percent of children from social classes I, II, and III, but in only 58 percent of children from social class V and parents who were unemployed. The reason for this difference is not stated, but presumably it has to do with such cultural factors as ability to read and follow rather complex instructions, familial organization and discipline, and willingness to devote time to the project.

Whatever the reason, the home dipslide method clearly discriminated against those of lower social class. What started out as a cost-effectiveness analysis of two methods to achieve the same end (finding cases of asymptomatic bacteriuria) turned out to reveal that policy makers really had two options: to find cases as efficiently as possible, or to give schoolgirls of all social classes a fair chance at being screened.

Every cost-effectiveness analysis involves two or more methods to purportedly similar ends. If the means have differential effects, the analysis can be restated as a comparison of two methods to two somewhat different ends. Often the most efficient method will not be the one that distributes the benefits among the recipients most fairly. Efficiency is the choice of those who would opt for a social ethic that merely maximizes benefits.

PROMOTING JUSTICE

The other possibility for a social ethic for medicine goes beyond merely striving to maximize aggregate benefits, to pay attention to who receives the benefits. This approach emphasizes the relationships among people within the moral community and the claim that each has only a fair share of the health resources. It is built on a principle—the principle of justice—that is analogous to the nonconsequentialistic principles of autonomy, veracity, and fidelity at the level of the individual. Just as at the individual level our society has opted for an ethic that provides benefits within the constraints of respect for the individual's autonomy, so at the social level we need an ethic that maximizes benefits within the constraints of the uniqueness of individuals as equals in their claim on social resources.

Whether we are willing to sacrifice some efficiency in producing aggregate or average good in order to treat people fairly will, I suggest, depend on one's understanding of a sense of moral community. The sense of community underlying the social ethic of justice presented here affirms the equal status of individuals. It is a uniquely Judeo-Christian view strangely at odds with both the Greek and modern libertarian views—views that have no difficulty treating people as intrinsically unequal. In fact it could be argued that John Rawls, Ronald Dworkin, and other secular philosophers advocating more or less egalitarian justice are simply bootlegging the Judeo-Christian vision of the moral community. [4]

If I am correct, it is a mistake to pose the problem as if our commitment to autonomy were in tension with our commitment to the community. Rather, the conflict over paternalism and autonomy that diverted our attention for a few years may provide a model for the real work of building a mature medical ethic that can handle social as well as individual ethical questions. At the individual level, the Hippocratist pulls us paternalistically to benefit patients even at the expense of violating their autonomy, while our Judeo-Christian heritage and its secular successors tell us to benefit, but only within the constraints of respect for autonomy. At the social level, the consequentialist pulls us to pay attention only to producing benefits—net benefits in aggregate—while our Judeo-Christian tradition and its secular successors tell us to strive for the common good, but only within the constraints of respect for the uniqueness of members of the moral community and their claims for a fair share of our social resources.

If I am right, the principle of autonomy is nothing more than a footnote to a full theory of medical ethics dealing with those rare cases where we can pretend that the community is limited to an isolated patient exercising his or her will unbounded by obligations to others. Autonomous individuals are self-legislating, but that means legislating only for themselves. If this is the case, autonomy's triumph is truly temporary. The real challenge in medical ethics is deciding which version of community should dominate when our ethic turns social. It is to these problems of social ethics in the professional/ patient relation that we now turn.

CHAPTER NINETEEN

DRGs and the Ethics of Cost Containment

The greatest strain on the patient/professional relationship of the past decade has come from pressures to contain health care costs. Clinicians are increasingly being asked to be cost-conscious and to reduce the unnecessary use of resources. The costs of medical care have reached a level that can no longer be ignored. In absolute dollar amounts, the figure has reached $1.5 billion a day in the United States.[1] Not only that, the percent of GNP devoted to health care has more than doubled, from 4.4 percent in 1950 to over 11 percent now.[2]

What makes matters worse, some of that care is at best marginally useful or even useless. It is inevitable that insurance planners, government officials, labor union officials responsible for health care benefit plans, and ordinary citizens are asking whether constraints based on economic considerations are acceptable.

CASE 13: COST CONTAINMENT IN THE CORONARY CARE UNIT

The utilization review committee of a major teaching hospital found that one cardiologist's patients suffering acute myocardial infarctions consistently had hospitalization expenses far exceeding those of his colleagues' patients. While the average stay at this hospital for such patients was 13.1 days, this physician's patients stayed on average 18.2 days. The average cost of hospitalization at this institution for acute myocardial infarction was $10,257, while this physician's patients averaged $14,132.

The hospital received prospective payment for Medicare patients under the Diagnosis Related Group (DRG) system that provides a fixed reimbursement based on diagnosis. The patients being reviewed were those falling into DRG group 122, "acute myocardial infarction without complications, discharged alive." The costs overruns from one member of the staff could jeopardize the financial stability of the entire program.

Their problem was whether and to what extent the committee should review the physician's care with the goal of reducing costs, bringing him into line with other physicians, and if so, on what ethical grounds it ought to proceed.

If a clinician has entered into a partnership with a patient in which he or she is constrained by a promise to protect that person's rights and welfare, it would appear that any pressure to have the clinician reduce expenditures is really a pressure to violate that promise. The problem is illustrated by this example of how clinicians are utilizing coronary care services for heart attack victims.

The initial problem raised in utilization review is the justification of outliers. While the term *outlier* often refers to patients who deviate substantially from mean resource consumption, a physician who consistently has such patients may also be termed an outlier. The question is raised whether outlier care should be reduced, and, if so, why? A working assumption in utilization review is often that the average amount of care given for a diagnosis group is the ideal amount of care. There is no reason to assume this, but deviations from the average are likely to require justification.

Let us assume that the utilization review committee has examined this physician's cases and determined that there are no special social factors of age, severity of disease, complications, or the like that immediately explain the deviation from the average. Should the hospital, stimulated by the DRG system, exert pressure on the physician to reduce the extent of his care, and if so, on what ethical grounds?

While considerable attention is being given to the technical aspects of operating the DRG system,[3] to ways of categorizing patients to produce a fair reimbursement,[4] and even to the impact that prospective payment will have on health care,[5] little analysis has been offered of the general ethical issues of cost containment. Some potential cost-cutting measures are ethically suspect. A hospital could, for example, adopt more rigorous intake screening and transfer costly patients more aggressively. Since criteria for admission, especially for nearly hopeless cases, are ambiguous and the practice of deciding not to resuscitate is gaining strength, a hospital could probably cloak cost-saving decisions in judgments not to admit or resuscitate. One hospital found that in DRG 386 (extreme prematurity, neonates), based on current average costs, it will lose $1,000 per patient. It could close its neonatal unit, cutting the loss. It could raise the minimal birth weight at which a resuscitation would be attempted, thus systematically eliminating the babies who, if they survive, would predictably generate the highest costs. While these strategies might eliminate the loss, that is not the response that the DRG system was intended to produce. Some more sophisticated ethical analysis is called for.

The initial premise of this analysis is that the DRG system or any other financing arrangement should be seen as an opportunity to allocate resources ethically. Patients will not be treated fairly if too few *or too many* resources are committed to them. While I am not denying that the weightings for DRG groups were originally based on empirical findings, I suggest they should be adjusted to reflect what constitutes an ethically acceptable portion of resources for each group. The weights should be seen as a scale of the relative claims of patients in different categories.

THE ETHICS OF REDUCING CARE

Four of the ethical principles I have discussed relate to the level of care given patients. The first two are patient-centered beneficence and autonomy. They are not directly related to cost containment, but honoring them may nevertheless reduce costs. These two principles would remain valid considerations even if they happened to increase costs. They are thus only indirectly related to cost containment.

The two other principles operate at the social level. These are social or full beneficence and justice. Unlike the patient-centered principles, these are directly relevant to cost containment. As long as public funds are limited, the following two questions arise: (1) how can we do the *most* good with the resources available (which the principle of full beneficence addresses), and (2) who should receive the benefits (which the principle of justice addresses)? These four principles, which are relevant to DRG and other cost containment decisions, are presented in diagrammatic form in Figure 1.

PATIENT-CENTERED PRINCIPLES

A rigorous application of traditional ethical principles that focus exclusively on the individual patient—the patient's welfare and self-determination—may actually reduce costs.

Patient-Centered Beneficence

The first ethical principle that may reduce the cost of care is a modified version of the traditional professional ethics of physicians. As we have seen, the physician's duty has traditionally been to benefit the patient according to

A Classification of the Ethical Principles
in Cost Containment

	consequentialistic	non-consequentialistic
individual	Hippocratic beneficence	autonomy
social	full beneficence	justice

FIGURE 1

his or her ability and judgment. However, if individual practitioners use their own judgment in trying to benefit patients, they will sometimes be mistaken, and may actually hurt patients. The outlier physician problem may be an example. The well-meaning clinician may wrongly conclude that extensive care is required when, in fact, some of that care could actually do more harm than good. Some argue that the Hippocratic principle should be modified so that physicians in such cases are instructed to yield to the best objective estimate of the patient's welfare. That would require them to serve the interests of their patients according to the best evidence that is available, not depending solely on their own judgments.

The result is still patient-centered beneficence, but now on a more objective basis. Most patients would not want a physician to try to benefit them according to his or her own judgment if that opinion differed substantially from the best possible judgment—at least not without careful and detailed consent. In the language of a contract theory of medical ethics, rational members of society in negotiating the second-level contract with the profession would never agree to authorizing clinicians to act on their own judgments when a more objective assessment of patient welfare would not support such actions.

The notion of "objective welfare" used here is a difficult one, however. While the Hippocratic tradition commits the physician to serving the patient's welfare (according to the physician's judgment), practitioners are not really equipped to assess all the elements thereof. As we saw in earlier chapters, welfare is a complex concept. It includes social, economic, aesthetic, and spiritual components as well as the organic. Surgery, for example, will have medical consequences. It will have an impact on morbidity and mortality. It will also affect the social, aesthetic, and economic well-being of the patient. A peer review panel should be capable of determining the medical consequences of health care interventions.

Two additional tasks are necessary, however, before those consequences can be determined to improve the patient's welfare. In neither of these tasks are physicians uniquely expert. First, the medical consequences of treatment need to be assessed. For example, if an intervention involved a slight increase in survival probability at the cost of great suffering and inconvenience, it is not clear whether it would be beneficial or harmful. Second, the medical consequences of treatment, once evaluated, must be compared to the other consequences. Any specialized group including physicians on utilization review committees may assign unique values to medical consequences of treatment. (They may give unusual emphasis to mortality over morbidity, for example.) They may also relate medical consequences to nonmedical ones uniquely. (They may be willing to pay an unusually high economic or aesthetic price to improve mortality or morbidity risks.)

A peer review system can be expected only to determine what is *medically* beneficial based on the values of health professionals. Such a professional assessment is probably a reasonable approximation of what other people would also find medically beneficial. We might, therefore, adopt a policy that limits medical care to interventions that are medically beneficial and use the health professional assessment thereof as an approximation.

The care provided in the myocardial infarction example can be divided into several components. Figure 2 illustrates these components with regard to the days of hospital stay. It shows schematically the aggregate net medical benefit of hospitalization plotted against the number of days of stay. The first day of stay is typically the most beneficial. Each succeeding day offers less benefit until a maximum is reached (here represented as occurring at day N). After that, some net harm might actually occur (taking into account the iatrogenic risks involved and possible psychological harms of remaining in the hospital), represented by the slight downturn in the curve. In order for a utilization review committee to examine such a problem, it must have some notion of the medically ideal stay (N). This will probably be close to the average days of stay, but not necessarily identical to it.

If the ideal (N) for DRG group 122 was thought by the utilization review committee to be about thirteen days (assuming no complicating factors), its members would see their outlier physician as providing five days too much care to his typical patient. Those five days would do the patient no net medical good and might actually harm him. Using the modified Hippocratic ethic, the committee might exert pressure to reduce care *in order to benefit the patient*. The unmodified Hippocratic ethic leads to provide $N + 5$ days of care; modified, it drives care back toward N days. The reduction is justified by patient welfare, not by cost saving.

Autonomy

We have seen, though, that the Hippocratic ethic has been challenged not only by those seeking more objective grounds for determining what counts as medical welfare, but more radically by those advocating the principle of autonomy. Many, myself included, have concluded that patients, who

Aggregate Net Medical Benefit as a Function of Days of Stay

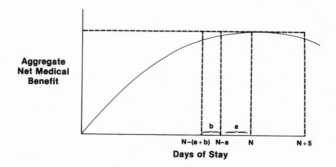

FIGURE 2

may have values and beliefs quite different from those of the medical community, have the right to refuse medical care even if that care is determined "as objectively as possible" to be in their best medical interests. In the terms of the ethical theory presented in chapter 6, the nonconsequentialistic principle of autonomy takes precedence over the consequentialistic principle of patient-centered beneficence.

Patients may evaluate the medical consequences differently or trade off the medical and other benefits and costs differently. They may, for example, place strong value on being at home with family, having home-cooked meals, being away from others who are ill, or simply having privacy. Patients may prefer simply to sacrifice their welfare for the welfare of their families. While none of these is a medical value, each might be taken into account in deciding whether to consent to care. The patient might, based on autonomy, decide to refuse certain care that is recommended to be in his or her best medical interest.

The days near the Nth day of stay are interesting in this regard. Patients may prefer to reject some part of the proposed care. In our example they might rather be home on the Nth day. They might consider some marginal increment (a) in Figure 2 expendable. If they should so choose, autonomy supports their right to reject the care in our example to leave the hospital early.

Costs of care on average might well be reduced somewhat if only hospitals rigorously affirmed the right to decline treatment—even treatment that is medically beneficial. The result of the autonomy principle is that a second component of care is eliminated. The basis is not cost containment; it is rooted in an ethical principle focused exclusively on the patient. In this case that principle is now patient autonomy, rather than welfare.

It might be argued, of course, that, given freedom to choose, for every patient who elects to go home a day early there will be one who chooses to stay a day extra. Those choosing $(N + a)$ days will cancel out those choosing $(N - a)$. However, while autonomy requires letting patients refuse care, it does not require that they be permitted to get care beyond some accepted standard. In this sense the implications of the autonomy principle are asymmetrical. The result is that the principle of autonomy—called for on independent grounds—has the pleasant side effect of reducing costs, even below what the standard of objective medical interests would require.

MOVING BEYOND THE PATIENT'S PERSPECTIVE

These patient-centered principles provide two independent grounds for reducing costs. The problem, however, is that these changes alone may not be sufficient. In the myocardial infarction case, the reimbursement was slightly below $7,000. If the outlier physician's patients were reduced to the average length of stay of the patients of the remaining physicians, costs for patients in group 122 would average $9,104. The hospital would still lose money.

One response of clinicians is to attack the DRG system itself for forcing them to compromise quality of care. They might be willing to eliminate care that is actually harmful and even care that autonomous patients refuse, but they cannot tolerate eliminating care that is beneficial to and desired by the patient. Yet that seems to be precisely what the DRG system requires. This leads to demands to adjust the reimbursement so that the ideal care (N days in Figure 2) or ideal care adjusted for patient autonomy ($N - a$ days) can be delivered. It leads to even more radical demands that the entire system be scrapped.

A more careful analysis requires close examination of the ethics of providing all care that would be delivered based on the criteria of patient-centered beneficence and autonomy. It seems reasonable to examine the ethics of eliminating marginally beneficial care that is very expensive in comparison to the benefits that it provides. Some increment of care—let's call it b—would be objectively medically beneficial and would be desired by patients, but nevertheless is not ethically justified because other uses of these resources are ethically more weighty. If autonomy reduces the average length of stay for myocardial care patients by a, then this additional factor may reduce care by b, thus leaving the average length of stay as $N - (a + b)$.

What is needed is an analysis of the ethical grounds for determining which, if any, of the marginally beneficial, expensive care should be eliminated between the $[N - (a + b)]$ and $(N - a)$ points. We should ask: "Would a reasonable person planning health insurance before knowing whether he or she would eventually need the service under consideration want such care included assuming that it would increase premiums and those funds could otherwise be used on some other worthwhile social or personal projects?" Surely, at least some such care would be eliminated. The reimbursement for various diagnostic groups, from this point of view, ought to be set so that adequate care is given but some marginally beneficial, desired, expensive care must be eliminated. Each DRG group weight should be a measure of the ethical claims of persons in the group. The weighting should be set so as to drive care below the ideal level and down to the ethically justified $[N - (a + b)]$ level. A social ethic of resource allocation will tell us the appropriate weighting on which to base fair reimbursement.

The two social ethical principles (full beneficence and justice) each provide a basis for deciding questions such as what the relative weights for DRG groups ought to be.

The Principle of Full Beneficence

Health planners might be inclined to ask the classical utilitarian question: "How do the net benefits from using resources in this manner compare with those of using them in some other manner?" The ethical principle of beneficence presses decisionmakers to maximize the net good done by one's actions. This version differs from the Hippocratic version of beneficence by requiring that the benefits and harms to all parties, not only the patients, be taken into account. Thus, this is *full* beneficence. This is the ethical principle underlying cost-benefit analysis and cost-effectiveness analysis as normally practiced.

In our example, at some point further days of stay become marginally beneficial while still about as expensive as other hospital days. If the net benefit of using the resources in this way is compared with other possible medical or even nonmedical uses of the resources, the marginally beneficial days will lose. It is only because the calculations are so complex that sophisticated techniques including computer modeling are sometimes used to make the benefit/cost comparisons. If this strategy were used by the insurance planners to set the relative DRG weights, the goal would be to arrange the weights so that the amount of good done in the system as a whole would be maximized. The marginal expenditures in each DRG group ought to be producing the same marginal increments of good.

If it turns out that the existing DRG weights are not doing this, a utilization review committee or a hospital administration might consider cost-shifting from one group to another in order to maximize the total amount of good it is doing as a whole. Thus if the acute myocardial infarction group (DRG group 122) gets only $7,000 reimbursement per patient, but the local experts consider that $9,100 worth of care is ideal, someone at the local level might ask whether the marginal dollars spent on other DRG groups could more effectively be used for myocardial infarction patients. Surely they would not want to appropriate funds to bring that care all the way up to the $9,100 mark, because as that ideal point is reached, the benefits get smaller and smaller to the point of being negligible. Certainly those funds could be used more effectively for some other purpose.

This is the implication of the principle of full beneficence for national and local decisionmaking. It may turn out that there are good reasons not to allow this principle to be overriding, especially not to permit local decisionmakers to cost-shift. We shall look more closely at the reasons for avoiding local cost-shifting later.

There are two common objections to using the principle of full beneficence to make these decisions. First, many object that the problems of quantification are enormous. For example, comparing the benefits of the eleventh day of hospitalization after a myocardial infarction with those of a comparable dollar investment in nursing home care for the Alzheimer's patient is extremely difficult. If benefits could be measured in a single statistic such as mortality rate, it would be easier, but a rich notion of benefit includes not only preventing death but relieving suffering, avoiding psychological trauma, and so forth. At best all that can be given is a rough approximation.

Although this argument should add humility to a cost-benefit analyst's work, it is not very convincing. In every policy decision some such comparisons have to be made. The defenders of systematic efforts to compare costs and benefits rightly point out that the only alternative to quantification of alternative outcomes is to leave important decisions to intuition or chance.

The second objection commonly made against the principle of full beneficence is much more serious. As I discussed in chapter 18, by aggregating all benefits and harms and then comparing them, the standard methods of cost-benefit analysis mask variations in distribution.[6] Furthermore, as the bacteria example in chapter 18 showed, the ethical problems caused by differences in distribution cannot be avoided by shifting to cost-effectiveness analysis. If full beneficence and the techniques of cost-benefit and cost-effectiveness analysis are used to determine the appropriate DRG weights, benefits may be distributed very unevenly among patients. It is theoretically possible that the most efficient way to maximize net medical benefits in the Medicare system is to assign very high weights to certain groups and very low weights to others. This result may be efficient but still unfair. Full beneficence should not be regarded as the sole principle of morality. This of course does not rule out its validity altogether. All things being equal, it does seem to be morally required to maximize good consequences. But to ensure fairness we need to turn to a principle of justice.

The Principle of Justice

Just as a nonconsequentialist principle (autonomy) provides an alternative to Hippocratic or patient-centered beneficence at the individual level, so we should explore the possibility that there is a principle at the social level that forces us to look beyond mere accumulation of good consequences. If the DRG system were ever extended to include a category for bacteriuria screening in schoolgirls, the planners would have to determine whether they wanted only enough funds to screen most efficiently (regardless of social class) or whether they wanted enough funds to screen in a manner that gave all schoolgirls an equal chance at having their cases found. The principle of justice must also be considered.

The meaning of the principle of justice has been open to serious scholarly debate, especially since the publication of John Rawls's A Theory of Justice.[7] Those attempting to identify justice as independent of either autonomy or beneficence emphasize equity or fairness in distribution, and normally this includes some version of a notion of equality. A pure, egalitarian understanding of the principle would have us distribute resources so as to produce opportunities for equality of welfare. In the health care sphere this often leads to striving for opportunities for people to be as healthy as others. With regard to the DRG weights, we would want them assigned in such a way that funds were available to give people in different diagnostic groups equal opportunities for health.

Three objections are raised to the egalitarian interpretation of justice as applied to health care. First, it is not clear whether the goal should be equality of health status or equality of welfare more generally. It seems that in an ideal world the egalitarian would in fact strive for overall equality. As a practical matter, however, the principle of justice might be easier to apply if health were treated separately from other goods.

A second problem with this egalitarian interpretation is that it leaves open what the relationship should be with the other principles. What should happen, for example, if striving for opportunities for health requires giving enormous weight to DRG group 386 (extreme prematurity, neonate), but this turns out to be a very inefficient way of maximizing aggregate net benefits? To answer this question, those involved in making cost-containment decisions need a theory that relates the various principles. Our medical ethics of treatment refusal has led many to the conclusion that the nonconsequentialist principle of autonomy takes absolute precedence over paternalistic patient benefit. At the social level as well, nonconsequentialist principles such as justice ought to be given priority status. If they are, then no amount of social benefit would ever justify inflicting enormous harm on individuals (such as in the Nazi experiments).

That still does not tell us how the nonconsequentialist principles would be related among themselves. I suggested in chapter 6 that we must revert to a balancing strategy with no one principle having priority. Often the proper weighting becomes clearer in the context of a real-life dilemma. In any case, this balancing problem is not unique to egalitarians.

A third and more serious objection is frequently raised against the egalitarian position. It is often argued that egalitarianism is impractical because it generates an infinite demand. Certain patients have very little medical welfare and would get high priority based on egalitarian theories of justice. If their conditions are hard to treat, they would generate demands that are virtually limitless, breaking the bank and leaving somewhat healthier people without any health care at all.

Several responses are available to this important argument. First, egalitarian justice itself sets some limits. If a person with a serious uncorrectable handicap such as blindness generated an infinite demand, eventually he would take so many resources that others in the society would be deprived of even the basics of health care. But as the others' opportunities for health declined, eventually they would become worse off than the blind person, and on the basis of justice, they would then take priority over him. Justice itself sets a first limit on the infinite demand.

Another limit comes from the principle of autonomy. In certain cases it might be prudent for the least well off not to exercise their right to opportunity for equality—in order, say, to keep others healthy enough to render them needed aid. The principle of autonomy gives persons the right to waive certain of their claims. In instances when it would not be in their interest for the least well off to exercise their right to opportunity for equality, they (or their agents) might waive their right in order to improve their lot. The result is something similar to Rawls's difference principle, except that in this formulation justice still requires equality. Autonomous actions of the least well off provide a moral counter to the claims of justice. In this formulation (though not in Rawls's) it is critical that it is the least well off (or their surrogates) who are approving the inequality. In such cases, health care resources could be diverted away from them thus placing another limit on the infinite demand.

A third limit is found in the possibility that promises have been made to those who are not least well off. If promise-keeping is a duty on a par with justice, then some balancing is required, and at least in some circumstances it would be in order to keep the promises of health care resources already made to those who are not least well off.

Finally, if these three means of overcoming the infinite demand problem are not satisfactory, one might have to revert to the idea that full beneficence can be balanced against justice, with each having an equal force. Doing so would easily explain why some resources would go to those who are better off. Making this move, however, opens some doors very wide—doors that seem to justify behaviors such as slavery and Nazi research, at least in principle. These are doors that are better kept closed if possible.[8]

PROBLEMS IN APPLYING THE PRINCIPLES
TO COST CONTAINMENT

We now have an ethical framework for thinking about cost-containment decisions such as those related to DRGs. Patient welfare and autonomy give us a relatively good basis for curtailing expenditures. Two additional ethical principles (full beneficence and justice) provide further grounds for limiting care. Although often they will lead to the same decisions, they are in fact very different and occasionally (such as in the bacteriuria example) lead to different policies and different DRG weightings. Several problems arise in the application of these principles to DRGs and cost containment.

THE ROLE OF CLINICIANS IN COST CONTAINMENT

One problem is the role of clinicians. When DRG reimbursement will not cover the average costs, a typical strategy is to encourage physicians to be more cost-conscious. Bulletin board posters may be displayed, for example, showing the costs of equipment and procedures. Since cuts based on either patient welfare or autonomy would not require such cost-awareness, the strategy of encouraging cost-consciousness must be rooted in the ethical concerns of justice and full beneficence.

Consider what would happen, however, if social policy encouraged each clinician to be more cost-conscious and to eliminate procedures that seemed marginal. Each physician would probably shift the level of care somewhat. The outlier physician now hospitalizing for eighteen days might drop to seventeen, while the physician at the other end of the spectrum might reduce his care somewhat as well. The result would be a slight shift in average cost, but with the outlier overtreating physician still providing excess care and the undertreating physician reducing care even further.

There are more subtle problems with this strategy. Physicians, in effect, would be determining what is a reasonable reduction below ideal care for their patients. Such an assessment would require comparing the health care under consideration with other goods that could be obtained with the resources. Clinicians would have to draw on their own beliefs and values to make these comparisons. Yet, as we have seen, this is a judgment about which professionals may predictably be atypical. It is not that physicians would overvalue health care for ulterior motives—say in order to increase income. It is rather that people who have given their lives to a profession should believe strongly in its value. Just as military officers might overvalue defense appropriations or philosophers might overvalue philosophy, dedicated health care professionals may predictably overvalue health care. When this is combined with the high incomes of physicians that would make extensive expenditures seem reasonable, it is quite predictable that clinicians would, if asked to determine what a reasonable level of care is, opt for more than lay people would choose.

Even more serious, asking the clinician to be cost-conscious in order to eliminate marginally beneficial care would require a major shift in traditional professional ethics. Physicians would be required to abandon traditional patient-centeredness. They would be asked to remove the Hippocratic Oath from their waiting room wall and replace it with a sign that read, "Warning all ye who enter here. I will generally work for your rights and welfare, but if benefits to you are marginal and costs are great, I will abandon you in order to protect society." It is not clear that either physicians or lay people really want clinicians to take that stand. A good case can be made that at the level of the second contract, professionals and other members of society would agree to a special moral norm for the professional when in a clinical relation with a client or patient.

In chapter 2 I developed the notion of role-specific duties, duties that are established by social contract to apply to those in particular roles. We might grant to clinical professionals a special "role-specific" ethic.[9] Just as parents or defense attorneys have special moral duties (to be advocates for their children or their clients), so clinical professionals might be asked to be advocates for their patients and exclude resource allocation and social welfare from their normal clinical agenda. Society would, if you like, grant health professionals a limited exemption from the responsibilities of social ethics so that they could fulfill important obligations to their patients. The professional/patient relation would then be one in which the parties could trust one another to focus exclusively on the relationship.

Of course, if cost containment is not on the physicians' agenda, it would have to be on someone else's. Since these are fundamentally nonmedical choices about maximizing net benefits or distributing benefits equally, it is appropriate that these decisions be made by the general public. Thus for DRG weightings the society as a whole, working through its representatives, should decide the relative merit of the claims of the members of various diagnostic groups. If health professionals are among those making these social ethical decisions, they should be there not as clinicians but in some other capacity. If clinicians' evaluation of the relative importance of health care and other goods is atypical (just as any other person's would be), then they should not be represented in such a policy-making body in numbers that exceed their membership in the general population.

This decisionmaking strategy has already come about for DRG group 103—heart transplants. The weighting for DRG 103 is 0.000; that is, no patient in the DRG system will receive reimbursement for a heart transplant. Moreover, that judgment was made by a political official. It was not based on the medical judgment that heart transplants would never benefit any Medicare recipient or that all rational candidates would exercise their autonomy to refuse such care, but on the judgment that it would cost the Medicare system a great deal. The decision was made that other uses of the funds were of higher priority. Surely it would make no sense to ask the individual cardiac surgeon or even cardiac surgeons as a group to determine whether heart transplants deserved the weighting they received.

The choice for clinicians is an awkward one. They must either adopt a social ethical perspective (involving some mix of full beneficence and justice) and in the process give up patient-centeredness, or accept a special role-specific duty to be a patient advocate and in the process yield any role in resource allocation and cost containment. I am increasingly convinced that the better case can be made for the latter alternative.

If this move is made, then the clinician should have no direct role in eliminating marginally useful care for cost-containment purposes. The planners of prospective payment systems should make judgments about the relative merit of the claims of people in various groups, taking into account the claims of justice both of those in other medical groups and of those who have needs that are not medical.

THE ROLE OF UTILIZATION REVIEW COMMITTEES

The dilemma of utilization review committees should now be clear. Such committees, made up of clinicians, face the same problems as do individual clinicians. If they make judgments about reducing marginally beneficial care, they will bring to bear atypical constellations of values. They will, at least in this role, have to abandon their patient-centeredness in order to promote social efficiency or fairness. While there is nothing logically inconsistent about asking clinicians to adopt one ethic in their patient care and another in their committee work (assuming they do not serve on committees when they review their own patients), the psychological transition between patient-centered clinician and societally centered committee member would be very difficult. Moreover, insofar as the committee establishes general policies that seek to eliminate marginally beneficial care (for example, a day limit on ordinary acute myocardial infarction hospitalization without formal review), the members would be generating policy decisions that affect their own patients. They could not work toward such an end while remaining loyal to their patients.

Another problem with using local utilization review committees for these tasks is that different committees would almost certainly make different trade-offs. One committee might reduce stay by one day, while another would do so by two days. It is unfair that patients be subjected to policies that compromise their interests at the margin by differing amounts solely on the basis of subjective variations of this sort. If cuts are to be made, it would be fairer to make them more uniformly. The weighting for DRG group 122 should be set uniformly so that the reimbursement would fund, for example, three days below ideal care.

The implications for establishing a standard of objective net medical benefit are more complex. There is some tendency to rely on the fact/value dichotomy, acknowledging that clinicians—even groups of clinicians—cannot answer questions such as whether the tenth day of stay in the hospital does more good than the same dollars spent on an Alzheimer patient, but then to give the clinician the supposedly factual task of identifying treatments that objectively do no good. I have argued that even identifying whether a treatment does any medical good necessarily requires evaluative judgments. It is in theory impossible for clinicians to determine medically whether any good is done, let alone whether the good is greater than that done with some other use of resources. Nevertheless, such judgments are so complex and require such detailed knowledge that I feel we are warranted in making a tentative presumption that if a peer review group decides that an intervention does no net medical good, in fact, it does not. This presumption that clinicians will evaluate treatments similarly to lay people should be open to dispute. The majority of lay people may rationally believe that some intervention produces a benefit even if all clinicians disagree. For example, many intensive care physicians tend to use whether the patient is discharged from the hospital alive as an end point for determining whether an ICU intervention has done any good. Some patients, however, may feel there is some benefit of an ICU intervention if it prolongs life briefly even if the patient is not discharged alive. Barring such specific cases where lay people overrule the clinical consensus because they hold different conceptual and evaluative commitments, I feel it is plausible to make a finding through peer review that a treatment offers objective net benefit a necessary condition for funding.

That is a judgment quite different from the finding that even though the treatment offers some chance of benefit, the benefit is so marginal that the resources are morally more appropriately used somewhere else. That is a judgment totally independent of medical science. It relies not only on the values of those doing the assessing, but also on answers to questions such as the correct moral relation between full beneficence and justice and exactly what is meant by justice. Those are issues about which medical professionals have no special expertise and which they cannot address without abandoning their commitment to their patients.

THE IMPLICATIONS FOR COST-SHIFTING

All of this has important implications for the morality of cost-shifting. Cost-shifting sometimes refers to shifting cost from patients insured by one system such as Blue Cross to another such as Medicare. It can also refer to shifting costs from one DRG group to another. It is the latter that is of particular relevance here. If, for example, the hospital finds that it has a loss in one DRG group and a profit in another, it has several options. It could eliminate the services for the losing group, increasing profits in the process. If it finds that morally objectionable, however, it might simply let one service subsidize the other.

The problem, however, is that this systematically circumvents the allocation that was envisioned when the weights were assigned. The weights make sense only if they reflect a fair resource distribution among the DRG groups as judged by a group authorized to represent society in making these judgments. Cost-shifting between groups—even if it is done on a nonprofit basis—circumvents this judgment. It is unfair to the group that generates a profit to have those resources used at the local hospital's discretion for care of some other group who will be getting care at a level above that envisioned by those who assign the DRG weights. Cost-shifting from one DRG group to another is difficult if not impossible to justify ethically.

ELIMINATING CARE WITHIN A DRG GROUP

One final practical problem remains. The DRG weights ought to be arranged so that a hospital committed to avoiding cost-shifting will discover that the costs of patients in DRG group 122 exceed somewhat reimbursement even after the elimination of useless care and care refused by autonomous patients. How should the institution go about reducing costs?

It is indeed unusual—a measure of society's faith in the medical community—that it simply sets a reimbursement level without specifying how much care should be delivered. It is unimaginable that the administrators of the food stamp program would give a grocery store a fixed dollar reimbursement and tell the manager to provide an adequate, unspecified amount of food that he or she considers reasonable. That is what the Medicare system is doing to hospitals, however. Only with enormous faith in the integrity and dedication of administrators and clinicians is such a system thinkable. The hospital is held in check only by malpractice laws, the fear of bad publicity, and the institution's own moral integrity and good will. Eventually there may have to be some broader societal participation in deciding how much care ought to be delivered for the reimbursement set for a given DRG group. In the meantime, local hospitals have been left with that task. It is therefore important to understand the ethical basis for such decisions.

Once a DRG weight is assigned and the hospital knows its resource limits, the resources must be allocated among patients within that DRG group. The goal can be either to maximize the benefit per unit of resources invested or to give patients an equal opportunity for health. If the goal is to maximize aggregate benefit (measured in mortality and morbidity statistics), then sicker and more elderly patients may get low priority because they consume more resources in producing comparable benefits. For example, if a young patient and an elderly patient are being treated for a comparable disease, the elderly patient may require a longer stay in the hospital. If, however, the goal is equality of opportunity for health, then it is irrelevant that more days of stay are invested in older, sicker patients and that aggregate mortality and morbidity statistics are not as good because of this allocation. An egalitarian view of justice clearly calls for the latter view.

Some confronting this position concede that for larger, macro-allocation decisions, the public should make the decisions. They should decide, for example, whether to include heart transplants in Medicare. But they argue that fine-tuning the application at the micro-level cannot be done by lay people. They could not, for instance, decide which heart attack victim should be dismissed from the hospital when resources cannot provide for all.

I am convinced that mechanisms are available for much greater public participation. HMOs, for example, could rely on consumer panels to determine which kinds of services they should include. Labor unions and other groups of workers should be given the opportunity to choose through collective bargaining which kinds of medical services they want to include in their coverages.

Still, the critics are right that these lay panels could not possibly adjudicate every dispute among prospective patients for scarce resources within a given service. What they can do, however, is articulate principles and rules by which the allocations ought to be made. They could tell a hospital cardiology department, for example, to arrange the resources available so as to obtain the greatest aggregate number of days of survival. They could tell it to arrange resources so as to minimize pain or to give the worst-off patients the greatest chance of surviving. If the aggregate reimbursement to the service provided 90 percent of the resources needed to deliver what was considered the medical ideal (N days of care in our example), the lay population could tell the professional staff to give each patient 90 percent of the resources needed to get to his or her individual ideal level of care. More plausibly it could tell the staff to give the worst-off patients more than their 90 percent share while giving much better off patients perhaps even less than 90 percent of their ideal level of care. Choosing among these guidelines requires a decision about the relation between full beneficence and justice as well as a decision about exactly what justice means. These are surely not decisions of medical science.

There is an additional problem: How will individual patients consume their allotment of resources? There is no reason based on justice why each patient must expend his or her resources on exactly the same mix of services. One might want to "trade in" one allotted day of stay for additional diagnostic tests. Surely even in an egalitarian health care system there is room for personal liberty and variation.

While justice would not require the same mix for each patient, it might be impractical to permit patients to choose different mixes. Administering such "intrapatient" resource shifts would be extremely difficult. Just educating the patient sufficiently to make knowledgeable decisions would be difficult (although every patient may need much of this knowledge in order to give an informed consent to the treatment). Another pragmatic problem is that were a patient permitted, on grounds of autonomy, to make such shifts, sometimes making the shift would leave the patient much worse off medically. While this would not matter to a lover of autonomy, provided the patient is not using up more than his just share of the resources, it could present a more complex problem. The patient who has become sicker because of such a shift would have had the opportunity for health and have refused it. Therefore he or she would have less of a claim on medical resources than other comparably sick patients.

Two possible solutions to this problem come to mind. First, anyone choosing to shift resources at the "intrapatient" level could be required to buy an insurance policy to cover the costs of additional care needed because of this free choice. Then further care needed could be covered out of a separate insurance pool. Second, and probably more practical, intrapersonal shifts could be banned, not on the grounds that they jeopardize patient welfare or that people should not be free to choose, but on the grounds that this would create enormous administrative problems.

The DRGs and the concern about cost containment provide an intriguing opportunity for us to reassess the ethics of medicine. Some patient-centered concerns may given us adequate leverage for curtailing costs, at least if patient benefit is considered objectively and is supplemented with patient autonomy. These alone, however, ought not to be adequate. Important cost-curtailing decisions ought to follow. Therefore, newer, more socially oriented ethical principles will have to be incorporated into our medical ethic. While a fuller commitment to beneficence is the more obvious candidate for an expanded ethic, justice may be the more legitimate principle for cost-containment decisions. DRG weights should be viewed as a scale of the relative ethical claims of patients in the different diagnostic groups. If these social principles become a central part of a medical ethics of the future, we shall have to decide whether health professionals in their clinical role should incorporate them into their ethics or whether they should be given a special duty to remain patient-centered. A good case can be made for the latter.

CHAPTER TWENTY

Justice and Economics: Care of the Terminally Ill, Persistently Vegetative, and Elderly

In the previous chapter I tried to make the case that even after objectively useless and undesired care is eliminated, it is wrong to deliver all the possible medical care that really could be beneficial to and desired by patients. I suggested that while clinicians should strive to deliver all such care, the social system ought to be arranged so that they cannot get all that would benefit. In particular, the society should arrange the insurance system so that certain marginally beneficial care that is relatively expensive is excluded.

One obvious target is health care for the terminally ill. Enormous amounts are spent for "heroic" interventions on patients who die soon after receiving treatment. Somewhere between 20 and 30 percent of health care expenditures are devoted to the terminally ill—depending on how one defines terminal illness.[1] For example, Lubitz and Prihoda found that 27.9 percent of Medicare expenditures went to patients during the last twelve months of life in spite of the fact that only 5.9 percent of that population dies in a twelve-month period.[2]

In discussing the ethics of the economics of terminal care, the definition of "terminal illness" will be critical. For our purposes it is defined in the same way as in the Hastings Center project on ethics and economics of the care of the termially ill, that is, as "an illness in which, on the basis of the best available diagnostic criteria and in light of available therapies, a reasonable estimation can be made prospectively and with a high probability that a person will die within a relatively short time."[3]

If it is inevitable that economic considerations will begin to generate questions about the acceptability of health care, it is equally inevitable that terminal care will be questioned with special rigor. Ethical questions about the legitimacy of using economic considerations to decide about providing such care will become crucial.

Relating ethics to economics in decisions about appropriate care for the terminally ill requires conceptual clarity about the problem and ethical clarity about the ethical principles relevant to public policy. Conceptual analysis alone will reveal two quite separate issues. One presents no serious ethical problems; the other poses an enormous ethical dilemma.

USELESS CARE VS. MARGINALLY BENEFICIAL CARE

In the previous chapter a distinction was made between care that is of no benefit at all and care that is really beneficial but not very helpful compared to the social and economic costs involved—between useless care and marginally beneficial care.

USELESS CARE

Some care can be identified as useless in the sense that it offers no medical benefit. This is a judgment requiring an evaluative assessment, so while normally, as I suggested, we can rely on professional peer review to identify such treatments there will be times when the lay public may disagree. These issues arise frequently in care for the terminally ill. For example, providing ventilatory support or blood transfusions may temporarily extend the life of an unconscious or semiconscious patient. The medical community may consider such transient extension of no use, but some lay people could consider it important. In such cases the lay population should retain the right to override the professional consensus and classify such treatment as useful. In the normal case, however, the peer review determination of uselessness should be an adequate approximation for public policy purposes.

We also saw in the previous chapter that some care that is labeled useful by peer review may nevertheless be of no use to individual patients. Again, since these judgments are particularly difficult and subjective in the context of terminal illness, we should expect that in many cases individual patients or their surrogates will consider interventions useless for them even though others would classify them as useful. Rational persons would not want care that they perceived as useless. Such treatments are prima facie a violation of the principle of autonomy and the legal requirement of an adequately informed consent, even though the appearance of consent may be present in a signed form.

The problems of useless care may be important, but the ethics seems straightforward when approached from the patient's perspective. This care violates the rational patient/physician contract. There are historical, sociological, legal, and psychological explanations why such care is given to patients, but none of those presents immediate or dramatic ethical problems. Not much is known about the dynamics of useless medical care, for instance, how extensive it is, or what proportion of total care for the terminally ill or of total expendable care it constitutes. There is anecdotal evidence about its sources—demands from family members and providers and even from misinformed patients—but not much else. It is rumored that such care is delivered because it is defensive medicine being practiced by physicians fearing lawsuits. If that is the case, the law may need to be changed so that physicians will not be in legal jeopardy for failing to provide useless care. It seems more likely that the law does not now require useless care and that the real problem is that physicians have unreasonable fears about their legal jeopardy. If so, physician education is needed.

It is perhaps not too early to begin thinking about some guidelines for the appropriate relationship of ethics and economics in decisions about terminal care. These might be used by health insurance planners, any future national health insurance or health service, health maintenance organizations, and professional review organizations as guidelines for policy formation. One guideline that is suggested by the notion of useless care is that "care judged by the competent patient (or the legal agent for the incompetent patient within the limits of reason) to have no net benefit or care provided without a valid consent should not be covered under health insurance and should not be reimbursable."

MARGINALLY BENEFICIAL CARE

The real ethical problems are raised not by useless care, but by care that is beneficial as assessed by the patient or surrogate, with caring advice from professionals and other advisors, but is so marginally beneficial on balance that an objective observer might question whether the cost is justified. From the patient's perspective, the potential benefits seem worth the risks. If the care is to be withheld, it will have to be either out of the patient's sense of altruism or from some claim that the person is not entitled to the care.

I begin with what I take to be obvious: some care for terminal patients has predicted benefits so marginal in comparison with social and economic costs that it simply must be—will be—forgone. Either we shall have to create a rational, systematic plan for excluding it, or we can rely on care providers to use good judgment in eliminating it, maintaining the fiction that no policy exists.

Having a terminal illness is directly relevant to the concept of marginally useful care since the terminal condition directly affects the extent of the predicted benefit. Having defined a terminal illness as one that can reasonably be predicted with high probability to lead to death relatively soon, we avoid the problem of placing economic limits on care offered to people who will, in fact, die in a short time, but who cannot predictably be said to be dying.

THE PHYSICIAN AND MARGINAL CARE

In the previous chapter, I suggested that it is dangerous to rely on the physician to make ad hoc decisions to restrict access. Such decisions are subject to the variability and dangers of subjective, nonsystematic action. Different caregivers will have different standards of what constitutes expendable care. They will hold different systems of value in relating their patients' unknowing sacrifice to the common good. Because of sociological variables, different patients will be treated differently and perhaps even discriminatorily. This is likely to happen even though we have every reason to assume that the individual caregivers will be acting with good will, trying to be fair.

Even if there were no practical problems of this kind, there is an ethical problem with relying on individual caregivers to eliminate marginally useful but expensive care. As we have seen, traditionally the Hippocratic physician's mandate has been to do what he or she thinks is in the patient's interest. There is no qualifier saying, "unless the costs are great in comparison to the benefits to be gained." The ethics of the Hippocratic physician makes yes or no decisions on the basis of benefit to a single individual without taking into account what economists call alternative costs. Yet when the alternatives are considered, it is clear that marginal benefits are at least problematic. We are in what Clark Havighurst has called the "quality/cost no man's land."[4] If physicians are asked to reject such care for their patients in order to serve society, they must abandon their Hippocratic commitment.

The solution proposed in the last chapter was to give the physician a special exemption from the general moral duty to be fair, just, and efficient in the use of social resources. Physicians would then be free to do all they could for their patients. However, then some person or group would have to have the responsibility of limiting the use of marginally beneficial resources.

A second preliminary guide that might be taken into account by health planners for decisions about relating ethics to the economics of terminal care is suggested: "Any physicians choosing to remain committed to their Hippocratic duty to do what they think will benefit their patients or what is right by their patients should be excused from, indeed, excluded from, the task of deciding to exclude care on grounds of social costs."

A corollary is in order to protect patients when physicians have decided to abandon their patient-centered perspective. That corollary recognizes the need for patients to be adequately informed when their physicians consider nonpatient interests: "Any physicians choosing to abandon their commitment to pursue only the rights and welfare of their patients in order to participate in decisions about the elimination of marginally useful care should inform their patients of this potential conflict of interest."

Whether we finally decide to include clinicians in the group deciding to limit marginally useful care for the terminally ill or exempt them from this task so they can become unencumbered advocates for their patients, some persons or groups will ultimately have this responsibility. They will need to have a set of social ethical principles to guide their decisions. While we often jump immediately to the principle of maximizing the total net good as the basis for making social ethical resource decisions, I have argued that justice offers an important alternative: it has radically different implications when it comes to decisions about marginally useful care for the terminally ill. Especially with the terminally ill, standard cost-benefit analysis is likely to lead to conclusions that benefits to be gained for specific patients do not equal the benefits to others if the resources were instead allocated to them. If human capital approaches are used to calculate the value of a medical intervention, by definition the human capital gained will be near zero.[5] If willingness-to-pay approaches are used,[6] commitments to the terminally ill again will be small, in part because many who are terminally ill will be unable to pay very much for a benefit, especially a marginal one, and in part because the healthy may not be able to empathize with the terminally ill. Cost-benefit analysis, and the principle of maximizing aggregate net welfare upon which it is based, will not lead to a morally satisfactory resolution of the problem of decisions about medical care for the terminally ill.

JUSTICE-BASED LIMITS ON TERMINAL CARE

Ethical social policy planning requires that a full range of ethical principles be satisfied, including the principle of justice as well as autonomy and efficiency in maximizing aggregate net benefits.

INSURANCE MODELS AND JUSTICE

An increasingly familiar approach to ethical problems of resource distribution involves insurance modeling.[7] We can ask what kinds of health insurance for terminal illness rational people would buy. Assuming they got the difference in the form of a lower premium, they would certainly exclude some care currently being provided for terminally ill persons. They would at least exclude care that they judge, based on their beliefs and values, to produce no net benefit, as well as care that they would refuse if only they knew enough about it.

Moreover, there is some care that rational persons would exclude even if it is judged by their own values to be of some benefit. They would exclude coverages whenever the marginal premium needed could be spent in other ways to produce greater benefit to them. Depending on the extent to which they are altruistic, they might even exclude coverages when the marginal premium would be of greater benefit to other persons, particularly other family members and loved ones.

Exactly what kinds of terminal illness care would rational insurance purchasers forgo? Most obviously, they would exclude care that was expensive and so experimental that it had a very low probability of success. They probably would also forgo care that would stave off death but leave one seriously debilitated—chronically in pain, permanently severely impaired, or seriously compromised mentally, unconscious, or vegetative. They would probably also exclude relatively expensive nonexperimental procedures with a low probability of success. These coverages would be forgone not necessarily because they would be counted as having no net benefit. Even a small chance of success may be better than none when one is dying. Rather, they would be forgone because they are not good insurance buys. The small chance of success of an expensive treatment would raise the insurance premium by an amount that would more prudently be spent on something else to buy even greater benefit.

On the other hand, there are other coverages that rational insurance buyers would be willing to pay for: pain relief and other palliative care—probably even if it is rather expensive; basic nursing care to provide cleanliness and dignity; and possibly widely accepted chronic treatments where costs are modest. These would be rational insurance purchases. Another group of rational insurance buys would be safe, simple, and sure treatments for acute illness, but these are, by definition, impossible in the case of terminal care.

Some people using the insurance model have incorrectly jumped to the conclusion that whatever rational, self-interested people would buy is what ethics requires. As those familiar with contract theories of justice such as those of John Rawls[8] and the application of those theories to health care by people such as Norman Daniels[9] are aware, in order for a health insurance scheme to be ethical (as well as politically feasible), certain additional constraints are required. First certain procedural requirements must be met.

PROCEDURAL JUSTICE

Generally, people are free to contract with one another and, under certain conditions, are bound by their contracts. Covenants are formed. The morality is one of keeping promises. Under certain special circumnstances, it would be reasonable for people to come together and agree to forgo certain marginal health care when they are terminally ill. But the ethical constraints on such agreements are severe.

Even advocates of free market solutions realize that certain conditions must be met to justify such an agreement. The absence of monopoly and the freedom of entry into the market for both suppliers and consumers are necessary, but neither is really the case in the world as we know it today. Health care suppliers dominate the planning of health insurance plans and reimbursements; the insured often have no real voice in deciding what coverage is provided.

Present insurance mechanisms lack procedural justice. It is the nature of insurance to limit available options—often only a single plan will be available from an employer. If that is the case, then these constraints require fair participation of all in the decisions about what insurance options are available. This suggests another guideline for health planners: "Any decisions made to place limits on health care coverage on the grounds of terminal illness must be made with full, fair, and equal participation of all insured in the insurance pool." At the very least, there ought to be full participation by socioeconomic, age, sex, and racial groups. Otherwise, on its face, the insurance protection will be unfair.

Of course, full and equal participation will be very difficult, perhaps impossible, to obtain. Perhaps this factor alone is an argument against any such scheme to make terminal illness a relevant factor in deciding about insurance coverage. But, even if it were possible, there would still be problems of substantive justice.

SUBSTANTIVE JUSTICE

Even if the voices of the poor, the elderly, and the sick were heard adequately in such a contracting process, it is still possible that the results would be unfair. We are interested in the *ethics* of the economics of terminal illness, not simply a social or political decision about public policy. If we were only pursuing a political policy decision, then some Engelhartian agreement reached among rational, self-interested contractors to limit insurance coverage for terminal illness would be sufficient. Ethics requires more than contractual agreement, however. It requires taking "the moral point of view."[10] The well-being of all parties must be given fair consideration in order for a policy to be ethical.

Even if all parties are given full and equal participation, that will not necessarily guarantee that they are given fair consideration. Some, especially those who are terminally ill, may not have the strength or power to ensure that their interests are adequately considered. This will in part be controlled by the fact that all persons can presume that even if they are not now members of the group, they one day will be. Thus in comparison with the interests of racial, ethnic, and gender groups who are politically weak, all can identify with the terminally ill when planning insurance coverage.

Still, there is reason to fear that the moral point of view will be lacking in such planning. For one thing, while all can assume they will one day be terminally ill, not all terminal illnesses will necessarily be fairly represented in such planning. The diseases of politically weak groups may not be adequately spoken for. All rational persons participating in the political process at least know they will not die of a disease of infancy. They may retain an empathic interest in such diseases insofar as they can envision their children, grandchildren, or relatives succumbing to them, but we should not assume that all terminal illnesses will automatically get ethically fair attention unless additional moral constraints are imposed.

Insofar as we want to know what is ethical in the economics of terminal illness, we must impose the constraints familiar to advocates of the hypothetical contract. An insurance scheme will be ethically (as well as politically) acceptable insofar as those participating in the planning process can approximate the characteristics of ideal contractors. They should be as knowledgeable as possible and have understanding of and empathy for the points of view of all parties. John Rawls goes so far as to say that a practice would be ethical if the parties had no knowledge of their particular interests, psychological idiosyncrasies, and positions in the social system.

In the real world, of course, such a hypothetical vantage point does not exist. Fortunately, it need not. It is a heuristic device for telling us the kind of perspective planners of insurance schemes ought to adopt insofar as they want their results to be ethical.

The critical question is whether such planners taking the moral point of view would accept limits on terminal care when that care is perceived by the patient or surrogate to be somewhat beneficial, but is very expensive in comparison with the net benefits. Given that some such care will offer very little benefit and those same resources could bring much greater good in other ways, it seems intuitive that persons taking the moral point of view who were not already terminal rationally would prefer the greater benefit while not terminal and would opt for some limits on terminal care. Thus: "In order for limits on terminal care to be just, they ought to be limits that reasonable persons would accept if they did not know whether they would be the ones who at some point would need the care."

A straightforward utilitarian should have no problem with that conclusion. For someone whose ethical theory includes a more robust independent theory of justice, it is a little harder to comprehend. The most important version of an independent theory of justice holds that the less well off have some special moral claims over and above those who would simply receive greater benefits from scarce social resources. For Rawls and other maximin theorists, this leads to the principle that practices should be arranged so that benefits redound to the least well off groups. For egalitarians, who are often perceived to be identical with Rawlsians but are, in fact, somewhat different, it leads to the principle that resources should be used in order to produce greater equality of well-being.

In either case the terminally ill are in a special position. They are potentially among the least well off groups. They seem to need more resources in order to create or restore more equality of well-being. The claim of maximin theorists and egalitarians is that social planners taking the moral point of view would (at least prima facie) arrange social resources so as to benefit the least well off or make them more equal in well-being to other groups. Does that not mean that the terminally ill, if they are plausibly the least well off group in our community, have claims on resources even if it is not efficient to use the resources in that way?

DECIDING WHO IS WORST OFF

It does, assuming the terminally ill are really the worst off. However, that assumption needs exploration. One problem in determining who is least well off is trying to establish an objective basis for interpersonal comparison of well-being. Some hold that objective interpersonal standards for comparing well-being do not exist and that preferences are all we can go on. That, however, leads to the strange conclusion that the healthy, wealthy member of an elite social group who claims to be miserable could be worse off than someone who is wretched and dying but tolerating his fate well. At least for purposes of public policies related to resource allocation, purely subjective expressions of well-being will be inadequate. If there is to be any moral basis for a health policy, it must be some pretense to objective interpersonal comparisons of well-being. Two very different perspectives are available for attempting such comparisons.

The Slice-of-Time Perspective

The most obvious is to have health planners contemplating different insurance coverages while taking the moral point of view attempt to determine which groups are worst off at the present time. From this *slice-of-time perspective*, it is quite easy to understand if such planners concluded that the terminally ill were among the worst off. If they are among the worst off, then planners emphasizing an independent theory of justice will have at least prima facie reasons for committing substantial resources to them even if greater good could come from using the resources on other, better-off groups. A group of utilitarians in the original position might opt for sacrificing the terminally ill, but not those striving for justice.

The Over-a-Lifetime Perspective

There is a second way that our hypothetical insurance planners might try to identify the worst-off groups, however. We might view persons as having continuity over their lifetimes. Social planners could strive for equality of well-being over their lifetimes.

This *over-a-lifetime perspective* might easily lead to the conclusion that some of those currently terminally ill are not the worst off in the society. While the terminally ill presently have low levels of well-being, their lifetimes taken as a whole may be quite good. Others suffering from chronic, debilitating diseases of childhood, or those who are simply miserably poor, may be leading lives that are much worse than the lives of those who are presently terminal. From the over-a-lifetime perspective, the terminally ill are not necessarily the worst off.

Is the slice-of-time perspective or the over-a-lifetime perspective the correct one for deciding how to create a just health care insurance system? In either case planners could strive for justice. The issue now is not the place of the principle of justice or which interpretation of that principle applies. It is, rather, a problem of trying to identify whether the terminally ill are necessarily among the worst off.

For some interventions, the slice-of-time-perspective seems appropriate. For the terminally ill cancer patient in excruciating agony who could be treated cheaply with morphine, it does not seem relevant that he has had a long, happy life with enormous well-being. For the terminally ill person in need of clean sheets or compassionate nursing support, the fact that he or she has experienced a long, happy life seems irrelevant. These are the interventions that rational contractors would include in insurance coverage for the terminally ill.

For other interventions, however, it is not so obvious. For the person inevitably dying comfortably who has had a long and good life, does it make sense to claim that aggressive, expensive resources ought to be devoted to life prolongation simply because the patient insists that adding days counts as a benefit? From the over-a-lifetime perspective, such a person is not as low on the scale of well-being as the homeless child or the adolescent in the agony of poverty who is not terminally ill. If that is the proper perspective for assessing this kind of terminal care, then even an egalitarian attempting to make social policy on a principle of justice rather than a principle of utility can—must—support limiting care. From the point of view of one who doesn't know whether he will be the terminally ill person who finds life prolongation a benefit or the non-terminally ill homeless child, it makes sense to conclude that the terminally ill are not necessarily the worst off. If so, justice, not utility, demands limits on this kind of terminal care. Another guideline is identified: "Insofar as the terminally ill can be seen as better off than others, justice requires that limits be placed on their care."

PROBLEMS

Using justice as a basis for limiting care for the terminally ill raises some problems with the logic of the justice argument.

TWO-TIER CARE AND THE RIGHT TO TRADE

With an insurance model for setting ethical limits on terminal care, some but not all terminal care will be available. Would this not simply create a market for a second tier of terminal care that the rich could buy with private funds or for which they could buy insurance? If, for example, hemodialysis were not available to those diagnosed as terminal, would not some wealthy patients simply buy dialysis or buy supplemental insurance for it?

Alternatively, would it not be rational for the very poor to sell part of their terminal illness coverage in order to buy medical or other goods that they value more? Would it not be prudent, for example, for a poor person to surrender basic nursing care and cleanliness while permanently unconscious in order to have some money to buy food while young and healthy?

These possibilities raise questions about whether the criteria of justice can determine a single level of terminal care that should be available for all—even those who would rather buy extra care or sell some in order to have other goods. The issues are not limited to terminal care allocations. They arise with particular drama, however, when the care that is being bought or sold has direct bearing on whether one lives or dies.

The argument is too complex to be pursued here in detail. There are good reasons why, from the point of view of justice, it will make no difference whether people sell their basic entitlement to terminal care or buy a luxury tier of care over and above the basic entitlement. The principle of justice requires providing opportunities for equality of well-being in general, not just medical well-being. If someone who is on the bottom could be a little better off by selling his terminal illness entitlement, why should he not be permitted to do so?

We could ask whether our hypothetical contractors would support the kinds of transactions we are considering. Permitting selling of basic entitlements in a world where resources are distributed justly does not seem controversial. Everyone would have a fair share of resources to start with and if two people wanted to swap with one gaining extra terminal illness care and the other a larger food allotment, who could complain in the name of justice? Limiting the sale on the grounds that the money would be spent foolishly rests on the doubtful empirical assumption that such persons would really be better off if they were forced to have the medical care allotted rather than something they think would make them better off. In any case it rests on pure paternalism.

On the other hand, there are pragmatic, nonpaternalistic reasons to prohibit such transactions. It would be socially offensive to have to watch the terminally ill suffer from lack of analgesics or lie in filth because they have sold their insurance right to nursing care. If terminal care entitlements could be sold, then presumably other care entitlements could be as well. If some patients had sold some of their entitlements, then two patients medically identical would have to be treated differently not only for their immediate medical needs but throughout their lifetimes, creating bureaucratic tracking nightmares.

In the real world where people will be bargaining with an initial unfair allotment of resources, it is not so evident that selling entitlements should be accepted. Some would hold that the planners of insurance should permit such trades whenever the lot of the least well off would be improved. Others would hold that the planners ought to strive to get at least some elements of social practices arranged the way they would be in an ideal, just society, even if they cannot get the entire system to be just. They might choose to arrange coverage for terminal illness so that persons had those things considered basic—those things justice requires in the slice-of-time perspective—and no more. Either arrangement could be defended.

Even if one concludes that *justice* requires that insurance planners taking the moral point of view prohibit selling one's basic entitlement or buying a luxury tier of terminal care, other ethical principles may support these practices. Even if justice requires banning transactions with terminal illness entitlement, autonomy may support them. It may even be overriding. In all likelihood these questions will be resolved not in the context of terminal illness care, but at the larger level of limits on transactions in social entitlements.

PERMANENT VEGETATIVE STATE

The justice-based argument for limiting terminal care has implications for other groups who may not be terminal. There is one special group that by my definition and by most legal definitions are not terminally ill whose entitlement to medical care should be examined here: those in a permanent vegetative state (PVS) or what we used to call, apparently inaccurately, coma.[11] Many in such a state would previously have concluded that further life support is of no value when one is forever to be unconscious. They should have treatment stopped based on their expressed values. Other PVS patients may be inevitably dying. Even if they have left clear indications they would consider such care beneficial, they might still have care stopped on the grounds that justice does not permit such care for the terminally ill. Many such persons are not terminal, however. Their lives can be prolonged indefinitely (although without restoration of consciousness). Assuming that they once did or their surrogates do now consider the care beneficial, is there any basis for stopping it?

A utilitarian can easily say that the benefit that accrues is very small in comparison with the benefit the same resources could bring to conscious persons. One committed to justice will have to ask whether these PVS patients are among the worst off in society, and if so, whether justice demands providing what they or their surrogates take to be a benefit for them.

The justice analysis developed for the terminally ill provides a foundation for approaching this problem as well. Some PVS patients have had substantial opportunities for well-being over their lifetimes. This suggests that they are not among the worst off after all. If this is so, then even if we can somehow construe life support for PVS patients to be a benefit, they would not necessarily have a claim of justice for such care. Alternatively, we can approach the question of benefit from continued life support. If we can conclude that there is no real benefit in spite of the patient's previously expressed views to the contrary, then we might also limit care even if we conclude that the patient is legitimately among the worst off among us. Either approach avoids introducing the principle of full beneficence and utilitarian reasoning to place limits on such care.

This justice-based analysis would support establishing a special new diagnosis-related group for PVS, which would provide only enough funds for confirmation of diagnosis and a short period to permit loved ones to accept the irreversibility. Then, at least for adults, justice would seem to require that funding of care cease. If care can reasonably be labeled useless, then that DRG should probably cover infants as well. The medical coverage provided by a health system or health insurance must be substantively as well as procedurally just.

THE ELDERLY

If we accept these justice-based limits on the terminally ill and persistently vegetative, does that not set up a moral logic that would also permit limiting health care on the basis of age? Could we not argue that justice requires assessing the entitlements to health care of the non–terminally ill elderly using the over-a-lifetime perspective? I am convinced that that is precisely what is required. This analysis of justice thereby provides a framework for setting age-based limits on all health care, even for those not terminally ill.

It is widely reported that in Britain patients over the age of sixty-five are excluded from hemodialysis. In fact, this is not official policy, but one study reported that 80 percent of United Kingdom dialysis centers excluded patients over sixty-five.[12] Whether official or not, the idea is horrifying to many Americans. Health care resources are limited, but excluding solely on the basis of age sounds wrong.

Americans may not be able to avoid age-based allocation, however. Until recently the DRG system had many groups divided by age, typically at age seventy. Identical patients of different ages generated different reimbursements. Medicare funding of heart transplants is likely to include an upper age limit. Already liver transplants are authorized on the basis of age. Congress's Office of Technology Assessment was so concerned that it commissioned a study of the social and ethical problems of distributing life-sustaining technologies, including the role of age in setting limits.[13] Two kinds of arguments are given defending age-based limits.

UTILITARIAN ARGUMENTS FOR AGE-BASED ALLOCATION

One bases cut-offs on the judgment that old people are no longer useful members of society. Dialyzing persons over age sixty-five takes resources away from younger, more useful members of the society—those who could lead productive lives. If that is the basis, defenders of age-based limits are in for considerable argument.

In the first place, it just is not true that persons over sixty-five are necessarily less useful. Some are still working efficiently in important jobs, including homemaking. Some younger persons are not terribly useful citizens Calculations would have to include more subtle value of older persons—as role models, loving caregivers, and compassionate grandparents. More fundamentally, most find the idea of allocating resources on the basis of usefulness simply repulsive. Scholars such as Jerry Avorn,[14] James Childress,[15] and Harry Moody[16] have all challenged the ethics of allocating resources to younger persons on this basis.

At this point defenders shift to medical usefulness. They suggest, for example, that medical risks make heart transplants contraindicated above age fifty-five. Age is only a marker of medical success, not blatant age discrimination per se. That sounds more acceptable, but raises questions. We simply cannot identify some specific age that is a clear indicator that an intervention will not work. Age, at best, is statistically related to success. Even if age is a predictor of success, there are still problems. Society is increasingly skeptical of using social indicators in allocating resources. For some medical interventions, men statistically do better than women, the rich better than the poor, or whites better than blacks. It seems wrong to use these sociological facts to eliminate those interventions for the social groups doing worse statistically. Medical usefulness based on a statistical prediction of usefulness is only a social criterion in disguise, not based on any evidence of success in the individual. If we reject the argument that only the social groups who do statistically better are entitled to treatment, would we not reject age as a social criterion for allocating resources?

JUSTICE

The defense of age as a predictor of usefulness is going to be a difficult one. Many doubt that the health care system should simply do as much good as possible independently of how benefits are distributed, even if it means, for example, eliminating care to whole age groups. Utility is not a good reason for using age to allocate resources. There is another basis for using age, one focusing more on fairness and justice. At least three different examples of this kind of reasoning have appeared recently. Daniel Callahan in his recent book *Setting Limits* reaches a policy conclusion similar to the one suggested here. He concludes that life-prolonging care for the elderly should be limited to relief of suffering, not life-extending technology.[17] His recommendation rests, however, on the notion that there comes a point when the life span is complete, when one has had the opportunity to experience life's major phases. He does not argue explicitly that justice places limits or that age has any implication for allocating resources other than at the critical boundary between those who have lived out their natural life span and those who have not. In practice this would seem to require one very sharp line in health resource allocations. Insurance would cover certain life-extending technologies for those who have not completed their life span and would not cover those over some critical age.

Callahan resists specifying a particular age. He mentions ages in the seventies. It would be impossible to administer Medicare, however, without having some clear age—say, seventy-five—at which persons would be said to have completed their normal lifespans.

Norman Daniels, a professor of philosophy at Tufts University, argues that aged-based allocation is fundamentally different from allocation based on sex, race, or other social categories.[18] He asks us to imagine ourselves trying to decide what portion of our resources we would want to allocate to health care at different stages of our personal life cycles. He suggests that the reasonable thing to do would be to provide enough care to have fair opportunities at each age range. What is needed for normal opportunity for adolescence is not the same as what is needed at old age. Daniels proposes that we would rationally want health insurance that would give us opportunities for functioning that are normal for different stages in the life cycle. This would mean different care for persons of different age groups not based on the usefulness of persons or even on medical effectiveness of interventions at different ages. According to Daniels, justice requires that a society adopt insurance schemes that provide such age-specific normal opportunities. Both Callahan and Daniels end up with moral defenses of age-based limits that are grounded more in what is just or fair than what is efficient or useful.

My own approach to establishing age-based limits in justice starts with the premise that people should be given health care necessary for them to have a chance for opportunities for equality. However, we have seen that there are two different ways to treat people equally. We could assess the medical needs at a moment in time. Two people of different ages suffering from equally life-threatening end-stage renal disease could, from the "moment-in-time" perspective, be said to have equal need. On the other hand, people could be entitled to the health care needed to give them equal opportunities over their lifetimes. From the "over-a-lifetime" perspective, an elderly and a young person suffering equally serious kidney problems are not at all comparable. The elderly person has had a lifetime of opportunity. By contrast, the younger person has much greater need in order to have a lifetime of opportunities. Treating them equally from this lifetime perspective means that the young person deserves priority.

My scheme provides a different theoretical basis for limiting care on the basis of age from that of Callahan or Daniels. Some people low on the scale of well-being at a given moment may nevertheless have had considerable opportunity for well-being over their lifetimes. Older persons generally have had a greater opportunity for well-being over their lifetimes than, say, critically ill infants. From that perspective, if one compares two critically ill patients, one an infant and the other elderly, the infant has much stronger claims on resources in order to have an opportunity for well-being over its lifetime comparable to the elderly person. The infant might be entitled in the name of justice to a much larger proportion of the resources regardless of any ambiguous and controversial notion of age-specific species-typical functioning. If so, justice would require that the resources go to the younger person. On the other hand, for those resources more appropriately allocated from the slice-of-time perspective such as pain relief, we could conclude that treating the two equally would require giving them equal relief at the moment.

This interpretation of justice thus seems to provide a basis not only for limiting certain kinds of terminal care, but also for using age—chronological age—as a criterion for allocating health care resources to the nonterminal as well. In contrast to Callahan's scheme, there would be no hard-and-fast line between those who have completed life spans and those who have not. Those just above the age of completed life span would have a stronger claim than those substantially above. Those just below would have substantially less claim than youngsters who have barely had any opportunity for well-being.

This justice-grounded allocation on the basis of age would not rest on any controversial concept of age-specific, species-typical functioning. While

Daniels' scheme seems to give persons of different ages an equal claim to the care needed for typical functioning at their age, my proposal gives persons priority in inverse proportion to age. Callahan's scheme draws a sharp division between those who have completed the major stages of the life cycle and those who have not. He provides no basis for distinguishing between those who have recently reached this point and those who have long since reached it. Likewise, he seems to provide no basis for assigning age-based priority between an eighteen-year-old and someone nearing the end of the life cycle (say, someone in his late sixties). Daniels' approach recognizes different ranges of normal opportunity at different life stages and could easily account for different allocations to the eighteen- and sixty-eight-year-olds. The over-a-lifetime view recognizes gradations of claims over the entire life cycle, thus avoiding Callahan's unrealistically sharp chasm between those who have completed their life cycle and those who have not, and Daniels' separation of claims into different age groups.

When age becomes the basis for allocating rather than terminal illness, there is an additional complication. Should safe, simple, and sure low-cost curative treatments be allocated on the moment-in-time or over-a-lifetime perspective? These are, by definition, impossible in the case of the terminally ill. Callahan says that even those who have completed their life spans should get such care, much as they get relief of suffering and basic nursing care. That seems intuitively correct, but does not seem to fit with allocation based on whether life span has been completed. My justice-based allocation formula would more easily support safe, simple, and sure remedies even for the centenarian, based on the claim that they should be allocated to provide equality for well-being using the moment-in-time perspective.

A theoretical basis for deciding which care is justly allocated on the moment-in-time perspective and which using the over-a-lifetime perspective has not yet been developed. It seems obvious which applies, but there should be an articulated theoretical basis. Some needs of persons are so immediate that they seem to command immediate attention without regard to the amount of well-being one has experienced over a lifetime. Intense pain and suffering is one such need. Basic nursing care is another. Intervening to provide an easy, cheap cure for an acute illness may well be a third.

This should not be taken to imply that there is no such foundation. That foundation need not be utilitarian either (although cost-benefit analysis might also lead to the same division of types of care). I am suggesting that whatever it is that leads us to invest enormous resources to rescue the child in the well without regard to utility calculations or the relative well-being of others who could benefit from our attention, that same sense of immediateness calls for the slice-of-time perspective in allocating certain care to the elderly as well as to the terminally ill. At the same time, egalitarian justice can also explain, using the over-a-lifetime perspective, why other kinds of care can be excluded based on age or terminal illness.

Ethical discussion of limiting health care is no longer a taboo topic.

People are realizing that resources are limited, that some criteria are needed for allocating health care—based not on social utility but on fairness. Age, at first, looks to be just another social vehicle for discrimination. More careful examination seems to be taking us in an unexpected direction. If we are reasonable and fair about planning what we would like for ourselves when we are elderly, some interventions should be excluded. This same approach will provide guidance for allocating care among different age groups, even for those not elderly. In chapter 22, we shall see its relevance to transplants and the artificial heart. Before turning to those issues, however, one additional element of the issue of justice, which I call the voluntary health risks problem, must be addressed.

CHAPTER TWENTY-ONE

Voluntary Risks to Health:
The Ethical Issues

In the previous chapters I presented arguments for allocation of health care resources based, at least in part, on an egalitarian principle of justice. Justice requires, according to this interpretation, that opportunities for well-being be distributed equally. In the sphere of health care, this implies that, at least as a practical matter, opportunities for health should be distributed equally as far as possible. Of course, justice is only one of several nonconsequentialist ethical principles. I have held that while these nonconsequentialist principles collectively take precedence over consequentialist ones, among themselves the nonconsequentialist principles are coequal. They should be balanced against one another.

One of these potentially competing principles is the principle of autonomy referred to in chapter 6. These two clash most conspicuously when people are in poor health because of voluntary lifestyle choices they have made. Autonomy would support their right to make such choices, yet what should be done if persons need health care because of those choices? Does egalitarian justice strive for equal health? If all that justice requires is an opportunity for well-being, it might be argued that those voluntarily risking their health have had that opportunity and have chosen not to take advantage of it. The problem of voluntary risks to health needs special attention as a footnote to an egalitarian theory of justice in health care.

In an earlier era, one's health was thought to be determined by the gods or by fate. The individual had little personal responsibility for his or her health. The modern medical model has required little change in this latter view. One of the primary elements of the medical model was the belief that people were exempt from responsibility for their condition.[1] If one had good health in old age, one would say he had been blessed with good health. Disease was the result of mysterious, uncontrollable microorganisms or the random process of genetic fate.

A number of proposals have been put forth that imply that individuals are in some sense personally responsible for the state of their health. The town of Alexandria, Virginia, refuses to hire smokers as firefighters, in part because smokers increase the cost of health and disability insurance (*The New York Times*, Dec. 18, 1977, p. 28). Oral Roberts University insists that students meet weight requirements to attend school; the dean said that the school was just as concerned about the students' physical growth as their intellectual and spiritual growth (*The New York Times*, Oct. 9, 1977, p. 77). Behaviors as highly diverse as smoking, skiing, playing professional football, compulsive eating, omitting exercise, exposing oneself excessively to the sun, skipping needed immunizations, automobile racing, and mountain climbing all can be viewed as having a substantial voluntary component. Health care needed as a result of any voluntary behavior might generate very different claims on a health care system from care conceptualized as growing out of some other causal nexus. Keith Reemtsma, chairman of the Department of Surgery at Columbia University's College of Physicians and Surgeons, has called for "a more rational approach to improving national health," involving "a reward/punishment system based on individual choices." Persons who smoked cigarettes, drank whiskey, drove cars, and owned guns would be taxed for the medical consequences of their choices (*The New York Times*, Oct. 14, 1976, p. 37). That individuals should be personally responsible for their health is a new theme, implying a new model for health care and perhaps for funding of health care.[2]

Some data correlating lifestyle to health status are being generated. They seem to support the conceptual shift toward a model that sees the individual as more personally responsible for his health. The data of Belloc and Breslow make those of us who lead a slovenly lifestyle very uncomfortable.[3] As Morison[4] has pointed out, John Wesley and his puritan brothers of the covenant may not have been far from wrong after all. Belloc and Breslow identify seven empirical correlates of good health: eating moderately, eating regularly, eating breakfast, no cigarette smoking, moderate or no use of alcohol, at least moderate exercise, and seven to eight hours of sleep nightly. These all seem to be well within human control, far less mysterious than the viruses and genes that exceed the comprehension of the average citizen. The authors found that the average physical health of persons aged seventy years who reported all of the preceding good health practices was about the same as persons aged thirty-five to forty-four years who reported fewer than three.

We have just begun to realize the policy implications and the ethical impact of the conceptual shift that begins viewing health status as, in part, a result of voluntary risktaking in personal behavior and lifestyle choices. If individuals are responsible to some degree for their health and their need for health resources, why should they not also be responsible for the costs involved? If national health insurance is on the horizon, it will be even more questionable that individuals should have such health care paid for out of the same money pool generated by society to pay for other kinds of health care. Even with existing insurance plans, is it equitable that all persons contributing to the insurance money pool pay the extra costs of those who voluntarily risk increasing their need for medical services?

The most obvious policy proposal—banning from the health care system persons who have medical needs resulting from risky behaviors—turns out to be the least plausible. For one thing, it is going to be extremely difficult to establish precisely the cause of the tumor at the time the patient is standing at the hospital door. Those who have carcinoma of the lung whether from smoking or from unknown causes should not be excluded.

Even if the voluntary component of the cause could be determined, it is unlikely that our society could or would choose to implement a policy of barring the doors. While we have demonstrated a capacity to risk statistical lives or to risk the lives of citizens with certain socioeconomic characteristics, it is unlikely that we would be prepared to follow an overall policy of refusing medical service to those who voluntarily brought on their own conditions. We fought a similar battle over social security and concluded that—in part for reasons of the stress placed on family members and on society as a whole— individuals would not be permitted to take the risk of staying outside the social security system.

A number of policy options are more plausible. Additional fees on health-risk behavior calculated to reimburse the health care system would redistribute the burden of the cost of such care to those who have chosen to engage in it. Separating health insurance pools for persons who engage in health-risky behaviors and requiring them to pay out of pocket the marginal cost of their health care is another alternative. In some cases the economic cost is not the critical factor; it may be scarce personnel or equipment. Some behaviors might have to be banned to free the best neurosurgeons or orthopedic specialists for those who need their services for reasons other than injuries suffered in a motorcycle accident or a skiing tumble. Of course, all of these policy options require not only judgments about whether these behaviors are truly voluntary, but also ethical judgments about the rights and responsibilities of the individual and the other, more social components of the society.

ETHICAL PRINCIPLES

There are several ethical principles that could lead us to be concerned about these apparently voluntary behaviors, and even to justify decisions to change our social policy about paying for or providing health care needed as a result of such behavior.

HIPPOCRATIC BENEFICENCE

The Hippocratic principle is committed to having the physician do what he thinks will benefit the patient. Based on it, one would approach the individual patient out of paternalistic concern about the medical welfare of the patient. This might lead to a conclusion that, for the good of the patient, this behavior ought to be prevented. As we have seen, however, the paternalistic Hippocratic ethic is suspect in circles outside the profession and is even coming under attack from within the physician community itself.[5] The Hippocratic ethic leaves no room for the principle of autonomy—a principle at the core of liberal Western thought. The freedom of choice to smoke, ski, and even race automobiles may well justify avoiding more coercive policies regarding these behaviors—assuming that it is the individual's own welfare that is at stake.

SOCIAL BENEFICENCE

The hyperindividualistic ethic of Hippocratism also leaves no room for concern for the welfare of others or the distribution of burdens within the society. A totally different rationale for concern is being put forward, however. Some, such as Tom Beauchamp,[6] have argued that we have a right to be concerned about such behaviors because of their social costs. He leaves unanswered the question why it would be considered fair or just to regulate these voluntary behaviors when and only when their total social costs exceed the total social benefits of the behavior. This is a question that we must explore.

JUSTICE

The principle of justice could also provide a very different moral basis for deciding how to pay for health care resulting from health-risky behaviors. Procedural justice requires that like cases be treated alike. Substantive justice, at least in its egalitarian form, requires opportunities for equality of well-being. If those needing health care as a result of voluntary lifestyle choices are different in a morally relevant way, then different moral conclusions would seem to be possible. If funding their care from common resources such as insurance pools means some will not get an opportunity to be as healthy as others, then such funding would be substantively unfair.

Clearly, the argument is a complex one requiring many empirical, conceptual, and ethical judgments. Those judgments will have to be made regardless of whether we decide to continue the present policy or adopt one of the proposed alternatives. At this point, we need a thorough statement of the kinds of questions that must be addressed and the types of judgments that must be made.

ARE HEALTH RISKS VOLUNTARY?

The first question, addressed to those advocating policy shifts based on the notion that persons are in some sense responsible for their own health, melds the conceptual and empirical issues. Are health risks voluntary? If these behaviors are not really voluntary, then the issue is moot. Several models are competing for the conceptual attention of those working in the field.

THE VOLUNTARY MODEL

The model that considers the individual to be personally responsible for his health has a great deal going for it. The empirical correlations of lifestyle choices with health status are impressive. The view of humans as personally responsible for their destiny is attractive to those of us within modern Western society. Its appeal extends beyond the view of the human as subject to the forces of fate and even the medical model, which as late as the 1950s saw disease as an attack on the individual coming from outside the person and outside his control.

THE MEDICAL MODEL

Of course, that it is attractive cannot justify opting for the voluntarist model if it flies in the face of the empirical reality. The theory of external and uncontrollable causation is central to the medical model.[7] It is still probably the case that organic causal chains almost totally outside human control account now and then for a disease. But the medical model has undergone so much reality testing in the last decade that it can hardly provide a credible alternative to the voluntarist model. Even for those conditions that undeniably have an organic causal component, the luxury of human innocence is no longer a plausible defense against human accountability. The more we learn about disease and health and their causal chains, the more we have the possibility of intervening to change those chains. Since the days of the movement for public health, sanitation, and control of contagion, there has been a rational basis for human responsibility.

Even for those conditions that do not yet lend themselves to such direct voluntary control, the chronic diseases and even genetic diseases, there exists the possibility of purposeful rational decisions that have an indirect impact on the risk. Choices can be made to minimize our exposure to potential carcinogens and risk factors for cardiovascular disease. Parents now have a variety of potential choices to minimize genetic disease risk and even eliminate it in certain cases. We may not be far from the day when we can say that all health problems can be viewed as someone's fault—if not our own fault for poor sanitary practices and lifestyle choices, then the fault of our parents for avoiding carrier status diagnosis, amniocentesis, and selective abortion; the fault of industries that pollute our environment; or the fault of the National Institutes of Health for failing to make the scientific breakthroughs to understand the causal chain so that we could intervene. Although there remains a streak of plausibility in the medical model as an account of disease and health, it is fading rapidly and may soon remain only as a fossillike trace in our model of health.

THE PSYCHOLOGICAL MODEL

While the medical model seems to offer at best a limited counter to the policy options rooted in the voluntarist model, other theories of determinism may be more plausible. Any policy to control health care services that are viewed as necessitated by voluntary choices is based on the judgment that the behavior is indeed voluntary. The primary argument countering policies to tax or control smoking is that the smoker is not really responsible for his or her medical problems. The argument is not normally based on organic or genetic theories of determinism, but on more psychological theories. The smoker's personality and even the initial pattern of smoking are developed at such an early point in life that they could be viewed as beyond voluntary control. If the smoker's behavior is the result of toilet training rather than rational decisionmaking, then to blame the smoker for the toilet training seems a bit odd.

Many of the other presumably voluntary risks to health might also be seen as psychologically determined and therefore not truly voluntary. Compulsive eating, the sedentary lifestyle, and the choice of a high-stress life pattern may all be psychologically determined.

Football playing is a medically risky behavior. For the professional, the choice seems to be made consciously and voluntarily. But the decision to participate in high school and even grade school competitive leagues may not really be the voluntary choice of the student. Then, if reward systems are generated from these early choices, certainly college-level football could be the result. The continuum from the partially nonvoluntary choice of the youngster to the career choice of the professional athlete may have a heavy psychological overlay after all.

If so-called voluntary health risks are really psychologically determined, then the ethical and policy implications collapse. But it must seriously be questioned whether the model of psychological determinism is a much more plausible monocausal explanation of these behaviors than the medical model. Choosing to be a professional football player, or even to continue smoking, simply cannot be viewed as determined and beyond personal choice because of demonstrated irresistible psychological forces. The fact that so many people have stopped smoking or drinking or even playing professional sports suggests that such choices are fundamentally different from monocausally determined behaviors. Although state of mind may be a component in all disease, it seems that an attempt to will away pneumonia or a carcinoma of the pancreas is much less likely to be decisively influential than using the will to control the behaviors that are now being grouped as voluntary.

THE SOCIAL STRUCTURAL MODEL

Perhaps the most plausible competition to the voluntarist model comes not from a theory of organic or even psychological determinism, but from a social structural model. The correlations of disease, mortality, and even so-called voluntary health-risk behavior with socioeconomic class are impressive. Data from Britain and from the Medicaid system in the United States[8] reveal that these correlations persist even with elaborate schemes that attempt to make health care more equitably available to all social classes.

In Great Britain, for instance, it has recently been revealed that differences in death rates by social class continue, with inequalities essentially undiminished, since the advent of the National Health Service. Continuing to press the voluntarist model of personal responsibility for health risk in the face of a social structural model of the patterns of health and disease could be nothing more than blaming the victim,[9] avoiding the reality of the true causes of disease, and escaping proper responsibility for changing the underlying social inequalities of the society and its modes of production.

This is a powerful counter to the voluntarist thesis. Even if it is shown that health and disease are governed by behaviors and risk factors subject to human control, it does not follow that the individual should bear the sole or even primary responsibility for bringing about the changes necessary to produce better health. If it is the case that for virtually every disease, those in the lowest socioeconomic classes are at the greatest risk,[10] then there is a piously evasive quality to proposals that insist that individuals change their lifestyles to improve their positions and their health potential. The smoker may not be forced into his behavior so much by toilet training as by the social forces of the workplace or the society. The professional football player may be forced into that role by the work alternatives available to him, especially if he is a victim of racial, economic, and educational inequalities.

If one had to make a forced choice between the voluntarist model and the social structural model, the decision would be difficult. The knowledge that some socially deprived persons have pulled themselves up by their bootstraps is cited as evidence for the voluntarist model, but the overwhelming power of the social system to hold most individuals in their social place cannot be ignored.

A MULTICAUSAL MODEL AND ITS IMPLICATIONS

The only reasonable alternative is to adopt a multicausal model, one that has a place for organic, psychological, and social theories of causation, as well as voluntarist elements in an account of the cause of a disease or health pattern. One of the great conceptual issues confronting persons working in this area will be whether it is logically or psychologically possible to maintain simultaneously voluntarist and deterministic theories. In other areas of competing causal theories, such as theories of crime, drug addiction, and occupational achievement, we have not been very successful in maintaining the two types of explanation simultaneously. I am not convinced that it is impossible. A theory of criminal behavior that simultaneously lets the individual view such behavior as voluntary while the society views it as socially or psychologically determined has provocative and attractive implications. In the end it may be no more illogical or implausible than a reductionistic, monocausal theory.

The problem parallels one of the classic problems of philosophy and theology: How is it that there can be freedom of the will while at the same time the world is orderly and predictable? In more theological language, how can humans be free to choose good and evil while at the same time affirming that they are dependent on divine grace and that there is a transcendent order to the world? The tension is apparent in the Biblical authors, the Pelagian controversy of the fourth century, Arminius's struggle with the Calvinists, and contemporary secular arguments over free will. The conclusion that freedom of choice is a pseudo-problem, that it is compatible with predictability in the social order, may be that most plausible of the alternative, seemingly paradoxical answers.

The same conclusions may be reached regarding voluntary health risks. It would be a serious problem if a voluntarist theory led to abandoning any sense of social structural responsibility for health patterns. On the other hand, it seems at least to apply to differentials in behavior within socioeconomic classes or within groups similarly situated. Admitting the possibility of a theory of causation that includes a voluntary element may so distract the society from attention to the social and economic components in the causal nexus that the move would be counterproductive. On the other hand, important values are affirmed in the view that humans are in some sense responsible for their own medical destinies, that they are not merely the receptacle for external forces. These values are important in countering the trend toward the professionalization of medical decisions and the reduction of the individual to a passive object to be manipulated. They are so important that some risk may well be necessary. This is one of the core problems in any discussion of the ethics of the voluntary health-risk perspective. One of the most difficult research issues is the implications of the theme for a theory of the causation of health patterns.

RESPONSIBILITY AND CULPABILITY

Even in cases where we conclude that the voluntarist model may be relevant—where voluntary choices are at least a minor component of the pattern of health—it is still unclear what to make of the voluntarist conclusion. If we say that a person is responsible for his or her health, it still does not follow that the person is culpable for the harm that comes from voluntary choices. It may be that society still would want to bear the burden of providing health care needed to patch up a person who has voluntarily taken a health risk.

To take an extreme example, a member of a community may choose to become a professional firefighter. Certainly this is a health-risking choice. Presumably it could be a relatively voluntary one. Still it does not follow that the person is culpable for the harms done to his health. Responsible, yes, but culpable, no.

To decide in favor of any policy incorporating the so-called presumption that health risks are voluntary, it will be necessary to decide not only that the risk is voluntary, but also that it is not worthy of public subsidy. Firefighting, an occupation undertaken in the public interest, presumably would be worthy of subsidy. It seems that very few such activities, however, are so evaluated. Professional automobile racing, for instance, hardly seems socially ennobling, even if it does provide entertainment and diversion. A more plausible course would be requiring auto racers to purchase a license for a fee equal to their predicted extra health costs.

But what about the health risks of casual automobile driving for business or personal reasons? There are currently marginal health costs that are not built into the insurance system, e.g., risks from automobile exhaust pollution, from stress, and from the discouraging of exercise. It seems as though, in principle, there would be nothing wrong with recovering the economic part of those costs, if it could be done. A health tax on gasoline, for instance, might be sensible as a progressive way of funding a national health service. The evidence for the direct causal links and the exact costs will be hard, probably impossible, to discover. That difficulty, however, may not be decisive, provided there is general agreement that there are some costs, that the behavior is not socially ennobling, and that the funds are obtained more or less equitably in any case. It would certainly be no worse than some other luxury tax.

THE ARGUMENTS FROM JUSTICE

The core of the argument over policies deriving from the voluntary health-risks thesis is what is fair or just. Regardless of whether individuals have a general right to health care, whether justice in general requires the social provision of health services, it seems as though what justice requires for a risk voluntarily assumed is quite different from what it might require in the more usual medical need. Two responses have been offered to the problem of justice in providing health care for medical need resulting from voluntarily assumed risks.

That Risks Are Involuntary

One response, given by Dan Beauchamp and others, resolves the problem by attacking the category of voluntary risk.[11] He implies that so-called voluntary behaviors are, in reality, the result of social and cultural forces. Since voluntary behavior is a null set, the special implications of meritorious or blameworthy behavior for a theory of justice are of no importance. Beauchamp begins forcefully with a somewhat egalitarian theory of social justice, which leads to a moral right to health for all citizens. There is no need to amend that theory to account for fairness of the claims of citizens who bring on their need for health care through their voluntary choices, because there are no voluntary choices.

It seems reasonable to concede to Dan Beauchamp that the medical model had been overly individualistic, that socioeconomic and cultural forces play a much greater role in the causal nexus of health problems than is normally assumed. Indeed, they probably play the dominant role. But the total elimination of voluntarism from our understanding of human behavior is quite implausible. Injuries to the socioeconomic elite while mountain climbing or skiing are not reasonably seen as primarily the result of social structural determinism. If there remains a residuum of voluntary action, then a theory of justice for health care will have to take that into account.

THAT UTILITY SHOULD BE THE BASIS

A second approach is that of Tom Beauchamp,[12] who goes further than Dan Beauchamp. He attacks the principle of justice itself. Dan Beauchamp seems to hold that justice or fairness requires us to distribute resources according to need. Since needs are not the result of voluntary choices, a subsidiary consideration of whether the need results from foolish, voluntary behavior is unnecessary. Tom Beauchamp, on the other hand, rejects the idea that needs per se have a claim on us as a society. He seems to accept the idea that at least occasionally behaviors may be voluntary. He questions whether need, whether corrected for voluntary choice or not, provides a plausible basis for deciding what is a right allocation of health care. He offers a utilitarian alternative, claiming that the crucial dimension is the total social costs of the behaviors. He argues:

> Hazardous personal behaviors should be restricted if, and only if:
> (1) the behavior creates risks of harm to persons other than those who engage in such activities, and
> (2) a cost-benefit analysis reveals that the social investment in controlling such behaviors would produce a net increase in social utility, rather than a net decrease.

These two conditions for imposing limits on voluntary health-risky behaviors first make clear that paternalistic controls are not justified. The behaviors must produce harm to others. Presumably the harm could be direct and physical (such as controlling driving while intoxicated) or could be financial (such as engaging in behaviors that will increase health insurance payouts and thereby predictably increase other persons' health insurance premiums). Tom Beauchamp thus limits the traditional utilitarian approach by insisting that the harm must come to third parties. He would not limit health-risky behavior even if doing so increased net social utility in cases where the increased good accrued only to the one being constrained. (Perhaps this is because he believes that, because of the disutility of paternalistic coercions, no such constraint will ever increase aggregate utility, or at least that the rule prohibiting such paternalistic coercions has more utility than any alternative rule.)

This antipaternalistic utilitarianism has a strange implication, however. Apparently, if an individual knowingly engages in a health-risky behavior that will harm others, but the harm to others is less than the benefit that will accrue to the risk taker, then no social policy to compensate the innocent third parties is justified. This is one of the classical flaws of utilitarianism. It is not only tolerable, but actually moral, for me to purposely harm others provided the benefits to me exceed the harm to them.

JUSTICE AS AN INDEPENDENT PRINCIPLE

I have suggested that there are nonconsequentialist ethical principles that also provide a basis for social practices, including those that affect health-risky behaviors. An approach rooted in these nonconsequentialist principles would also avoid paternalistic controls on such behaviors. It would avoid them not based on the problematic claim that paternalism is likely to have bad consequences (although it might). Rather, it avoids paternalistic limits simply on the grounds that respecting autonomy is the right thing to do. Likewise, not all harms to others necessarily justify policies related to health-risky actions, only those called for by justice.

A totally independent, nonpaternalistic argument is based much more on the principle of justice. This approach examines not only the impact of actions, but also questions of fairness. It asks if it is fair that society as a whole should bear the burden of providing medical care needed only because of voluntarily taken risks to one's health. From this point of view, even if the net benefit of letting the behavior continue exceeded the benefits of prohibiting it, the behavior justifiably might be prohibited, or at least controlled, on nonpaternalistic grounds.

Consider the case where the benefits accrue overwhelmingly to persons who do engage in the behavior and the costs to those who do not. If the need for medical care is the result of the voluntary choice to engage in the behavior, then those arguing from the standpoint of equity or fairness might conclude that the behavior should still be controlled even though it produces a net benefit in aggregate.

Both Beauchamps downplay a secondary dimension of the argument over the principle of justice. Even those who accept the egalitarian formula ought to concede that all an individual is entitled to is an equal opportunity for a chance to be as healthy, insofar as possible, as other people. Since those who are voluntarily risking their health (assuming for the moment that the behavior really is voluntary) do have an opportunity to be healthy, it is not the egalitarian dimensions of the principle of justice that are relevant to the voluntary health-risks question. It is the question of what is just treatment of those who have had opportunity and have not taken advantage of it. The question is one of what to do with persons who have not made use of their chance. Even the most egalitarian theories of justice—of which I consider myself to be a proponent—must at times deal with the secondary question of what to do in cases where individuals voluntarily have chosen to use their opportunities unequally. Unless there is no such thing as voluntary health-risk behavior, as Dan Beauchamp implies, this must remain a problem for the more egalitarian theories of justice.

In principle I see nothing wrong with the conclusion, which even an egalitarian could reach, that those who have not used their opportunities fairly should receive inequalities of outcome. I emphasize that this is an argument in principle. It would not apply to persons who are truly not equal in their opportunity because of their social or psychological conditions. It would not apply to those who are forced into their health-risky behavior because of social oppression or stress in the mode of production.

From this application of a subsidiary component of the principle of justice, I reach the conclusion that it is fair, that it is just, if persons in need of health services resulting from truly voluntary risks are treated differently from those in need of the same services for other reasons. In fact, it would be unfair if the two groups were treated equally.

For most cases this would justify the funding of the needed health care separately in cases where the need results from voluntary behavior. In extreme circumstances where the resources are scarce and cannot be supplemented with more funds (e.g., when it is the skill that is scarce), then actual prohibition of the behavior may be the only plausible option, if one is arguing from this kind of principle of justice.

The other situation in which actual control of behavior would be justified is when it is the behavior itself—rather than the economic or social consequences of the behavior—that injures others. On this basis voluntary consumption of drugs, such as amphetamines or alcohol, that can lead directly to harm to others should be controlled. In more typical cases, however, it is only the social and economic consequences of the behavior that harm others. In those cases all that is necessary to satisfy this kind of a principle of justice is to arrange things so that those who engage in the behavior pay the full costs including the medical costs. This can often be done most easily by placing a health fee on those behaviors that are public and monitorable.

THE CLINICIAN AND HEALTH-RISKY BEHAVIORS

It has become fashionable to encourage clinicians to focus on health-risky lifestyles and to attempt to get patients to be more health-conscious. Some even go so far as to claim that it is inherent in the role of the physician to do what is possible to get patients to lead healthier lives. I have tried to make clear that the implications for the clinician are not that obvious. The clinician who set out purposely to promote the health of the patient by getting him or her to change to a more healthful lifestyle might be acting paternalistically. That might be good Hippocratic medicine, but it is an affront to the partnership model of the physician-patient relation. I have suggested that clinicians are not necessarily even very good at determining what maximizes patients' medical well-being, let alone their total well-being. No rational patient will want to lead a lifestyle that would literally maximize health. It would be a boring, painful, unaesthetic existence that required sacrificing all other aspects of the good life for one important but very limited one.

The partnership model would surely require clinicians to inform patients of the possibility of learning about a lifestyle that leads to better health. To the extent that the patient wanted to learn of those changes, autonomy supports the effort. The patient and clinician can then become limited partners in an enterprise for which they share a common goal. No health promotion beyond that agreed to by the patient can be justified in the partnership model, however.

The main basis for limiting health-risky lifestyles is not promotion of patient welfare but promotion of justice to others. In particular, policies are necessary to limit the effects of such lifestyle choices when they do not deserve social support and when others are burdened by the voluntary choices of the individual. The social costs per se justify limits on actual behavior whenever the behaviors are directly harmful or when the resources used to treat the injured patient are scarce. Otherwise it is the injustice of making others bear the economic costs that is critical. Justice simply requires that individuals bear those costs themselves through taxes on the behaviors or through separate insurance risk pools.

In either case, by the time the health-risking patient seeks clinical help, the key ethical work will have been done. In rare cases the society will have limited the behavior directly. More frequently it will have collected funds to pay for the care needed. In the normal case, the clinician need not treat the patient any differently because the need for care may have resulted from voluntary choices on the part of the patient. The clinician should simply render care without having to take on the difficult and ethically troublesome task of trying to determine whether this care is needed as a result of lifestyle choices. To the extent that it is, the individual already will have paid for the needed care. The clinician's job will be making sure the patient is aware of the link between lifestyle and health and offering an opportunity for assistance in changing that behavior of it is desired. The clinician need no longer be a priest or a policeman. He or she is a partner in pursuit of mutually agreed-upon goals within the constraints of the first two social contracts that set limits on a few behaviors and generate justice-based obligations to make sure that people pay for the costs of their voluntary choices.

THE MONITORING CRITERION

This essentially egalitarian principle, which says that like cases should be treated alike, leaves us with one final problem under the rubric of justice. If all voluntary risks ought to be treated alike, what do we make of the fact that only certain of the behaviors are monitorable? Is it unfair to place a health tax on smoking, automobile racing, skiing at organized resorts with ski lifts, and other organized activities that one can monitor, while omitting the tax on failing to exercise, mountain climbing, skiing on the hill on one's farm, and other behaviors that cannot be monitored? In a sense it may be. The problem is perhaps like the unfairness of being able to treat the respiratory problems of pneumonia, but not those of trisomy E syndrome or other incurable diseases. There may be some essential unfairness in life. This may appear in the inequities of policy proposals to control or tax monitorable behavior, but not behavior that cannot be monitored. Actually some inge- nuity may generate ways to tax what seems untaxable—taxing gasoline for the health risks of automobiles, taxing mountain-climbing equipment (as- suming it is not an ennobling activity), or creating special insurance pools for persons who eat a bad diet. The devices probably would be crude and not necessarily in exact proportion to the risks involved. Some people engaged in equally risky behaviors probably would not be treated equally. That may be a necessary implication of the crudeness of any public policy mechanism. Whether the inequities of not being able to treat equally people taking comparable risks constitute such a serious problem that it would be better to abandon entirely the principle of equality of opportunity for health is the policy question that will have to be resolved.

COST-SAVING HEALTH-RISK BEHAVIORS

Another argument is mounted against the application of the principle of equity to voluntarily health-risking behaviors. What ought to be done with behaviors that are health-risky, but that end up either not costing society or actually saving society's scarce resources? This question will separate clearly those who argue for intervention on paternalistic grounds from those who argue on utilitarian grounds or on the basis of justice. What ought to be done about a behavior that would risk a person's health, but risk it in such a way that he would die rapidly and cheaply at about retirement age? If the concern is from the unfair burden that these behaviors generate on the rest of society, and if the society is required to bear the costs and to use scarce resources, then a health-risky behavior that did not involve such social costs would surely be exempt from any social policy oriented to controlling such unfair behavior. In fact, if social utility were the only concern, this particular type of risky behavior ought to be encouraged. Since our social policy is one that ought to incorporate many ethical concerns, it seems unlikely that we would want to encourage these behaviors even if such encouragement were cost- effective. This, indeed, shows the weakness of approaches that focus only on aggregate costs and benefits.

REVULSION AGAINST THE RATIONAL, CALCULATING LIFE

There is one final, last-ditch argument against adoption of a health policy that incorporates an equitable handling of voluntary health risks.

Some would argue that, although the behavior might be voluntary and supplying health care to meet the resulting needs unfair to the rest of society, the alternative would be even worse. Such a policy might require the conversion of many decisions in life from spontaneous expressions based on long tradition and lifestyle patterns to cold, rational, calculating decisions based on health and economic elements.

It is not clear to me that that would be the result. Placing a health fee on a package of cigarettes or on a ski-lift ticket may not make those decisions any more rational calculations than they are now. The current warning on tobacco has not had much of an impact. Even if rational decisionmaking were the outcome, however, I am not sure that it would be wrong to elevate such health-risking decisions to a level of consciousness in which one had to think about what one was doing. At least it seems that as a side effect of a policy that would permit health resources to be paid for and used more equitably, this would not be an overwhelming or decisive counterargument.

PART
IV

Special Problem Areas

CHAPTER TWENTY-TWO

The Ethics of Organ Transplantation

One of the most critical areas involving the social ethics of medicine and the allocation of resources is the transplantation of human organs and tissues. As long as transplantation is the best means available for treating some patients with critical or life-threatening illness, as long as part of one person's body is deemed essential to the welfare of another, medical ethics will necessarily be social ethics. When there are not enough of those body parts to meet the needs of those in the moral community, the social ethics of justice and resource allocation will come into play.

The bioethical debate over organ procurement goes back at least to the first kidney transplants in 1954. The current generation of controversy, however, can be dated from December 3, 1967, when Christiaan Barnard transplanted the first human heart into the chest of Louis Washkansky. While organ procurement from living donors, especially related donors, appears to be acceptable in cases where the transplant would be life-saving for a recipient and would not be life-threatening for the donor, there is widespread disapproval of using living donors when the the removal of the organ would be life-threatening.[1] There has been debate over this issue, especially in the case of anencephalic infants. Some have proposed that laws be changed to permit organ procurement from these special groups.[2] Their position seems to be mistaken on two grounds, however. First, they have repeatedly referred to anencephalics as "brain-absent." This simply is not true. Anencephalic infants who are plausible candidates for organ procurement clearly have some living brain tissue present. They are not dead according to any current law defining death.

Second, while proponents of the use of organs from these groups may ultimately be correct in their conclusion, they seem wrong in their analysis. If one or more groups (such as anencephalic infants) should be deemed acceptable as organ sources, advocates should be able to describe in general terms the characteristics that make them so. The plausible characteristic is irreversible loss of any capacity to feel, perceive, or have interests, that is, permanent vegetative state or some similar diagnosis and prognosis. This characteristic is precisely what some are advocating as the standard for a revised definition of death. I suggest that it is because some of us believe that such individuals are actually dead (or have never been alive) that we find organ procurement acceptable. If so, then the proper stance is to continue the battle for a further revision of the definition of death, rather than advocating that certain classes of living individuals be accepted as organ sources.

PRELIMINARY ISSUES

The definition of death involves a debate that extends far beyond the transplantation of organs. Suffice it to say that as long as we limit organ procurement from those who meet current definitions of death focusing on irreversible loss of all functions of the entire brain, there is widespread acceptance of such a definition. While there is some objection among Orthodox Jews,[3] rabbis from Conservative and Reformed traditions have endorsed the use of brain criteria for death pronouncement,[4] as have Catholics.[5] The only reservations come from those often associated with the right-to-life position who fear that acknowledging that a person is dead based on brain criteria might indirectly lessen respect for those who are still living.[6] Protestants, both conservative[7] and liberal,[8] accept brain-oriented definitions of death. Likewise, secular philosophical, legal, and public policy commentators have shown widespread acceptance of such definitions. Most of the serious debate today centers on whether someone may be dead even if lower brain functions such as brainstem reflex functions remain.

More significant, there is substantial ethical agreement on the second preliminary ethical question, removal of cadaver organs. There has in general been no objection among either the secular or the religious bioethical community to the removal of organs for life-saving purposes from human bodies once it is established those persons are dead. Protestant and Catholics have raised no serious opposition provided appropriate respect is shown for the deceased and appropriate permissions are obtained.[9]

Jewish thought poses a weightier question, since in Judaism there are religious obligations to bury the dead with organs intact.[10] This obligation is superseded when a cadaver organ can save the life of another identified person in need. Thus all major religious traditions accept the legitimacy of removing cadaver organs for life-saving transplantations. Some may insist on more conservative heart-and-lung-oriented criteria for death, and some, especially Orthodox Jews, may object to organ removal for research or educational purposes, but the two preliminary ethical problems pose no insurmountable obstacles for cadaver organ procurement. In fact, they all place a high value on the saving of human life, so that while the state may not be authorized to salvage organs routinely, individuals bear at least a moral obligation to facilitate organ procurement for life-saving purposes.

GIVING VS. TAKING

This brings us to the two more critical and controversial core ethical issues. The first is the controversy over the two basic alternatives for organ procurement, donation vs. salvaging. Under salvaging schemes, such as that proposed by Dukeminier and Sanders, cadaver organs would routinely be made available as needed as a social resource.[11] Normally, advocates of salvaging would permit individuals to object in writing while living or even permit relatives to object in cases where the individual had not expressed his or her wishes.

The second alternative, donation, has been favored by virtually every writer within the Judeo-Christian tradition and by every religious group speaking on the subject.[12] The reason is fundamentally that according to the Judeo-Christian tradition, our respect for the individual and the rights associated with that individual does not cease at death. Obligations of respect—for the wishes of the deceased and the integrity of his or her earthly remains—must continue. In the Judeo-Christian tradition, as opposed to much pagan Greek thought, the body is affirmed to be a central part of the total spiritual being. Any scheme that abandons the mode of donation in favor of viewing the cadaver as a social resource to be mined for worthwhile purposes will directly violate central tenets of Christian thought and create problems for Jews as well, especially in a state not based on Jewish law. It will, more pragmatically, predictably produce vociferous, agitated opposition. While I cannot predict street riots comparable to those sparked in Israel after the passing of autopsy laws permitting routine violation of the corpse,[13] it is safe to say there would be sustained and vocal opposition.

At the same time there is uniform support in all major traditions for not only the ethical acceptability of donation, but the actual moral obligation to take organ donation seriously. Especially within Orthodox Judaism, the priority of the duty to preserve life can actually lead to the conclusion that there is a moral duty to procure organs for transplant. It is not clear whether that moral duty would be translated into a law permitting routine salvaging against the wishes of the deceased expressed while competent or those of the next of kin. This suggests that while, for practical and theoretical reason, there is widespread opposition to salvaging, the main traditions of Western culture would look favorably upon public policies facilitating donation. Given the fact that these religious traditions all support organ donation in at least some circumstances and in fact consider it a morally weighty obligation, they would favor public policies making it as easy as possible to express a willingness to donate organs for life-saving purposes.

The public policy implication is that the correct solution to the controversy is maximum encouragement of donation, provided this does not subtly coerce those unwilling to donate or does not trick them into doing so unintentionally. Thus various routine inquiry laws have gained substantial support recently. These laws mandate initiation of conversations asking the patient or next of kin to donate organs. They come in two forms: postmortem required request of next of kin and routine inquiry of persons while they are still living and competent.

For some reason, postmortem required request laws have gained favor in state legislatures. They create real problems, however. Families must be approached during time of severe trauma and stress. Consent to use organs has not risen dramatically, perhaps because some relatives are offended by the requests. More serious, postmortem required request is a second-best strategy ethically. The real commitment of those who have opted for donation is to respecting the wishes of the patient expressed while competent. Sometimes the next of kin may know the patient's wishes and be willing to express them, but at other times he or she may not. We know that people say they are more willing to donate relatives' organs than their own. Some have even advocated required request of relatives in order to increase the yield of organs. But that would be statistically a purposeful evasion of the patient's own wishes.

Especially since postmortem required request is not working very well, it seems wise to try the second alternative: routine inquiry of persons while competent. Most states now give people an opportunity to donate on their driver's licenses, but many people do not bother to answer. We could go one step further, requiring an answer, even if it is "I don't know." In addition, questions on federal documents, especially those already computerized for easy retrieval such as income tax or social security records, would seem appropriate. The ideal for of the question about willingness to donate would permit three responses—yes, no, and no response—thus not creating any presumptions or pressures on any respondents. This strategy seems far preferable to continental European public policies authorizing routine salvaging unless objection has been registered.[14] It is even preferable to the scheme endorsed by the British Working Party of the Health Departments of Great Britain and Northern Ireland, which would give a designated government or hospital official the power to remove organs in cases where no objection has been registered and relatives cannot be located.[15] This group who die alone, without relatives available, is sufficiently small and sufficiently vulnerable that those formulating public policies should bend over backwards to avoid abusing their right to be treated with maximum respect.

ALLOCATING ORGANS

This brings us to the final critical question: fairness in the distribution of organs to transplant recipients. While those standing within the traditions I am attempting to summarize would be concerned about efficient distribution, I think it is clear that they would place at least equal emphasis on fair distribution. The problem arises when there is a head-on conflict between an efficient and equitable allocation of an organ. For example, if two patients need a kidney, one may be expected to get the greater medical benefit from the organ, whereas the other may be said to need it the most. One such conflict is seen in current efforts to increase benefits from organ transplantation for tissue-typing potential recipients. It is now well known that better tissue matches are likely to lead to longer graft and patient survival. For this reason substantial efforts are being made to match up donors and recipients.

A serious ethical question is posed, however, when one realizes that racial minorities such as blacks and Hispanics are harder to tissue-type. A policy of maximizing tissue match in order to maximize the benefits of a transplantation program is de facto a whites-first policy. Equity seems to require that members of all racial groups have an equal chance at receiving organs. Especially if they contribute to the organ pool and need organs through no fault of their own, there should be equitable allocation, even if it means decreasing the aggregate benefits of the program.

MARKET MECHANISMS

One controversial basis of allocation uses direct market mechanisms to permit buying and selling of organs. Other schemes may not be so blatant. Current Medicare policy prohibiting funding of heart transplants under government health insurance has a similar impact of discriminating against the needy.[16] It is my sense that the critics of inequity are realists. They recognize that the government cannot make a commitment to pay for all possible medical care. They do, however, share with the President's Commission for the Study of Ethical Problems in Medicine and Biomedical and Behavioral Research the conviction that there should be some floor level of heath care under which no one ought to fall.[17] In the allocation of scarce organs for transplant, at least in cases such as hearts, kidneys, or livers, where the organs are literally life-saving, allocation is simply unfair if it is based on ability to pay. If anyone has access, all should have an equal chance, by some lottery system, by random assignment of organs to those in equal need, or by the randomness of having each wait in line for needed organs. No one should get an organ for transplant (or an artificial organ for implant) until there is a fair, nondiscriminatory allocation system in place which gives everyone in equal need an equal opportunity of access.

Recently we have discovered even more subtle problems of fair and efficient allocation. Some individuals with particular skills in reaching the medical profession or the mass media have been able to procure organs for themselves or their family members. Those supporting a small child in need of a liver transplant even, according to a fundraising campaign for a local radio station, convinced President Reagan to volunteer Air Force One to transport any donated liver. No one can possibly criticize them for fulfilling their obligations to their loved ones to do everything reasonable to serve their needs. In fact, they probably increase efficiency in organ procurement by reaching organs that may otherwise go to waste and by increasing public awareness of the need for organs. Society, however, should view with skepticism the use of such techniques of personal charisma and persuasion to obtain organs. It is unfair to those who lack the power or access to these means of obtaining organs. A much more systematic, institutional response is called for, one that in a disciplined way makes available every organ within reach donated by the patient or the responsible next of kin in a manner that gives all people of equal need an equal opportunity of access.

Voluntary Risks and Age in Allocating High Technology

One of the most fascinating problems in allocating organs for transplant arose by the close juxtaposition of two dramatic and controversial transplant efforts. Both led to cries that health resources were being used irresponsibly. Aside from some unsuccessful attempts in the 1960s, Baby Fae was in 1984 the first human to receive an organ transplanted from an animal of another species. This was followed in a few weeks by the implantation of an artificial heart into the chest of William Schroeder. The details of the two cases are as follows:

Case 14: Baby Fae: The Heart of a Baboon

> After a moratorium of two decades, Dr. Leonard Bailey of Loma Linda Medical Center created an uproar by transplanting a heart into an infant who became known to the world as Baby Fae. On October 12, 1984, Baby Fae was born a victim of hypoplastic left heart syndrome, a congenital deformity invariably fatal, usually within the first weeks. Treatment alternatives available included a human-to-human transplant, no treatment, or the Norwood procedure, a two-stage palliative procedure in which the first stage has a 45 percent success rate. Two of four patients who have undergone the second stage have survived. Prior to Baby Fae's birth, Loma Linda University's internal institutional review board had considered for fourteen months Dr. Bailey's request to perform baboon-to-human heart transplants. It had given final approval a week before Baby Fae's admittance to the university's medical center. Baby Stephanie Fae was the first case of a cardiac xenotransplantation in a neonate.
>
> The parents gave written consent to the procedure. It has been suggested that, because of their lack of schooling, their unmarried status, and encounters with the law, they were vulnerable to manipulation or coercion. In December 1984, a site visit was conducted at LLUMC by NIH's Office of Protection from Research Risks, and two nongovernmental consultants concluded that Loma Linda's review of Dr. Bailey's proposed procedure had been "appropriate and sensitive to the social and ethical issues." The report also concluded that the consent explanation was thorough and was without coercion or undue influence. Three shortcomings were found, though, in the consent document itself, which (1) failed to mention whether compensation and medical treatment were available if

injury occurred, (2) overstated expected benefits from the xenograft, and (3) did not include the possibility of searching for a human heart.[18] The surgery was performed on Baby Fae when she was fourteen days old. After initially doing fairly well postoperatively, she died twenty days after surgery.

CASE 15: WILLIAM SCHROEDER: IMPLANTING THE ARTIFICIAL HEART

William Schroeder, fifty-two, was the second recipient of a mechanical artificial heart, following by almost two years the highly publicized implant given to Barney Clark. Schroeder was a retired quality-control specialist at an army munitions facility, married with six children. He suffered from coronary artery disease, which led to deterioration of his heart. Schroeder, a smoker, was near death when he was rushed to surgery. On November 25, 1984, Surgeon William C. DeVries at Humana Hospital in Louisville, Kentucky, implanted a modified Jarvik-7 heart in a seven-hour operation. The 323-pound system was designed to replace Schroeder's heart function permanently. The option was available of switching to a portable unit for up to three hours a day. Two days later he was conscious and alert. His first request was for a can of beer.

The juxtaposition of the cases of Baby Fae and William Schroeder cries out for comparison. Some may argue that both are immoral tampering with nature or irresponsible use of resources. Others may affirm both as heroic but required efforts to preserve human life whenever we can. I am inclined to look for the differences and have tentatively concluded that, especially if one approaches the problem from the standpoint of the ethical theory I am using, one procedure is far more likely to be justified than the other.

Baby Fae's surgery involved transplantation from a baboon using procedures never before successfully attempted in humans, and involved controversies stemming from the use of other animal species. Some would object in principle to xenografts because of the religious or moral problems of cross-species transplantation or because of the violation of the purported rights of the animal from which the heart was taken. Some would identify this as the key moral difference between Fae and Schroeder. I suggest, however, that these are not necessarily insurmountable ethical problems with xenografts.

Some have argued that the critical difference is that Baby Fae could not consent to the experiment attempted on her, while William Schroeder could. The parental permission to operate has been questioned. Everyone would agree that any shortcoming in the consent process would have to be corrected in order for the procedure to be ethically acceptable. The parents would have to be told what they reasonably would want to know about the surgery, including, presumably, the items mentioned by the NIH panel.

Some have gone on to argue that even if the parents did have adequate information, they would not have the right to volunteer their child for a procedure so experimental that it could be said to be undertaken for the knowledge gained rather than for the benefit of the patient. However, the parents' conclusion that the xenograft best served their child's interests does not strike me as totally unreasonable.[19] Although their most reasonable decision might have been against the surgery on the grounds it did not serve their baby's interests, I am not persuaded that the decision the parents did make was so unreasonable that it should have been overridden. Thus I am not persuaded by any of the arguments supporting Schroeder's implant over Fae's transplant.

That brings us to the argument about the ethics of resource allocation. This I take to be the most critical moral problem. A number of people have suggested that even if the animal rights issues and consent problems are solved, it is unethical to spend hundreds of thousands of dollars on exotic, high-technology care when others in our society are doing without the basics of preventive care, maternal and child health services, and other basic medical needs.

I am increasingly convinced that such arguments rest fundamentally on a cost-benefit reasoning that is insensitive to basic questions of social justice raised in part III of this volume. Assuming it is true that the resources currently invested in high-technology, expensive medical interventions could do more good if they were spent on primary care, it does not follow that care should be so diverted. The hidden moral premise is that net utility in aggregate should be maximized as a matter of social policy even when aggregating utility masks any consideration of the distribution of benefits and harms. While that may be a good act of utilitarianism, I am convinced that it violates important moral insights conveyed in the principle of justice. This has led me to cautious support of Baby Fae's transplantation.

According to egalitarian justice, primary care would get priority only if those who did not get it would be worse off than those needing, but not receiving, the high-technology interventions. What would that mean for the Fae and Schroeder cases? It might be argued that both Baby Fae and William Schroeder were inevitably dying without surgery and that therefore they each had the highest possible priority for medical interventions under an egalitarian principle of justice. However, I think it is possible that that argument is wrong on two grounds.

Voluntary Risks to Health

First, the egalitarian justice principle requires equal *opportunity* for health, not equal health status. It is possible that Schroeder had considerably greater opportunity to avoid cardiac problems than Fae. This requires an examination of the reports that serious lifestyle problems, including considerable alcohol consumption, led to his heart condition. One of Schroeder's first requests after removal of the tracheal tube was for permission to have a beer. It may be that this peculiarly urgent desire had bearing on whether he had had an opportunity to be healthy in life. In chapter 21 I argued that if a patient can be shown to need medical care because he has voluntarily exposed himself to health risks, then he has had an opportunity to be healthy. We do not have enough information to say whether this was the case with Mr. Schroeder. If it was, however, his squandering of the opportunity to be healthy surely should have affected his claim for scarce medical resources.

Age and the Justice of Allocation

There is a second way in which Schroeder had opportunities for health beyond those of Baby Fae. On this point I am much more sure of the facts. Schroeder was fifty-two years old at the time of the surgery. Most of that time he had reasonably good health. He suffered from diabetes, but until shortly before his surgery, it apparently had not been debilitating. Baby Fae, on the other hand, had lived only a few days before surgery. From that standpoint Schroeder had considerably greater opportunity for health than Baby Fae.

If the egalitarian principle of justice requires equality of opportunity for health at any given moment in time, Schroeder and Fae may have had an equal claim, but then so would a one-hundred-year-old who is dying of heart failure. If, on the other hand, the egalitarian principle of justice requires opportunities for equal well-being over a lifetime, then Schroeder was considerably up on Fae. This form of the equality principle leads to the policy conclusion that priorities should be arranged in inverse proportion to age.[20] I am convinced that only this interpretation explains our intuition that if a ninety-year-old and a thirty-year-old could both gain five years of life from a hemodialysis machine, we would be inclined to give the machine to the thirty-year-old.

I am led to the conclusion that there are potentially two critical differences between Fae and Schroeder when it comes to the ethics of resource allocation based on an egalitarian principle of justice. First, insofar as Schroeder's need for a heart was the result of voluntary lifestyle choices over which he had control, his priority was lower. If health risks are truly voluntary, they should be taken into account in allocating resources. Second, Schroeder had lived many good years while Fae had not. Each was among the worst off medically and deserved priority over those who could gain marginal benefits from primary health care interventions even if those interventions would yield greater net aggregate utility. In comparing Fae and Schroeder, however, there is no question that Fae's well-being, viewed over a lifetime, was substantially lower than Schroeder's. As such she had a greater claim of egalitarian justice for the heart surgery.

CHAPTER TWENTY-THREE

The Technical Criteria Fallacy:
The Case of Spina Bifida

The partnership model rests on the fundamental observation that medical decisions necessarily require a set of beliefs and values as well as a set of relevant empirical data and that there is no reason why the beliefs and values used should be those of the clinician rather than the patient or patient surrogate. There is no area in which this insight has revolutionized health care more than in the care of the terminally and critically ill. In this chapter I shall provide an example of how beliefs and values necessarily penetrate the decisionmaking process in the care of critically ill patients. Then, in the next chapter I shall provide a more extended analysis of why the lay people in the partnership—the patient and family or other surrogates—ought to be brought into the decisionmaking.

The area of terminal and critical care that has generated the most controversy has been the care of severely afflicted newborns. Much of that discussion has centered on infants with spina bifida with myelomeningocele, a serious malformation of the spinal column that leaves the spinal cord exposed, leading to infection as well as spinal fluid drainage problems that can cause serious brain damage. With surgical correction, infants will have varying degrees of physical and mental impairment, but have a good chance of surviving. Without surgery, the infants have a very high likelihood of dying. The prognosis is dependent upon the location and seriousness of the spinal lesion as well as the degree of hydrocephalus. There have been efforts to establish norms for selection of infants for treatment or nontreatment.

Several sets of criteria have been developed to aid in the selection process. The most widely known example is the Apgar score used in the delivery room to predict outcomes for babies suffering from respiratory or other severe problems.

A number of lists of criteria have been proposed for spina bifida infants, of which John Lorber's has received the most attention.[1] These lists can be helpful in gaining a rapid and accurate prognosis for the infant. But there is a danger. We may become so infatuated with our technical abilities to accumulate data and tally scores that we run the risk of seriously misunderstanding the nature of the difficult decisions that must be made. We may succumb to what might be called the "technical criteria fallacy."

Some of these lists have implied that infants with spina bifida can be screened for treatment on the basis of objectively measurable criteria. At least with regard to one of his lists, Lorber has said bluntly that "infants who have any one or any combination of the following should not be given active treatment."[2] He includes such precise measures as "grossly enlarged head, with maximal circumference of 2 cm. or more above the 90th percentile related to birth weight."[3] G. Keys Smith and E. Durham Smith have proposed a list with slight differences.[4]

Sherman C. Stein, Luis Schut, and Mary D. Ames take strong exception to Lorber's criteria. They find that 52 percent of those who had major adverse criteria present nevertheless had a "satisfactory outcome" according to their criteria of IQ equal to or greater than 80 and a handicap that is moderate or less.[5] Their proposal, however, is not to abandon the search for criteria for selection for treatment, but rather to perfect them. The criteria they use (the presence of both lacunar skull deformity and multiple adverse physical findings or those children with associated gross congenital anomalies), however, are just as debatable as Lorber's. The authors have an empirical problem because even under their presumably more accurate criteria, 1 baby out of 53 with a so-called satisfactory outcome was not recommended for treatment, and 15 out of 110 recommended for surgery had an outcome considered unsatisfactory. They also have a theoretical problem because they offer no argument why their standard of satisfactory outcome ought to be definitive rather than, say an IQ of 75 (or even of 20, or a more-than-moderate physical handicap as long as mental function is above a certain level).

Perhaps some of those who advocate treatment for all babies with spina bifida are also committing the technical criteria fallacy. Some of their defenses do not make clear the basis of the policy being advocated.[6] One reason sometimes given for this policy is that it is impossible to predict outcomes accurately, at least with the present state of knowledge about prognosis. According to this argument, division of these infants into treatment and nontreatment groups on the basis of technical measures would be acceptable if only we had accurate technical measures. Another argument might be that it is always wrong (morally or legally) not to treat.

In principle it is a mistake to assume that any set of technical criteria will be able to definitively separate babies who should be treated from those who should not. If some decisions not to treat are acceptable—an assumption apparently made by Lorber, Smith and Smith, and Stein, Schut, and Ames—it seems plausible that there must be some range of cases for which discretion based on particular religious, cultural, or personal values is appropriate. At the very least, parents who want treatment for a child who falls within the group of those who have "contraindications for active therapy" should be permitted to act on their moral convictions.

It is not the precise content of the list which is important. Rather, it is the concept that any set of objectively measurable criteria can be translated directly into decisions about selection for treatment. Presumably the lists being proposed are meant to be reasonably accurate measures of prognosis. Yet the presumption that the treatment or nontreatment decision rests solely on prognosis is surely contestable. The decision must also include evaluation of the meaning of existence with varying impairments. Great variation exists about these essentially evaluative elements among parents, physicians, and policy makers. It must be an open question whether these variations in evaluation are among the relevant factors to consider in making a treatment decision. When Lorber uses the phrase "contraindications to active therapy," he is medicalizing what are really value choices.

Even those who are willing to concede that the criteria for selection may vary may frame the question in excessively technical terms. The British Working Party set up under the auspices of the Newcastle Regional Hospital Board emphasizes that "these criteria change and should be subject to constant scrutiny in the light of medical advance and in the conflict of ethical principles referred to in this report."[7] But they still seem to think the decision can be made on the basis of technical indicators rather than parental, societal, or other more universally grounded values that may vary from case to case. They thus hold that, at least for the present, Lorber's set of criteria "provides a sufficient basis for such selections." Consultation may be important to provide "a means of support for those involved in the decision-making and the subsequent emotional adjustment," presumably not to modify the choice on the basis of parental or other values. The technicalizing of the decision is supported by their strongly worded statement that it is the doctors' responsibility to make the decisions in individual cases. A similar fallacious generalizing of the physician's expertise to matters of moral and other value choices is seen in Herbert Eckstein's claim that "the decision to treat or especially not to treat must be taken at the consultant level."[8]

An alternative way of approaching the treatment decision would be to consider the evaluations of relevant decisionmakers to be only partially dependent upon technical measures of prognosis. Raymond Duff and A. G. M. Campbell conclude that the family must be the crucial decisionmaker, with society and health care professionals providing only general guidelines.[9] Whether the family's ethical judgments are the decisive ones is the question to be addressed in the next chapter.

I am convinced that even if there were complete agreement about diagnosis and prognosis of a seriously afflicted spina bifida infant, there would be only slightly more agreement about what we ought to do in a particular case. Prognosis cannot be the sole determiner of moral choice. The partnership model of medical ethics rests on the claim that these clinical choices necessarily incorporate ethical and other evaluations that must come from outside the medical sphere. It is that fact that gives the lay part of the partnership—the patient and his or her surrogates—standing to be active participants in the clinical decisionmaking. It is to the moral basis and limits on that lay participation that we now turn.

CHAPTER TWENTY-FOUR

Limits of Guardian Treatment Refusal: A Reasonableness Standard

One of the real challenges of doing medical ethics in a contractual mode, or in any system grounded in liberal political philosophy with its emphasis on autonomy, arises when the patient, such as the spina bifida infant, is not competent to be an active partner in the decisionmaking process. The question is especially difficult when the treatment, if rendered, may preserve life, but if refused would certainly mean death. Since the *Saikewicz* decision,[1] two seemingly irreconcilable approaches for refusing treatment on behalf of an incompetent patient have emerged. The prominent voices in the debate belong to lawyers and physicians.[2] The legal community has emphasized the essential role of a judicial decision mechanism,[3] whereas physicians have stressed the importance of the judgment of medical professionals.[4] Meanwhile, the judiciary, in decisions such as *Quinlan*,[5] *Saikewicz*,[6] and *Dinnerstein*,[7] has articulated conflicting legal standards for deciding when treatment may be refused on behalf of an incompetent patient.

Few of the commentators on this subject have properly emphasized the role of the guardian in formulating the initial decision whether to refuse treatment.[8] If we are going to take seriously a partnership between clinical professionals and lay participants in medicine, there will have to be a clearer role for guardians in making such decisions on behalf of incompetent patients. The medical professional must formulate his or her own conscience and withdraw from clinical partnerships when no meeting of the minds is possible with the patient or the patient's surrogate. Otherwise the professional's role should be limited to advising guardians and to initiating judicial and other review when guardians appear to have abused their discretion.

STANDARDS FOR REFUSAL OF TREATMENT

The principles governing when guardians can refuse treatment for an incompetent patient are related to, but not identical with, those supporting the right of patients to decide against treatment for themselves. The standards applicable to competent individuals refusing medical treatment provide a helpful beginning for a discussion of decisionmaking by guardians.

REFUSAL BY COMPETENT ADULTS

The treatment decisions of competent adults may be examined both legally and ethically. As a legal matter, a competent patient has a right to refuse any treatment that is proposed for his or her own good.[9] The right may be premised on a right of privacy,[10] a right to control one's body,[11] or a right of personal autonomy,[12] all of which have found their way into both constitutional and common law. Courts today never intervene to authorize treatment for a competent adult's own welfare when the patient has expressly refused it.[13] This general rule is limited to be compatible with two difficult situations: (1) it requires that the patient be legally competent; and (2) it permits treatment to be ordered when another's welfare is jeopardized by the decision.[14] Not all legal acts are ethical, however. For a competent adult's decision to refuse medical treatment to be ethical, there must be some attempt at justification. One proposed criterion is that a patient accept treatment whenever it may be useful. According to Orthodox Judaism[15] and one branch of physician ethics,[16] it is obligatory to preserve life whenever possible, regardless of the quality of the life preserved and the pain involved. According to this view, there are no justifiable reasons for refusing a treatment once it is established that it would be useful.

Most schools of medical ethical thought, including Roman Catholic, Protestant, and much Jewish theology, secular humanistic and philosophical analysis, and mainstream physician ethics, reject this approach, recognizing no absolute moral obligation on the part of a competent patient to accept a treatment simply because it would prolong life. The person refusing the treatment has an obligation not to do so frivolously, but other people should not have to find the reason rational or compelling.

What kinds of reasons have traditionally been found to be good ones? Unfortunately, we have inherited from several areas of the medical ethics tradition the language of "ordinary" and "extraordinary" means. That language is so confusing and misleading that it must be abandoned. The distinction is more effectively captured by the terms *reasonable* and *unreasonable*—reflecting the notion that there is good reason to accept some treatment but not others. We are still left, however, with the question of what count as good reasons. Two criteria have emerged: uselessness and grave burden.

While a treatment should not be required simply because it is useful, certainly if it is useless it ought to be morally expendable. Before uselessness can be adopted as an ethical criterion, however, two issues must be resolved. First, it is necessary to determine the goal of the treatment. The objective may simply be to preserve life, or it could be to restore something beyond basic metabolic processes. Choosing the goal involves a value judgment. Second, we need to determine whose values should be employed in making the judgment. Since the competent patient's right to refuse treatment arises out of an autonomy right, each individual should have an opportunity to apply his or her own values in choosing the objective of the treatment.

Although people may consider a treatment to be useful in achieving some objective, under certain circumstances they may still ethically refuse it. The definitional ambiguities that had to be resolved in discussing the uselessness criteria must also be resolved in this context: what is a grave burden, and whose values will be employed in determining its gravity? Again, the individual's own values must be decisive.

Refusal on Behalf of Incompetent Patients

This right of competent patients to refuse treatment for any good reason does not imply that guardians should have the same open-ended discretion to refuse treatment on behalf of their wards. The decision made on behalf of an incompetent patient should be measured by the uselessness and grave-burden criteria. The uselessness criterion appears to be easily transferred to incompetent patients. If a treatment would be useless, there is no ethical reason for the guardian to require it. However, since even judgments of uselessness involve subjective evaluative choices, some decisionmaking procedures for those choices will have to be established. Those limits will be discussed below. Before grave burden can be adopted as a criterion for treatment refusals on behalf of incompetent patients, similar judgments will have to be made.

Parents and other guardians have a moral and a legal obligation to serve the interests—especially the medical interests—of their wards. It is on this basis that Jehovah's Witnesses lose custody of their children when they attempt to refuse blood for them. But it is a valid presumption that the interests of incompetent patients in avoiding grave burdens are similar to those of competent patients. The law and many ethical traditions recognize that some medical treatments inflict such a grave burden that it would be in a competent patient's interest to refuse them. Likewise, surrogates should have the authority to refuse such treatments for their wards.

Admittedly, what counts as a grave burden may differ for incompetent individuals. Anticipation of agony may be crucial for a competent patient, but not relevant to an infant who cannot anticipate. Inability to continue one's life plan may be central to the competent adult's refusal of skin grafts after major burns, but irrelevant to an individual who has not yet formulated a life plan.

Assuming that grave burden can sometimes be a legitimate reason for refusing treatment, should the guardian be allowed to consider the burdens to persons other than the patient? If a competent adult wants to refuse a final life-prolonging cancer operation because it would consume family resources that are needed to put a child through school, most people would find nothing objectionable about the refusal. In fact, it seems a morally noble decision. If parents, however, decide to omit clotting-factor injections for their hemophilic son because it would jeopardize the financial interests of other members of the family, the matter is much more complex.

The simplest resolution would be not to take benefits and burdens to others into account when considering treatment decisions for one's ward. But this is too simplistic a rule. These other factors unavoidably influence treatment decisions, though the platitude of doing only what will benefit the patient is maintained as the official policy.

The grave-burden justification for refusing treatment on behalf of an incompetent patient should focus almost exclusively on the burden to the patient; however, there are exceptional situations where the door must be opened to consider the burden to others. It would be unrealistic not to recognize such exceptions.

CASE 16: TRADING OFF CHILDREN:
PARENTAL REFUSAL OF TREATMENT TO SERVE OTHERS

> Consider the situation of a family with moderate means consisting of husband, wife, and three children, including an infant with a severe immune deficiency. The infant is not expected to live, but the physician advises that if it were flown immediately across the country to a research facility, there would be about one chance in one thousand that the baby would survive. The treatment would not be painful to the child. The cost of the transportation and care would be approximately $100,000. The family has net worth, including equity in their house of $60,000, but they could borrow the remainder.

Most reasonable people would say that the parents are under no moral obligation to borrow the money to provide the infant this slim chance of survival. Yet, if only benefit to the patient were considered, they ought to be required to do so. There are several possible explanations for the moral sense that the family is not obligated to provide the treatment when doing so burdens others severely. One is that it is somehow really in the infant's interest not to have the treatment. The infant might live in such a financially deprived environment as to be "better off dead," or might live with such guilt when learning of the extent to which the treatment has deprived its siblings that the treatment would actually pose a grave burden to the infant later in life. A court used this logic in a less extreme case to justify transplanting kidneys from a mentally retarded incompetent man to his brother.[17] But it must be conceded that this reasoning is rather contrived.

An alternative rationale incorporating burden to others is the classic utilitarian analysis.[18] Utilitarians would argue that benefits to others, not merely benefits to the individual, are relevant. If great benefits to others are forgone by providing a small chance for benefits to the incompetent individual, then, on balance, the treatment ought not to be rendered.

These are not the only options, however. It is a mistake to assume that medical ethics must focus exclusively either on the individual patient or on aggregate benefits and harms, sacrificing the individual's rights for the good of society. Instead, we could adopt a position that permits a more sophisticated evaluation of what individuals owe to each other. The most straightforward example consistent with the contract theory used in this volume is cases where justice requires sacrifice for the good of others who are worse off. Even some terminally ill patients—especially older patients—may be better off than others if we are in situations where the over-a-lifetime perspective developed in chapter 20 is appropriate. Of course, such reasoning is less plausible in this case in which the patient is an infant. Only in rare circumstances would justice require sacrificing an infant's interest in order to serve the welfare of others who are worse off.

Without the individual's consent, society can reasonably impose an obligation to sacrifice for only certain other individuals. Independent of the individual's ability to formulate and express desires, there are some benefits to others that all individuals ought to desire. This is merely the extension of the argument advanced by Richard McCormick that there are certain minimal risks that can reasonably be imposed on children, provided certain safeguards are maintained.[19] This is a more honest justification for the parents' decision in the hypothetical case not to invest their life savings and thereby jeopardize the welfare of their other children for the extremely slim chance that their third child might survive. It is a much more satisfactory justification than the pretense that the incompetent patient was benefited by the guardian's refusal of treatment.

Having determined that the ethical guidelines of uselessness and grave burden are the appropriate criteria for treatment refusal on behalf of an incompetent patient, we confront a second problem. We need to determine who the substitute decisionmaker should be. Traditionally, physicians made decisions for such patients just as they did for those who were competent. But the decision whether to accept treatment necessarily involves value judgments. The recognition that health professionals making treatment decisions on behalf of patients are influenced by their own values has led many commentators to consider alternatives to the traditional approach. This is the impetus behind recent proposals for decisionmaking by the courts and guardians. All of these strategies have been unsuccessful, in large part because they do not draw a distinction between two different types of incompetent patients and between two different types of guardians. Until these lines are clearly drawn in law and in ethics, no further progress will be made in understanding the appropriate role of the guardian in treatment refusal decisions.

Types of Incompetent Patients

There are currently two legal approaches to making treatment decisions on behalf of incompetent patients. They are distinguishable according to whether evidence of the patient's own wishes is available. The first, called the substituted judgment standard,[20] applies to a patient who, while competent, expressed an opinion concerning life-saving medical treatment. The second standard, the best-interest standard,[21] applies to those who have never indicated their wishes concerning life-saving treatment, those who were never able to communicate a preference or simply did not do so.

Those with Known Views—The Substituted Judgment Standard. When a formerly competent patient has previously expressed a choice regarding treatment, it is possible to effectuate the patient's desires by substituted judgment. Persons who have executed living wills or documents mandated under state statutes now existing in thirty-nine states and the District of Columbia fall into this first category. Other patients may have left a clear record of their preferences even though they did not execute a standard document. The substituted judgment standard apparently applies under common law even in those states that have no living will statutes. When the patient's desires regarding treatment are overt and unambiguous, the substituted judgment is the mere execution of a decision made while the individual was competent. If the patient expressed wishes clearly enough, the guardian need only perform a purely administrative function.

Unfortunately, expressed wishes are rarely so evident. Typically the guardian is left with evidence of an array of general values and beliefs from which the patient's desires pertaining to treatment must be constructed.[22] In making the decision whether to refuse treatment, the guardian must attempt to make the choice that the patient would have made based on the criteria of uselessness and grave burden. Both decisions are subjective, based to the extent possible upon the beliefs, values, and desires believed to be held by the patient.

The substituted judgment standard is a logical extension of the principle of autonomy, which justifies the legal and moral right of competent patients to make such judgments for themselves. This role for the guardian merely extends the use of the subjective calculation of uselessness and grave burden, with the guardian offering a substituted judgment for the values and beliefs upon which the patient likely would have relied. A problem with the substituted judgment standard arises when the guardian did not have a relationship with the patient that preexisted the patient's incompetency. Such a guardian has difficulty gaining the requisite insight to interpret the patient's wishes properly. A second problem arises because, realistically, it is impossible for the guardian's own biases not to influence his interpretation of the patient's wishes. The legitimacy of that influence is considered below.

Those without Known Views—The Best-Interest Standard. When a patient has never expressed desires concerning life-saving treatment or left a record of values upon which a judgment can be based, it is not possible to judge by reconstructing his or her intentions. The best-interest standard is appropriate for individuals in this category.

Many discussions of guardian decisions end at this point, failing to recognize that we need to determine whose opinion governs what counts as the incompetent one's best interest. There seems to be no reason to turn to the idiosyncratic assessment of the clinician. One obvious criterion is that the best-interest determination must be the most reasonable one possible. In that case a reasonable-person criterion is in order. Alternatively, guardians could be permitted to draw on their own personally held values in deciding what counts as the patient's best interest. In order to decide which criterion is appropriate, we need to distinguish two types of guardians.

Types of Guardians

The distinctions between the two types of incompetents and between the two standards for judgment that relate to them—substituted judgment and the best-interest standard—have been noted by commentators. What they have failed to emphasize is that there are also different types of guardians available to make these judgments. Some guardians are appointed by the court or step into a decisionmaking role by virtue of holding some public or private office; there is no preexisting bond with the patient. These are "nonbonded guardians." By contrast, "bonded guardians" have a bond with the patient that preexisted the guardian-ward relationship. Bonded guardians fall into two categories: (1) family bonded guardians, and (2) nonfamily bonded guardians. Most often bonded guardians are the patient's next of kin or some other family member, but some are close friends. A close friend can become a guardian either because the patient, while competent, designated the guardian, or because the friend sought court appointment to make the treatment decision on the patient's behalf.

As a guardian for an incompetent patient, an individual bonded to the patient should be favored over a nonbonded individual. An agent designated by the patient or, absent such designation, the next of kin should be presumed to be the appropriate choice. Furthermore, in making the treatment decision, bonded guardians should be allowed greater discretion than nonbonded guardians. A nonbonded guardian should have no discretion in deciding what the patient would have wanted or what is in the patient's best interest. If the patient's views are known, the nonbonded guardian should have to choose what objectively appears to be the choice that the individual would have made if competent. If the patient's views are not known, the nonbonded guardian should have to choose what objectively appears to be in the individual's best interest. There is no basis for allowing the nonbonded guardian's subjective views to influence the decision.

On the other hand, a bonded guardian should be given some discretion to decide what the formerly competent patient who has expressed some views relevant to the decision would have wanted. If those views are unknown, the bonded guardian should be given some discretion in deciding what is in the best interest of the patient. Such guardians should be able to choose from among the reasonable available treatment choices and should not be constrained to choose the most objectively attractive option. The decision must be a reasonable one, but we should not insist upon the single most reasonable one.

Justifications for a Heightened Role for Bonded Guardians

Of course, the bonded guardian is not the only possible choice as the guardian of preference; both public officials and attending physicians readily present themselves as suitable candidates for this role. However, public officials or the attending physician cannot be presumed to have values that coincide with those of the patient. In fact, they not only may hold no special qualifications to make moral judgments on behalf of the patient, but also may have professional interests that are antagonistic to the patient's interests.

The best person to make the initial decision concerning treatment would be someone who has a preexisting bond with the patient. The courts, of course, would retain ultimate authority to review the bonded guardian's decisions to ensure that they did not exceed the realm of reasonableness. This scheme of limited discretion protects the patient, acknowledges the importance of familial responsibility, and avoids involving the courts in most routine cases.

There are numerous justifications for preferring bonded guardians over nonbonded guardians and for according discretion to bonded guardians. The specific justifications depend on whether the bond between the guardian and the patient is familial or nonfamilial.

Nonfamily Bonded Guardians. Some bonded guardians are designated by formerly competent patients in advance. Such a designated agent usually would have discussed questions of terminal care with the patient and, presumably, is in the best position to know the individual's beliefs, values, and desires. The key justification for authorizing guardian discretion in these cases is that the patient designated the guardian for this role while still competent.

Family Bonded Guardians. Two legal arguments have been offered for allowing family guardians discretion in deciding to refuse medical treatment. One is an extension of the right of autonomy of the competent patient. The other is premised on the basic rights of the family unit.

The extension of the patient's autonomy to the bonded guardian is the basis of several court decisions, including the Quinlan decision.[23] This, however, requires not only that the patient expressed wishes while competent, which is not always true, but also that it makes sense to speak of a surrogate exercising a right to autonomy (or privacy) on behalf of another. At least in the case of the never-competent patient, this is impossible.

A superior argument for according family members discretion in treatment decisions is based on the inherent rights of the family unit. The family is a fundamental institution in our society. Parents are permitted to make most decisions for their wards, and society gives them considerable discretion to make unpopular choices. We permit them to choose military schooling, in spite of the fact that most adults reject the values that lead to that choice. We permit them to choose private and parochial schools, some of which are established specifically to teach values that the broader society rejects. We permit parents to socialize their children into deviant values—the authoritarianism of the radical right, the machismo ideology of sexism, the aggressive achievement orientation of parents who want their child to go to medical school, or the egalitarian communalism of the utopian collectives. We permit parents to teach their children the treatment refusal theology of Jehovah's Witnesses in spite of the fact that we do not permit those parents to refuse blood for their children. Our society treasures pluralism in religious and ethical values, and we support families that transmit to their wards our wide range of beliefs and values.

The family unit's right to autonomy should not only support a presumption in favor of family guardianship, but also create a presumption in favor of the family guardian's decision. The values of society as a whole have no claim of moral superiority to justify displacing the role of the family in applying its own values. The significance of shared values is slightly different for each group of incompetents under the guiding standards. Under the substituted-judgment standard, appropriate for individuals who while competent voiced a treatment choice, the family guardian has an intimate understanding of the beliefs and values upon which the patient would make the decision were he still competent, and therefore can best interpret the patient's probable desires. Under the best-interest standard, appropriate for never-competent patients and those whose views are unknown, family guardians are permitted to draw upon their own values and beliefs in the absence of evidence of the incompetent individual's preferences. This is justified by the autonomy of the family unit.

A reasonableness standard must limit the discretion of bonded guardians substituting their judgment for that of a formerly competent patient and of bonded guardians attempting to further the best interests of a never-competent patient. Judgment in many of these cases necessarily incorporates the guardian's unique system of beliefs and values. Nevertheless, a family bonded guardian's decision should be given substantial deference.

A bonded guardian should be permitted to use discretion that incorporates his or her own beliefs and values or, alternatively, be forced to adopt the most objectively reasonable determination of the patient's best interest. If bonded guardians are forced to choose the treatment that objectively is considered the best course, they, in effect, have no decisionmaking authority at all. They are subordinated to the person(s) with the authority to determine that course—the judge or whoever is assigned that role.

Suppose several treatment options are available for a never-competent patient and that two of these are considered by all involved to be reasonable courses of action. Under similar circumstances, reasonable persons reflecting on their own care might choose either of these courses. The remaining options would generally be viewed as implausible, although small minorities of competent patients within the population might choose them. Suppose further that judges, physicians, and a large percentage of the general population consider one of the two reasonable courses to be the best. A judge or a nonbonded guardian deciding for a never-competent patient should be required to choose this single best course. Once it is established that one course is the best for serving the patient's interest, there is no reason to permit deviation, even to the other reasonable course. On the other hand, a bonded guardian holds a special position in relation to the patient and should be permitted to choose between the two reasonable alternatives.

THE SCOPE OF BONDED GUARDIAN DISCRETION

Bonded guardians should not be permitted open-ended discretion to depart from the single best course; if they could exercise such discretion, their wards would risk having their interests seriously compromised. Just how much discretion should guardians have in applying the uselessness and grave-burden criteria?

As a general rule, family guardians should not be allowed to deviate too far from the most reasonable course. They may choose alternative schools for their children, but they cannot choose no schooling at all.[24] Similarly, society ought to accept the reasonable views of bonded guardians in treatment refusal decisions even where objectively they are not the singularly best views. Bonded guardians should have discretion to deviate from the most reasonable course, provided their judgments about what is in the patient's interest or what is consistent with the patient's desires can be tolerated by the reasonable person. In short, bonded guardians' decisions should be reviewed under a reasonableness standard. Under this standard, an unreasonable application of the guardian's admitted values and beliefs or a decision based on an unreasonable set of values and beliefs would be impermissible. A decision would not be unreasonable simply because it lacked popular acclaim; substantial leeway must be given decisions soundly based on tolerable values and beliefs.

THE ROLE OF MEDICAL PROFESSIONALS

Along with this development of explicit roles for various guardians and the standard of reasonableness placing limits on those roles, we must consider the roles of other significant actors in these crucial decisions. Physicians and other health professionals obviously must play a significant part in the treatment decision. If they do not fulfill their roles in this regard adequately, they may be subject to civil or even criminal liability.[25]

The recent literature on the question of decisions about the care of incompetent patients remains ambiguous regarding the proper role of the physician and other health care professionals. Arnold Relman implies that the physician should be the key decisionmaker even in those cases where patients may have expressed their wishes while competent and/or family members are available as responsible guardians.[26] For example, he says that "the traditional responsibilities of the physician demand that he make judgments to treat, or not to treat, which in effect will determine whether, and for how long, and in what condition, the patient is likely to live or die."[27] He goes on to say that "there is nothing more crucial to a physician's professional role than the making of such decisions."[28] It is this apparent emphasis on the primary role of the physician that has generated charges of paternalism from Charles Baron and others who want to deemphasize the role of the medical professional.[29]

When Relman is careful, he makes clear that the emphasis on the primary role of the guardian is compatible with his position. He says, for instance, that the physician is "obliged to confer with his patients or their next of kin, to keep them fully informed, and to be guided by their wishes."[30] While sometimes he implies that the physician should merely consult with the family and remain the primary decisionmaker, elsewhere he speaks of "recommending" a course of action to the family.[31]

If the initial decision to accept or refuse treatment is made by a bonded guardian, two important functions remain for medical professionals to fulfill.[32] First, physicians may be advisors to patients or guardians responsible for making decisions. Even then they should be wary of the persuasive weight of their recommendations. With that proviso, physicians should provide care, compassion, consultation, advice, and wisdom, but should not assume the role of ultimate authority. Bonded guardians should arrive at independent decisions, and medical professionals should help them identify relevant considerations. Of course, as a practical matter, physicians' values will unavoidably influence guardians' decisions. In addition, patients might press physicians for moral guidance in lieu of, or in addition to, the advice of clergy, lawyers, relatives, and friends. Physicians should not suggest that their advice is superior to these other sources. Indeed, they should affirmatively suggest consultation with such other moral counsel as may be available to the guardian.

Second, in the role of advisor, physicians may occasionally encounter cases where they believe that patients' guardians are making unreasonable choices. In such cases, they should not take it upon themselves to disregard those decisions. Instead, they—like any citizens—should assume the responsibility of seeking ethics committee or judicial review of the competency of the patient or the reasonableness of the guardian's decisions. Physicians are particularly suited for this role because they will often be in the best position to learn of the decision and evaluate its reasonableness. This role shifts to the courts some of the burden of second-guessing the patient or guardian.

The remaining question is what standard should guide physicians in their decisions to seek judicial review. Should they seek such review whenever the decision is counter to their personal morals, or when it is counter to what they consider within reason or tolerable morals? Superficially, it would be most efficient for the physician to anticipate the standard which the court will use, i.e., seek review whenever the guardian's decision seems beyond reason. However, doing so could mean that some decisions that should be reviewed will not be. Some decisions that may seem within reason to the clinician may actually be deemed beyond reason by judicial authorities or public opinion. Alternatively, the physician could seek review whenever he believes the guardian has made less than the best decision. That would lead to erring on the side of review. Even then occasionally some case might not be reviewed that should be. Some physicians may consider a guardian choice the best when the courts or the society would consider it actually beyond reason. This has, in fact, occurred in several Baby Doe–type decisions. In making decisions about seeking review, physicians should realize that, should they concur in a parental decision that is, in fact, beyond reason, they share moral, and perhaps legal, responsibility for the results.

This interpretation of the physician's role differs from others in its effort to shift responsibility away from the clinician and toward the guardian. The *Dinnerstein* court spoke of the physician's responsibility to make decisions with the concurrence of the family.[33] Relman asserts that "unanimity of opinion between family and physician" obviates the need for judicial intervention.[34] My approach gives primary authority to the bonded guardian, with the physician responsible for the important roles of advising the bonded guardian and seeking judicial review when a question arises as to the propriety of the guardian's decision.

HOSPITAL ETHICS COMMITTEES

Some commentators have suggested a central role for hospital ethics committees. This notion will be explored in detail in chapter 26, but it is important here simply to indicate the limited role such a committee might play in reviewing questionable guardian decisions.

In treatment decisions made on behalf of incompetents, hospital committees could play four possible roles short of primary decisionmakers. First, a committee need not be involved in the ethics of treatment refusal decisions. Its task could be confined to double-checking any factual medical conclusions of the attending physician pertinent to a guardian's decision to accept or refuse treatment. The committee would therefore be composed primarily of experts and would not have an interdisciplinary membership. Such a committee should be carefully distinguished in name from hospital ethics committees to avoid unnecessary confusion.

Second, a hospital committee could share the attending physician's advisory role. It could advise the physician or, more plausibly, offer advice directly to the patient. In such a role, an interdisciplinary committee membership would serve well to promote a diversity of considerations and thereby dilute any single viewpoint. This could, for example, reduce the risk of undue influence by the attending physician.

Third, the committee could share the physician's role as initiator of judicial review. One of two models could be followed: (1) to decide whether to seek judicial review only upon the physician's request, or (2) to intervene actively to make all decisions to seek judicial review for patients in the hospital, regardless of the physician's recommendation. Again, in this role an interdisciplinary membership would be appropriate.

Finally, while a hospital committee should not take it upon itself to act as the primary decisionmaker, the state legislature might consider giving such committees ultimate reviewing authority. That is, the legislature might shift the reviewing function of the courts to a hospital committee. While this might alleviate some of the courts' burden and perhaps expedite the decisionmaking process, it is not a desirable plan unless the committee becomes a public body functioning as an agent of society with public review of appointments, due process, and other protections to ensure that it does not represent a hospital's idiosyncratic perspective.

THE ROLE OF THE COURTS

Although the initial decision to accept or refuse treatment should be made by the guardian, the court should continue to have a significant role in the process. Courts should be required to intervene in treatment decisionmaking at three points. First, in those cases where the competency of the patient itself is in dispute, the court should remain the arbiter of the decision to declare incompetency. Second, once it is agreed that the patient is not competent, a bonded guardian should assume the role of primary decisionmaker, supported and advised by the physician, other health care professionals, and other trusted advisors. The court should monitor the selection and function of the bonded guardian in cases where these are problematic.

Finally, in those most difficult cases where the patient is incompetent and there are no bonded guardians available to make the initial decision, the court should assume the primary responsibility by working through its normal due process to determine as objectively as possible what is most reasonable in that individual's interest. In performing this last function, the court may see fit to delegate authority. It might, for example, appoint a nonbonded guardian or even a committee to determine what course is in the best interest of the patient. Any such designee, however, would be functioning as an agent of the court and would be accountable to the court in a way not directly analogous to family guardians. The designee would have to do what is most reasonably determined to be in the best interest of the patient, not something that is simply within the realm of reasonableness. Thus, the court's role should necessarily depend on whether the decision is being made by a bonded guardian or by a guardian who was previously a stranger to the patient.

Bonded and nonbonded guardians should have fundamentally different roles, and their decisions should be reviewed in a fundamentally different manner by courts. Treatment decisions for incompetent patients with bonded guardians available should be primarily the guardian's responsibility with minimal judicial supervision. Treatment decisions for incompetent patients with nonbonded guardians should be primarily the responsibility of the courts or their designated agents.

The standard-of-reasonableness approach establishes an influential and frequently determinative role for family members and guardians with pre-existing bonds to the patient without granting unlimited discretion. It also provides a framework in which other participants in the treatment decision-making process—nonbonded guardians, health professionals, hospital ethics committees, and judges—may effectively operate.

CHAPTER TWENTY-FIVE

"Do Not Resuscitate" Orders:
An Ethical Analysis

The moral logic outlined in chapter 24 suggests that decisions of patients or their surrogates to refuse treatment should be based on subjective assessment of the uselessness and the burden of the proposed intervention. Increasingly these assessments are being made for such routine treatments as antibiotics, medically supplied nutrition and hydration, and cardiopulmonary resuscitation. One manifestation of this new ethic is the "do not resuscitate order," the "DNR," or the "no code" order. These refer to the decision not to provide resuscitative intervention for cardiac or respiratory arrest—including maintaining a patent airway, providing artificial ventilation, providing artificial circulation by external cardiac compression, and supplying fluids, drugs, and defibrillation.[1]

These decisions are being codified into protocols governing the "DNR order." The name *DNR order* is problematic on two grounds. In chapter 4 I suggested that it is unacceptable to refer to decisions, especially decisions by physicians, as "orders." That implies an authority relation inappropriate for the partnership mode of medical relations. Furthermore, later in this chapter I shall suggest that there is a conceptual problem with negatively labeling the instruction as an order not to resuscitate. I prefer to refer to decisions by patients or their surrogates to consent to resuscitation or to refuse consent to resuscitation. The importance of this linguistic distinction will become apparent in due course. Regardless of the label, it is nevertheless encouraging that health professionals are recognizing that there are cases when aggressive resuscitative efforts are inappropriate. Still, there may be reason to be concerned. If guidelines are not carefully constructed, problems can result.

A grand jury strongly condemned one New York hospital for permitting "nonresuscitation orders" using decisionmaking processes and means of communication inadequately documented, including placing detachable purple stickers on patients' file cards.[2] No one could tell whether physicians consulted with patients or whether they made the decisions at all. In one study, Bedell and Delbanco found that only 19 percent of patients studied had discussed resuscitation before the decision, and the physicians' perception of what was in the patients' interest differed in some cases from the patients'.[3] Even the hospital ethics committee guidelines on so-called DNR decisions may not have been examined adequately and may, in certain cases, pose dangers.

To gain a better understanding of the concept of deciding not to resuscitate, I studied thirty-three sets of guidelines. Some cover broader decisions to forgo life-sustaining treatments. Although many hospitals have written unpublished DNR guidelines and many individual authors have published their personal recommendations regarding DNR policy, these thirty-three sets of guidelines constitute all the published guidelines accessible to me that have official or quasi-official status within the institutions where they were prepared. They were prepared by committees or administrative officials in individual hospitals, state medical societies, state governments, and federal government agencies. What follows reports and evaluates what was found.

THE PATTERNS IN THE DNR GUIDELINES

Five problems emerged that are warning signs of potential areas of controversy. They do not appear in all the guidelines analyzed. My purpose is not to provide statistical data on the frequency of these patterns or to identify for criticism any of the institutions that have contributed to the guidelines. It is to identify the potential problems that may arise. Even when most guidelines examined avoid a problem, it is still important to point it out where it arises.

The documents were clearly written by people sensitive to the limits of medical care. The authors were attempting to show compassion and protect patients' rights and welfare. Yet, extreme care must be taken to avoid exposing patients to unexpected serious risks.

DNR AS AN ACT

The first problem is conceptual. We have recently seen what might be called the reification of the decision against resuscitation. Not performing resuscitative interventions is increasingly thought of as a thing we do to patients. It is something actually thought of as an act. We "trach" or ventilate a patient; now we DNR or no-code as well.

Some actually conceptualize DNR as a procedure to which a patient or surrogate might consent. We get informed consent for medical procedures; now we get consent for "DNRing" or "no-coding" as well. One guideline speaks of requiring "consent for DNR orders" from family members.[4] Another says that "a DNR order may be written upon the patient's informed consent."[5] Recently proposed legislation speaks of obtaining the "consent" of a patient or surrogate prior to issuing an order not to resuscitate.[6] At least six other examples of this idea of consenting to nontreatment were found.

In reality DNR is a decision to forgo a particular group of treatments. That calls not for consent but for refusal. The underlying legal and ethical rubric is not invading another's bodily integrity without permission. The decision not to resuscitate is one a patient or surrogate should reach in consultation with significant advisors, including the physician. It should lead to a refusal or withdrawal of consent.

Of course, resuscitation, like other procedures, may be initiated in emergencies based on presumed consent. Or the consent may be implied when it is obvious the patient would want it. However, presumed or implied consent is not acceptable when resuscitation is problematic and when there has been ample time to discuss treatment interventions in advance. Then the appropriate course is to discuss the alternatives, giving an opportunity to consent or refuse.

DNR as a Single Act

The decision against resuscitation is thought of not only as a positive action, but as a single act. Somehow the complex, diverse set of procedures subsumed under the rubric of resuscitation have been drawn together as a single all-or-nothing procedure. Deciding to nonresuscitate someone can become a *single* act. It can be charted in a single sentence, communicated by a three-letter code. Published guidelines generally do not take seriously the possibility that a patient might want some resuscitative interventions, but not others. One envisions a single decision that excludes all possible cardiopulmonary measures.[7] Another specifies that "'resuscitation' will be defined as any extraordinary or 'heroic' means employed to maintain . . . life . . . including any *one* of the following: intubation, ventilation, closed chest cardiac massage, and defibrillation."[8] Another includes all of these plus lab work, vasopressors, dialysis, transfusions, and transfer to critical care units.[9] It explicitly prohibits "half codes." This prohibition is an important and legitimate provision if it eliminates the practice of purposeful omission of some procedures in order to let the patient die while creating the appearance of resuscitation for legal purposes. It potentially infringes on patient autonomy, however, if it forecloses refusing some procedures while accepting others. Resuscitation might take place for many possible reasons. Some patients may want some procedures, but not others; they may want them for some conditions, but not others.

Reifying DNR treats patients as if they can be divided into two camps, those who choose resuscitation in all its complexity and those who choose none of it. Patients, however, are much more complex than that. In fact, studies have shown that often there is not documentation in the chart of exactly which interventions should be offered and which withheld.[10] Several critics have found wide disparity in what is actually provided or withheld in such circumstances. [11]

Resuscitative interventions are, in principle, no different from any other medical treatments. We cannot presume that patients want either all forms of resuscitation or none. Any sophisticated policy will allow patients to select specific interventions rather than treat the decision against resuscitation as a single phenomenon. Only broader guidelines, such as set from Presbyterian University Hospital, Pittsburgh, and St. Joseph's Hospital, St. Paul, Minnesota, begin to recognize this selectivity. They permit such designations as "limited therapy" and "comfort measures only," or they provide an explicit recognition that supportive care plans must be individualized to meet a patient's specific needs. Even they apparently treat resuscitative measures as an all-or-none phenomenon. They establish the designation "all but cardiac resuscitation"[12] or speak of applying "do not resuscitate guidelines"[13] as if resuscitative measures were a single phenomenon. By contrast, the "Standards and Guidelines for Cardiopulmonary Resuscitation (CPR) and Emergency Cardiac Care (ECC)" recommend that if specific types of intervention are desired, they should be written. Examples such as "lidocaine for VT" and "resuscitate short of intubation" are given. [14]

DNR AND PATIENTS' RIGHTS

The analysis thus far suggests that the so-called DNR order should be conceptualized as an omission rather than a positive act; it should acknowledge that there are a wide range of resuscitation treatments and that different treatments will be appropriate for different patients.

The same social patients'-rights revolution that gave rise to our awareness that sometimes some kinds of resuscitation are inappropriate also led to an awareness that patients (or their agents) must be the primary decisionmakers about their own care. Thus any decision not to resuscitate will be ethically unacceptable if it is generated by the physician. Bedell and Delbanco reported that eight out of twenty-four who could respond stated unequivocally that they had not desired resuscitation, even though all but one of the physicians caring for them did not perceive the patient's wishes this way. [15] Of course, data were not available on the views of patients who were not resuscitated, but a similar misperception of the patient's wishes would be disastrous. In a recent study Bedell and her colleagues found that only 22 percent of patients were involved in decisions about resuscitation. [16] Most, but not all, of the others were deemed incompetent. They raise the question, however, whether these patients could have been consulted earlier in the course of their illness. There are strategies to ensure that patients are given timely opportunity to express views about terminal care. [17] Even more critical, they found that in five cases where patients had been consulted, the patients had expressed a desire to be resuscitated that was reversed by family and physician after the patient had become unresponsive. This was done without a court order. It seems clear that if the procedures and principles outlined in the previous chapter were used, this would not be permitted.

Except for presumed consent for unanticipated crises, no physician should ever decide for or against resuscitation. It is remarkable how consistent the professional literature is in referring to the nonresuscitation decision as a choice the clinician faces.[18] Almost every one of the thirty-three guidelines reviewed for this chapter has at least one sentence implying that the physician is the one who decides on resuscitation. Sometimes the implication is subtle, even buried within text appearing to affirm the patient's role. For example, one says, "Before the [no code] order is written, the patient, if competent, will be consulted."[19] While affirming some patient role, it is a role of mere consultation. This is what elsewhere I have referred to as damning with faint authority.

The Veterans' Administration guidelines that were in effect from November 20, 1979, until August 24, 1983, are somewhat more blunt in their affirmation of the physician as decisionmaker: "The choice to 'code' or 'no code' will remain one of professional judgment on the part of the appropriate health care provider. . . ."[20] Another says that a DNR order "is written when the patient's physician believes that CPR is not indicated. . . ."[21] Then it damns with faint authority by adding, "before a DNR order may be written, it is the responsibility of the physician to ascertain and be guided by patient wishes. . . ." Another says, "The attending physician should determine the appropriateness of the DNR order for any given medical condition."[22]

The Special Committee on Biomedical Ethics of the American Hospital Association report states clearly that "if a patient does not agree to the proposed DNR order, it should not be written."[23] There is still, however, the presumption that the attending physician "must determine if resuscitation is likely to provide any medical benefit to the patient." It goes on to say that physicians "should not make these decisions in isolation," simultaneously affirming a presumption of the physician as decisionmaker and the need for patient involvement.

The American College of Physicians assigns "ultimate responsibility" for the decision to the physician.[24] It goes on to specify that under certain conditions "the physician decides that the disease process or other medical condition that the patient has would not positively be affected by the initiation of resuscitative efforts. . . . then a decision to write a do-not-resuscitate order is ethically proper."[25] It includes no reference in this paragraph to the patient or the patient's approval, in spite of the fact that elsewhere it affirms that the mentally competent adult can decide whether he wishes to be resuscitated when faced with a terminal event.

The "Standards and Guidelines for Cardiopulmonary Resuscitation and Emergency Medical Care" frequently slip into the language of the physician as the decisionmaker. They say, for example, "If the decision not to initiate CPR is made by a medical professional functioning in the professional capacity, it must be based on acceptable medical standards."[26] Elsewhere they say that such specific instructions should be written if "desired by the physician." The presumption that it is the professional's choice is often combined with a "recognition" that this is a difficult burden for the physician.[27] Even the literature most sensitive to the role of the patient as primary decisionmaker still slips into language implying that role for the physician. The Hennepin County guidelines talk of the ward team determining "the appropriateness of the do-not-resuscitate order for an individual patient," and of a decision "reached consensually by the patient and the physician" even though it is acknowledged that the resuscitation will not be forgone if the patient disagrees.[28] It is not clear what happens should the patient want no resuscitation when the physician considers it appropriate. The document states, however, that "until a public consensus is reached, physicians have a responsibility to use reasonable judgment and, if necessary, persuasion to limit the use of expensive life support to those patients in whom recovery to a meaningful existence is possible."[29]

The most frightening formulations speak of cases in which the patient need not be consulted before a decision is made. One, for example, states that "if in the opinion of the attending physician the competent patient might be harmed by a full discussion of whether resuscitation would be appropriate . . . the competent patient should be spared the discussion; therefore, if the physician and the Chief of Service deem a DNR order appropriate and the family members are in agreement . . . the DNR order may be entered by the physician."[30] Likewise, a state legislative proposal incorporates a "therapeutic privilege" provision permitting physicians to omit resuscitation of a patient without consulting that individual even if the patient has the capacity to consent if he or she would "suffer immediate and severe injury."[31] The authors must believe that some patients would so clearly be "better off dead" by means of nonresuscitation that they can have resuscitation withheld without their knowledge. Another guideline permits avoiding informing patients when it would be an "immediate and serious threat to the patient's (or surrogate's) health or life."[32] This amounts to paternalistically choosing death for competent patients. If arrangements are on the horizon whereby physicians, even with the approval of family members, are permitted to omit resuscitation of a still-competent patient without that patient's knowledge, then it is hard to avoid the conclusion that the "do not resuscitate" concept can be a dangerous innovation, very dangerous indeed.

Of course, hospitals have their own beliefs and values. Under certain circumstances, they should be permitted to act upon them. It could be that a hospital's guidelines reflect its underlying religious heritage. We should not object to that, provided that every patient and every health professional who enters such an institution knows what its values are and is given an opportunity to refuse. It is doubtful that any hospital could successfully function after publicly announcing a policy of having clinicians make decisions against resuscitation without informing the patient or surrogate.

Sometimes even the family is apparently excluded or overridden. One set of guidelines provides that "the wishes of the immediate family must be given very great weight" rather than any more definitive authority.[33] Another speaks of treating over a family's objection.[34] A third says, "If the surrogate and the physician do not agree, mechanisms for institutional review, such as an ethics committee, should be available." It also says that "a DNR order should never be written without the knowledge of the competent patient or the family of or surrogate for the patient."[35] This leaves open the possibility that resuscitation could be forgone against family wishes without judicial review. Another says, "When the patient is incompetent the appropriate member(s) of the patient's family should usually be closely involved in the decisionmaking process."[36] While meaning to affirm the role of patient and family, these guidelines condone judgments made without their approval.

The physician should not simply be passive. Deciding about resuscitation requires integrating medical and other facts with a set of beliefs and values that determine whether the proposed treatment is worth it. The physician must be active in supplying the medical facts (the diagnosis, prognosis, etc.) and contributing knowledge of other facts when possible. Moreover, he or she should discuss the plausible treatment options, including nonintervention. There is nothing wrong with recommending a course of action provided both physician and patient realize that the recommendation is necessarily based on what the physician thinks is *worth* pursuing, that is, on a personal value judgment. In this sense the resuscitation decision is no different from any other medical intervention.

Patients should seek guidance on these decisions from those whose beliefs and values they trust: their family, friends, clergy, and other moral advisors. In many cases the physician will be among them. Some patients, as well as some professionals, may not realize that the decision about resuscitation (or any other treatment) *requires* these ethical and other value judgments that cannot come from medical science. It is the physician's job and the job of the writers of guidelines to make sure patients understand the value component in resuscitation choices.

ETHICS COMMITTEES AS DECISIONMAKERS

The patient-centered perspective also has implications for hospital ethics committees (HECs). The role and function of hospital ethics committees will be explored in more detail in the following chapter. Here, however, it is important to observe their role in decisions pertaining to resuscitation. Sometimes the HEC is seen as the decisionmaker for or against resuscitation. One document states that "the [medical ethics] committee will act as a decision making and review committee on matters relating to DNR orders. . . ."[37] Of course, many guidelines avoid the problematic language. The point is that some groups, when writing guidelines, include language the implication of which they may not realize. Any guidelines that give the

HEC rather than the patient, surrogate, or court the authority to make actual resuscitation decisions would face the problems raised here.

In fact, HECs have no legal or moral authority to authorize treatment or nontreatment, grant immunity from prosecution, or override the patient's or agent's decision. As we shall see in the next chapter, even getting these cases to a committee may involve violation of confidentiality, where the patient or the agent has not authorized disclosure to the HEC.

While these committees can play an important role in helping patients and surrogates, they have no authority to make decisions about treatment. If these decisions are inherently subjective and based on the beliefs and values of the patient, then, in principle, no committee can make a definitive substantive choice.

I argued in the previous chapter that in cases involving patients who have never expressed their own beliefs and values, an emerging consensus favors granting guardians limited discretion based on familial beliefs and values subject to review and override by the courts.[38] If these trends are correct, then in principle no committee can ever determine objectively whether a resuscitation should be attempted. Some of the newer guidelines recognize this by explicitly including committees only in consultation and mediation.

GUIDELINES PROVIDING SUBSTANTIVE ANSWERS

This means that no substantive resuscitation guidelines are ever possible. Guideline writers should distinguish substantive from procedural guidelines. Procedural guidelines recommend actions before resuscitation decisions are made final. Physicians should, for example, discuss with the patient if competent, with the next of kin if the patient is not competent, etc.

Substantive guidelines specify diagnoses or prognoses under which resuscitation would be inappropriate. A substantive guideline might say that it is inappropriate to resuscitate if the patient is in a permanent vegetative state. However, certain patients might hold beliefs or values that would require resuscitation even in that condition. Clinicians should not override the patient's decision without formal public due process. There is no substantive condition for which resuscitation should *never* or *always* be attempted.

Nevertheless, several groups have drafted classificatory schemes sorting patients into treatment categories for or against resuscitation. The first to appear was from a conference held in 1973 by the American Heart Association and the National Academy of Science—National Research Council. It concludes, for example, that "cardiopulmonary resuscitation is not indicated . . . in cases of terminal irreversible illness where death is not unexpected or where prolonged cardiac arrest dictates the futility of resuscitation efforts."[39] The Massachusetts General Hospital[40] and Mt. Sinai[41] schemes have similar substantive categories and are thus in principle unacceptable.

A number of guidelines limit consideration of nonresuscitation to conditions that are terminal or "lethal." This excludes a patient's decision in cases where chronic, severely burdensome treatment might justify refusal.

Legislation proposed by the New York State Task Force also imposes a substantive guideline limiting surrogate resuscitation refusals to cases where the patient is terminal or irreversibly comatose, or where resuscitative measure "would probably be unsuccessful and would only serve to prolong the dying process."[42] That apparently prohibits refusal of resuscitation for a nonterminal, noncomatose, severely senile, suffering dementia patient.

By contrast, the Hennepin County guidelines are procedural. They tell some basic procedures, including getting a comprehensive evaluation of the patient's condition and giving priority to that individual's decision when he or she is competent.[43] If committees want to propose a set of substantive conditions under which they believe resuscitation would be wise, and another set in which it seems pointless, this could be helpful provided the lists are labeled as suggestions based on the value consensus of the committee, but they should not be treated as binding for patients and clinicians.

CONCLUDING RECOMMENDATIONS

Resuscitation guidelines should emphasize procedure. They might be based on the following principles:

1. Resuscitating a patient should be thought of as comparable to any other medical procedure. It requires the consent (express, implied, or presumed) of the patient or agent. Nonresuscitation should not be thought of as something done to a patient.

2. Resuscitation should be viewed as involving many different procedures, some, all, or none of which may be appropriate for the patient, based on his or her medical condition, beliefs, and values.

3. The competent patient should be viewed as the primary decision-maker with regard to his or her own resuscitative and other care whenever that care is proposed for the patient's own welfare. The patient should have the opportunity to discuss the options with family, friends, and clergy, as well as physicians and other health professionals. When there is the slightest doubt that the patient's consent to resuscitation can be presumed, resuscitative treatment options should be discussed with him or her to elicit consent or refusal.

4. Whenever there is doubt about competency, the patient must be presumed competent until adjudicated otherwise by a legitimate body such as a court. Only when the patient is obviously incompetent to all involved should incompetency be presumed without adjudication. Whenever the patient is clearly incompetent, the immediate task must be to determine who the surrogate decisionmaker should be.

5. The first priority for the surrogate should be someone legally designated by the patient while competent (using a living will or durable power of attorney). If instructions to that agent are available (such as might be con-

tained in a living will), they should be binding. If not, the agent should attempt to determine what the patient would have wanted regarding various resuscitative efforts. If no one has been so designated, then the agent should be presumed to be the next of kin as specified by state law. (Such laws currently exist in Arkansas, New Mexico, and Virginia. Blanket authorizations exist in all jurisdictions for parents of minor children to serve as agents in consenting to or refusing to consent to treatment including resuscitation.) Courts have the authority to override the next of kin who is acting unreasonably. Hospitals and health professionals should, when no legally designated agent exists, turn to the next of kin, normally the closest family member, for that role. (The legal justification of this presumption is not clear at the present time. Some commentators, however, are satisfied that decisions by next of kin regarding treatment are legally sufficient.)[44]

6. When no agent is available or when health professionals believe the agent has made a decision so questionable that it must be reviewed, judicial review should be sought.

7. Once the patient or agent has decided for or against a problematic resuscitation, the responsible physician should record that decision in the patient's chart, including the types of resuscitation accepted or refused.

8. While any concerned lay person or professional may seek such review of problematic decisions by agents, a hospital might find it appropriate to form an institutional ethics committee to review questionable agent decisions for the purpose of deciding whether to seek judicial review. Neither health care professionals nor ethics committees should think of themselves as having the authority to change the resuscitative decisions of the patient or the patient's agent.

9. From time to time as each case develops, the patient or agent, with the support of lay and professional advisors, should decide which treatments are appropriate and consent to them. This should include sorting resuscitative treatments and consenting to those that are appropriate.

CHAPTER TWENTY-SIX

The Ethics of Institutional
Ethics Committees

In the previous two chapters I argued that ethics committees should never be in the position of making decisions for or against resuscitation or other treatments. At this point some additional ethical questions pertaining to health care–delivery institutions are in order. One of the most important involves these hospital ethics committees. The problems go far beyond resuscitation treatment decisions.

One of the most significant ethical developments in the institutions delivering health care is the evolution of the institutional ethics committee. It is striking, however, how far removed the patient can be from the working of such committees. A partnership model for lay-professional relations cannot tolerate the distancing of the patient from the decisionmaking process in the way the typical ethics committee functions. The time has come to ask how an institutional ethics committee would function if it took seriously the centrality of the patient as an active partner in the decisionmaking process.

Hospital ethics committees (HECs) deal with ethics. They are created to confront some of the most difficult ethical questions patients and their agents face. They often see themselves participating in ethical dilemmas faced by physicians, nurses, and other health professional decisionmakers as well. What quickly becomes apparent to any participant in an HEC is that the committees themselves pose ethical questions.

The idea of hospital ethics committees has been with us for over a decade. [1] After this period of development, it makes sense to pause and see if we can gain some understanding of the ethical mandate that governs these committees and the ethical problems they may confront in bearing out their mission. This, then, is the beginning of an ethic for ethics committees.

Some of the problems are pretty close to the surface. The committees have often been created to deal with the problems of caring for terminally ill patients. Any such committee will soon be in the thick of controversies over the ethics of euthanasia, over whether there is an ethical difference between stopping a treatment and not starting it in the first place, over whether it is as justifiable to stop an IV or antibiotics as to stop some complicated gadget like a ventilator or a hemodialysis machine. Those, of course, are issues that patients, families, and health care professionals faced long before committees ever existed. When a committee speaks on one of these issues, however, it may give a false sense of closure to questions that are really not yet settled in the moral community. It may even relieve other decisionmakers of a sense of responsibility for the questions they face.

San Antonio physician Karen Teel offered as one justification for such committees the fact that they might diffuse the awesome burden of responsibility that is placed on an individual decisionmaker.[2] The committee in effect might leave no one with the sense of responsibility for the way a patient dies. Upon reflection, it is not so clear that such an effect, if it occurs, is good or morally acceptable.

Confidentiality is the second ethical question raised by any committee that deals with individual patient decisions about care. The idea of a hospital ethics committee often conjures up the image of a large, amorphous, often anonymous group of health professionals and even lay people who are reviewing the details of an individual patient's case. Often committees include members from outside the hospital and health care system. They may have access to the patient's record. Confidentiality problems are likely to arise at two points—when the committee gains access to information about the patient, and when the committee approaches family members and others for clarification about the decision. All of the contemporary professional and lay codes of medical ethics are in agreement that confidentiality is a right of the patient or the agent for the patient.[3] That means that committee members have no business having access to information about a patient's case without the patient's approval. Any scheme that involves hospital ethics committees without the knowledge of the patient is a clear violation of this moral standard. Moreover, there is logically no way that the committee can consult with the family about decisions for a patient unless the patient or the patient's agent has approved the disclosure of information about the case. Hospital ethics committees, like computerized information retrieval systems, should be added to the list of newfangled technologies that pose new kinds of threats to the confidentiality of the patient-physician relationship.

These are important ethical problems, but problems that in principle can be overcome. The committee should be alert to the possibility that it may have the effect of lessening the sense of responsibility of patients and health professionals for the moral decisions they make, but a committee sensitive to this problem need not have that effect. Committees need to be aware that when they gain information about individual cases, they are gaining privileged information. They have the right of access only with the patient's permission and can transmit it to others such as members of the patient's family only with further permission. Still, in principle, those are ethical requirements that a good committee should be able to meet.

HECs also raise ethical questions at a somewhat different, more profound level. Any institutional ethics committee, if it is to function well, must understand consciously and explicitly how its mission relates to what I call a theory of medical ethics. It must have in place, and consciously orient to, a set of general ethical principles that will guide its actions and shape its decisionmaking. The closest cousin to the institutional ethics committee, the institutional review board for the protection of human subjects, must by federal regulation adopt a set of ethical principles under which it operates.[4] The same kind of formal commitment to a set of principles is going to be required for an HEC.

In fact, for ethics committees I want to go even further. I want to suggest that an ethics committee cannot carry out its various tasks without some ethical frame of reference in front of it. When we examine how a set of ethical principles might operate, I think we will quickly discover that the tasks that are often assigned to ethics committees are simply incompatible with any plausible set of ethical principles that a committee might adopt. More critically, and more practically, once a committee has adopted a set of principles, it may discover, if it constitutes itself to fulfill one set of tasks oriented to certain ethical mandates, that it will be that very fact be incapable of fulfilling other tasks. Let me suggest what such an ethical framework might look like and then examine the impact it would have on the way the committee constitutes itself and goes on about its tasks.

ETHICAL PRINCIPLES FOR HOSPITAL ETHICS COMMITTEES

An immediate problem is faced by anyone analyzing the nature of an ethical framework under which an ethics committee might operate. Some people working in medical ethics have begun with the assumption that a professional group may generate its own code of ethics. I suggested in chapter 2, however, that this presents serious problems. Professional groups may well hold unique ethical positions on the ethics of professional obligation not shared by lay people with whom the professionals will be interacting. Any unilateral imposition of a set of principles may disenfranchise the patient population, the very group who will be most affected by the ethical code being adopted. A philosopher or professional analyst of ethical systems is not in a much better position to articulate a set of principles for the lay-professional relation. He or she may also stand in a special tradition or hold special commitments. This has forced many to the conclusion that the framework for a medical ethic must be generated by a complex process involving the active participation of both lay people and health professionals. Hence the triple contract or covenant that underlies the partnership model.

Any such set of principles will include the recognition that the health care team, including the ethics committee, should strive to serve the welfare of the patient. That is simply good old-fashioned Hippocratic ethics. However, we now recognize that the old Hippocratic ethic of benefiting the patient must be placed within severe constraints. To paraphrase the opening of a now-famous book by Robert Nozick, patients have rights, and there are certain things that health care professionals and hospital ethics committees cannot do to them without violating their rights.[5] Hence the principles outlined in chapter 6, including autonomy and justice—and probably truth-telling, promise-keeping, and avoiding killing as well.

When a hospital ethics committee sits down to adopt a basic set of ethical principles for its deliberations, when it consults with patients, health care professionals, and members of the community for guidance about what its core ethical framework ought to be, it will adopt such a set of principles. The real question then becomes, what does this set of ethical principles mean when an institutional ethics committee sits down to work?

ETHICAL PRINCIPLES AND THE TASKS
OF ETHICS COMMITTEES

One hospital-based ethics committee could have before it this full agenda of ethical principles, moving from task to task balancing autonomy and justice on one occasion, truth-telling and patient welfare on another. That turns out, however, in the eyes of most people, to create real, probably insurmountable problems. It is the nature of ethical problems that different tasks will emphasize different principles. Hence I have already suggested that clinicians should normally be exempt from the duties of justice.

The problem is related to one that Weberian sociologists would recognize as legitimation. If an institutional ethics committee is to function effectively within a health care setting, it will have to be conscious of its legitimation, of its claim to be taken seriously as having the appropriate skill and authority to deal with the tasks at hand. Should a small concerned group within the hospital simply appoint itself to be the institutional ethics committee and proceed to press its ethical agenda on the institution, it is likely to face serious problems of legitimation. Patients and health care professionals are likely to ask who these people are and where they think they got the authority to pronounce on ethical issues. For the institutional ethics committee to be viewed as legitimate, that is, as having appropriate authority to carry out its function, it must be able to demonstrate that it has the necessary skills and moral stature for the task at hand. It must be able to show that it was duly authorized for this task by those holding the authority for the decisions to be made, whether that be the patient, the health professional, the administration, or the general public. It will also have to show that it can avoid any serious conflicts of interest that would compromise its ability to carry out its task.

I am increasingly convinced that institutional ethics committees can plausibly be legitimated for only one ethical task at a time. Some committees may be so constituted that they take as their task the assistance of patients in making autonomous decisions. Others may take on the ethical responsibility of promoting justice in resource allocation. Still others might face the complex task of balancing the welfare of the patient and the welfare of the society in decisions about research involving human subjects. It is very difficult, if not impossible, for a single institutional ethics committee to have more than one ethics agenda.

The idea of committee legitimation is closely related to the question of to whom the committee is accountable. If the committee is accountable to physicians on a hospital staff, then it will take on the ethics agenda of that staff. It will be viewed as legitimate to the extent that the physicians believe it is really helping the medical staff make decisions based on its ethical framework. On the other hand, if the committee is accountable to patients, then it will turn to patients for its legitimation. Other committees might see themselves as accountable to the administration of the hospital, the board of trustees, or the broader community that has created the hospital, whether that be a city government or a church.

In order to see how these things might play themselves out in different ethical tasks of institutional committees, let me take three significantly different ethical mandates for ethics committees, each of which requires a different ethical principle as the guiding principle for the committee's work. These three different ethical mandates could cut across the four major functions of committees: education, consulting, guideline formation, and case review.

We can structure different possible mandates for hospital ethics committees by looking more carefully at the ethical principles that place constraints on the old Hippocratic ethic. One of those constraints would remain patient-centered. It insists that those in clinical roles recognize the rights as well as the welfare of the patient as primary. It would see clinicians as operating under a mandate of respecting persons—promoting their autonomy, keeping promises, dealing with them truthfully, and so forth. Thus one ethical mission for ethics committees might be simply to extend this patient-centered ethical mandate, acting so as to promote the rights of the patient.

AUTONOMY AND INDIVIDUAL PATIENT DECISIONS

No matter how much we would like to escape it, the first task people think of for an institutional ethics committee is participation in individual patient care decisions. The usual problem involves a terminally ill patient where the ethical question is whether it is appropriate to stop treatment. Exactly the same moral structure would apply for any other kind of individual case-oriented clinical decision. The early suggestions for hospital ethics committees such as that made by Karen Teel and that in the Massachusetts General Hospital Committee all saw the committees participating in clinical decisions, either making the actual decision or providing advice and counsel to the decisionmakers.

In the simple and straightforward case, these are fundamentally patient-centered problems. We want to know how not only to promote the welfare of the patient, but to do right by the patient. If we begin by considering the competent patient or the formerly competent patient whose wishes are known, these are fundamentally problems of autonomy and the related ethical principles needed to preserve autonomy, that is, truth-telling and promise-keeping. If there is an ethical problem at all, it is over whether the health care professional or someone else is ever justified in infringing upon the autonomy of the individual patient as a decisionmaker about his own health care. I am for the moment not considering cases where we might want to restrict medical care for purposes of conserving scarce resources, but only those cases where the welfare of the patient is the decisive consideration. The ethical problem is whether some other decisionmaker might on paternalistic grounds attempt to promote the welfare of the patient in violation of the patient's own autonomy.

I take it as a conclusion of both law and ethics resulting from the last decade's debate that in such a simple case the principle of autonomy must dominate. The competent patient has the right to consent to treatment or refuse treatment on any grounds whatsoever provided that treatment is offered for his or her own good. Thus one possible ethical mandate for a committee is to be patient-centered, not focusing exclusively on the welfare of the patient in Hippocratic fashion, but on the rights of the patient as well as helping the patient retain autonomy in decisionmaking.

The implications for an institutional ethics committee are radical. If the principle of autonomy is the dominant ethical principle, and the patient is the primary decisionmaker, then the institutional ethics committee for this kind of case must be accountable to the patient and must function as his or her agent, helping to clarify the alternatives available and the ethical justifications for and against the treatment alternatives under consideration.

Several implications follow. First, any committee that enters a patient's case without the knowledge of the patient is surely in violation of its mandate. If the health care professional, the physician, the nurse, chaplain, or social worker, believes that the case is complex enough that assistance from an ethics committee is called for, that individual should approach the patient and ask permission to bring the committee in contact with the patient.

Second, the composition of the committee should be governed by the task at hand. People should be placed on it for their skills in counseling and analyzing ethical alternatives in making clear to the patient what the medical and social implications are of alternative therapies being considered. Since patients are unique and operate with distinctive systems of beliefs and values, a standing committee at the hospital may discover that some of its members should step aside to be replaced by trusted counselors and advisors the patient might introduce to the committee. For example, if the standing committee included the hospital chaplain, it might be appropriate for the chaplain to step aside in favor of the patient's own clergyperson so that the spiritual counsel received could be based upon the patient's own religious heritage.

Third, insofar as the promotion of autonomy is the ethical mission of the institutional ethics committee, in principle there can be no protocol created that would provide substantive guidance for hospital staff about when to treat or when to stop treatment. The old Massachusetts General Hospital scheme that would classify all patients in four treatment groups solely on the basis of diagnosis and prognosis makes no sense.[6] Attempting to classify patients on the basis of medical criteria alone violates their autonomy. As we saw in the previous chapter, any protocol to decide which patients should be resuscitated would be ethically unacceptable if it attempted to make substantive judgments based solely on medical criteria of diagnosis and prognosis. Any guidelines created for HECs performing the task of promoting patient autonomy will necessarily be procedural. The guidelines might indicate who should be consulted, at what points patients should be asked to consent or refuse to consent to DNR and "no-code" orders, etc. They should never, however, spell out substantively which patients to treat and which not to treat.

JUSTICE, SOCIAL ETHICS, AND RESOURCE ALLOCATION DECISIONS

A second, radically different, task is sometimes envisioned for an HEC. It requires the abandonment of the exclusively patient-centered perspective. The second kind of ethical constraint on the Hippocratic ethic of benefiting the patient grows out of social considerations of the welfare of others in the society and the promotion of justice in the distribution of goods. A committee at New Britain, Connecticut, General Hospital was formed out of these concerns.[7] Suppose, for example, that a hospital needed to decide whether to spend a large bequest to build an expanded intensive care unit or to open a walk-in holistic preventive medicine clinic. This kind of question raises ethical issues that might be referred to an HEC. It is obvious, however, that the ethical principle of autonomy will not get us very far. Presumably, patients who are candidates for an ICU would favor the intensive care unit, whereas those in the local community who are active promoters of holistic health care would autonomously decide for the preventive medicine clinic. A hospital ethics committee that takes on these kinds of questions is in the realm of justice and social welfare.

The same kind of ethical question arises when a committee is asked to participate in decisions about allocation of scarce medical beds or to create guidelines about such allocation. These are questions that surely cannot be answered by asking individual patients and assisting them in expressing their autonomous decisions. It is important to realize that this ethical mandate rooted in the principles of justice and social welfare would not necessarily limit a committee to larger questions of hospital policy and macro-allocation. A justice problem would arise if a committee were asked to participate in decisions about when to limit expensive but marginal medical care for terminally ill patients. For example, whether to permit a ninety-three-year-old comatose patient in end-stage renal failure to be dialyzed is not a question to be answered under the rubric of the principle of autonomy; it is a problem of justice.

The HEC problem is whether it can promote the rights and welfare of the patient and simultaneously be expected to make judgments of social ethics based on justice and social welfare in which the rights and welfare of the individual patients must be compromised. It is sometimes maintained that individuals can operate from time to time under two different moral mandates, shifting hats, as it were, as the role dictates. A physician may, for example, be patient-centered while delivering clinical care and then abandon the patient-centered perspective when administering a clinic or research program. Others have argued that it is extremely difficult psychologically for individuals to shift moral mandates in this way. It is, in fact, impossible to act faithfully on both mandates at the same time.

If it is difficult for an individual to shift ethical principles, it is even more difficult for a committee—a corporate person—to do so. If an ethics committee is to take on these questions of justice and social welfare, it must be accountable to a much larger social unit. It needs to be accountable to the hospital as an institution, and ultimately to the moral community to whom the hospital itself is accountable, that is, to a government or church or other sponsoring agency.

If an ethics committee is to take on these questions of justice and social welfare, different skills will be required. The committee not only will need expertise on the technical aspects of medicine and nursing involved in the decision, but also will have the capacity to represent the ethical and other values of the group to which the committee is accountable. By contrast, a committee whose purpose is to facilitate autonomous patient choice has much less reason to be so representative. In fact, for choices rooted in the moral principle of autonomy, we could say that if the committee successfully reflects the moral consensus of the community and thereby entices the patient into a choice based on that consensus, it has failed. The committee charged with responsibilities requiring choices based on justice and social welfare, on the other hand, may not want simply to mirror the community values, but it surely must be very conscious of them, and it should articulate its sense of what is just in communication with them.

I am forced to the conclusion that it is extremely difficult, if not impossible, for one committee to work under the conflicting mandates of promoting patient-centered rights and promoting justice in the distribution of resources simultaneously. At the very least, if the committee sees as its task the placing of limits on patients' rights and welfare in cases where justice requires devoting scarce resources to others, the patient has to be informed of that.

An IRB for protecting human subjects is in many ways like these ethics committees involved in determinations of social welfare. It is clear that its sole ethical responsibility is not—in spite of its name—the protection of human subjects. If that were its only task, it could simply ban all non-therapeutic research and thereby provide maximum subject protection. It must trade off the welfare of the subject against the welfare of the society, determine whether subjects are treated justly, and decide whether the risks of research so violate the ethic of the institution that the collective moral sense cannot tolerate them. This is social ethics much like the resource allocation questions in hospital policy planning, hospital bed allocation, and cost containment. The IRB (rather than the hospital ethics committee dealing with individual clinical decisions emphasizing the principle of autonomy) might be a better committee for these problems. On the other hand, while the perspective may be similar, the IRB may require different specialized skills—people with expertise in research methodology, statistics, and the like. In the end a social ethics committee may be as different from an IRB in its ethical task and skill requirements as it is from the clinically oriented committee whose ethical mandate is autonomy promotion.

INCOMPETENTS AND PATIENT-CENTERED BENEFICENCE COMMITTEES

This leads us to a rather startling conclusion. There is virtually no area of work for which a committee should take as its mandate making a choice that will most benefit the patient. Promotion of patient autonomy is one legitimate ethical mandate. Much committee education work will be justified under this rubric, as will counseling with patients and families as well as health professionals. Promotion of justice and social welfare is also a legitimate ethical mandate for some committees. Neither of these committees, however, should see itself as making substantive decisions to benefit individual patients.

There is, however, one case where patient-centered welfare might appear really to be the ethical mission. That is when someone has to make individual patient care decisions and the patient is incompetent to participate as an autonomous decisionmaker. Here someone else must make a decision. In those cases where we have no idea what the patient would prefer—when he has not expressed himself while competent—the only basis for the decision is what someone else considers to be for the welfare of the patient. Is it here that the ethics committee is finally able to act on the classical Hippocratic principle of doing what it can to try to benefit the patient? Perhaps, but even here only in a most attenuated way.

Normally an incompetent patient has someone designated to be his or her agent. By a law in the state of Virginia, any competent person may designate someone for this role.[8] In several jurisdictions, by law the next of kin is the presumed agent in cases where no one has been so designated. In other cases, such as that of a parent, there is a presumption of guardianship whereby the agent—but not necessarily an ethics committee—has the task of attempting to make a decision that will serve the interest of the patient. As we saw in chapter 24, however, this patient-agent does not have unlimited discretion. As in the case of the Jehovah's Witness parent attempting to refuse to consent to a life-saving blood transfusion, any interested party has the right to seek judicial review to determine if the agent is being reasonable. Physicians or hospital administrators often take on this task, not directly acting on what they determine to be the patient's best interest, but attempting to get a court authorization to have someone else legitimated to give the consent.

The present arrangement is admittedly a bit chaotic. Anyone may seek review. If an individual physician chooses not to do so, however, there has been no due process, and his or her judgment may be idiosyncratic. It might be nice to have some committee specially responsible for determining whether to seek judicial review. In such a role, the committee would at least indirectly be acting out the ethical principle of promoting the welfare of the patient. It would not have the authority to authorize reversal of the agent's decision, but it would have formal responsibility for taking the first step to see if the courts would reverse it.

The committee might appear to be making this decision on the basis of the ethical principle of attempting to promote the incompetent patient's welfare. That is certainly the ethical charge to the parent or other agent who is the initial decisionmaker. While the committee would evaluate the case in terms of the patient's welfare, it is clear that it would not want to seek judicial review at just any point the agent's decision appeared to deviate from the best interest of the patient. The deviation would have to appear to be substantial; it would have to be intolerable. Otherwise we would have committees, and eventually courts, second-guessing parents on every decision they make. The agent's decision would have to appear beyond the realm of reason.9 Thus while the agent for the patient would strive to choose what is in the patient's best interest, a committee (or an individual health professional) would seek to initiate review only if the agent's decision appeared to be beyond the limits of reason. This still leaves open the ethical problem of how a committee would have access to such cases without the patient's or agent's consent and whether such access would constitute a violation of confidentiality. Presumably, those agents who were contemplating decisions so controversial that an ethics committee might feel compelled to seek judicial review might not readily grant consent to have the committee review their cases.

A related question is whether the committee could be given quasi-judicial authority to overrule the agent or to affirm the agent's decision, thus granting legal protection against charges of neglect. While some such arrangement might appear attractive, it poses some problems. The committee at best will reflect the moral consensus of the institution and its sponsors. That may not be the same as the moral consensus of the broader community, however. In fact, it is conceivable that a small minority of physicians could become aligned with a small minority of parents and other agents in approving decisions that most reasonable people take to be seriously contrary to the patient's interest. If those physicians were clustered in a small number of hospitals, it is possible that a committee (even if it were representative of the medical staff) would also express deviant moral judgments. If even a dozen hospitals nationally had committees that routinely approved grossly deviant decisions, and if agents and professionals favoring grossly deviant decisions clustered together at those hospitals, serious ethical infringement on the rights and welfare of patients could occur.

If the committee were so constituted that it could reflect the reasonable judgment of the community and operated under rules of due process, a judgment by the committee not to have an agent's decision reviewed by the court could be taken as supportive evidence that the parents were acting within reason. Here at last the committee might begin to approach the ethical mission of making a decision out of concern for the patient's welfare.

Here, then, we might have the beginnings of an ethic for ethics committees. Such an ethic will not only have to deal with more mundane problems of euthanasia, confidentiality, and committee integrity. It will also have to determine whether it is dealing with decisions that raise primarily problems of autonomy, of justice and social welfare, or of patient benefit. For the most part the traditional committee involved in terminal care clinical cases will have as its ethical responsibility the promotion of patient autonomy. In other cases the primary ethical issues will be justice and social welfare. Only in rare cases where the patient is incompetent and the patient's agent appears to have exceeded the limits of reason will a committee possibly find for itself a limited role in making a decision to try to benefit the patient. Even here it will not be directly to overrule the parents, but to determine whether the hospital should initiate a formal judicial review of that decision. To keep clear about these diverging ethical responsibilities, ethics committees ought to begin thinking about adopting a set of ethical principles to guide their work, and they ought to determine which of those principles ought to govern the particular tasks they are undertaking.

PART
V

The Future of the Partnership

CHAPTER TWENTY-SEVEN

Contemporary Bioethics and the
Demise of Modern Medicine

This completes my exploration of the contractual mode of medical ethics and its implications for the patient-physician partnership. Viewing the patient as an active, full participant in the relation means that patients no longer can be viewed as passive recipients of the benevolent paternalism of the Hippocratic physician. The Hippocratic Oath may have made sense for those living in the context of a minority Greek scientific/religious cult of the fourth century B.C., in which very few were educated and it was believed that transmitting knowledge to those who were not initiated into the cult was dangerous. When that mentality has been transferred into what can be called modern medicine, the result has been a moral and scientific disaster. Not only have patients been abused and their rights violated; they have been given versions of the medical facts necessarily distorted by conceptual misunderstandings about the nature of medicine and the medical decisionmaking process.

To clinicians continuing to practice medicine within this understanding, the challenge from contemporary bioethics has been disturbing. It started with institutional review boards to govern human subjects research. Karen Quinlan meant that the courts and the press were keeping physicians from using their own judgment about what they thought was good medical care. Since then philosophers and theologians have constantly pressed theories about informed consent that have led to a radical disruption of the traditional physician-patient relationship. Lawyers and courts have taken a lot of the blame, but bioethicists have taken their share of the criticism. One physician has even suggested that bioethicists are contributing to the demise of modern medicine.

The more I think about it, the more he seems to be right. The exploration in this volume of the partnership model of clinical relation and the contractual model of medical ethics upon which it is based leads me to a bold, perhaps radical, conclusion: contemporary bioethics and its bedfellows in philosophy of science are bringing to an end what we can call the era of modern medicine. The conceptual framework that contemporary bioethics brings to health care is so radically stretching the foundations of modern medicine that it will become increasingly difficult for clinicians in the modern medical paradigm and those working in the postmodern or contemporary world of bioethics to understand one another.

Let me suggest an analogy. I introduce it solely to try to convey the kind of paradigm shift of which I speak. A middle-aged, poorly educated, sickly woman comes to her primary-care physician having been diagnosed as having carcinoma of the breast. She tells him that her aunt had the same thing. She had taken large doses of vitamins and had been cured. The patient wants the same vitamins.

The clinician at this point might well be discouraged. He realizes that he has an enormous communication problem. It is not just a matter of persuading her that the vitamins will not cure her cancer. He must discover how to communicate with a patient whose very conceptual framework is different from his own. He must communicate with a patient who is not schooled in the notions of empirical evidence, statistically valid controlled trials, and the scientific mentality. The conceptual shift that takes place when one abandons the mentality of the anecdote and begins to think like a practitioner of modern medicine is fundamental. It is something akin to a Kuhnian paradigm shift. [1]

As radical as that shift is, I am convinced that contemporary bioethics and its siblings in the philosophy of science are presenting to modern medicine a paradigm shift that is equally radical. Just as the scientifically trained modern physician can no longer communicate well with or share the thought processes of the cancer patient who is impressed with her aunt's anecdote, so, I am suggesting in this volume, one who understands the patterns of thought emerging in contemporary bioethics can no longer communicate well with or share the thought processes of practitioners of modern medicine. If I am correct, the very essence of medicine as we know it in the modern West is in jeopardy. The most basic concepts are no longer meaningful. The most basic practices no longer make sense. The notions of "clinical judgment," of treatments being "medically indicated" or "treatments of choice," of the "medically correct thing to do," of "medically safe and effective," the practice of writing prescriptions and of ordering treatments—they all collapse in a conceptual muddle.

THE CHARACTER OF MODERN MEDICINE

Some clarification is in order. I use the term *modern medicine* to refer to the mainstream of orthodox Western medicine of the twentieth century. It has its roots in the Hippocratic emphasis on astute empirical observation, rationality, the demystification of disease, and what can be referred to as the scientific mentality. Over many centuries, but especially in the modern era, an attitude has evolved that grounds medicine in science, in empirical observation, and, by the twentieth century, in controlled clinical trials.

This has led medical practitioners and many sophisticated lay persons to look with skepticism at an individual who believes in the efficacy of a treatment based on a single experience or even a group of anecdotes, provided they are not collected and reported using accepted scientific method. At the same time, modern medicine places great emphasis on what is commonly called "clinical judgment." The applications of the science of medicine are so complex and patient situations vary so greatly that it is widely believed that individual practitioners who are skilled in the art of medicine can make clinical decisions in a manner that outperforms an algorithm or computerized diagnostic program.

For the purposes of this analysis, I am not interested in the dispute between those who believe that clinical decisions are best made by a skilled practitioner and those who believe they can be made better by algorithm.[2] I am interested in what those two views have in common: the idea that there is a medically best choice. A core presupposition of what I am calling modern medicine is that there is a medically best course of action for a given patient in a given situation. This concept is given various names such as "treatment of choice," "the medically indicated treatment," or sometimes "the technically right course."

The concept of "medically best course" can, of course, be case-specific. In fact, most clinicians would insist that it must be. The idea is that given a patient with a particular diagnosis, prognosis, medical history, and biomedical profile, it is a presupposition of modern medicine that a "good clinician" can figure out what the best course of action is for that patient. This is what stands behind the search for the good clinician, as well as behind such pop phrases as "Doctor knows best."

Medicine as a Science

There have been two different manifestations of this notion in modern medicine. The first was closely linked to the idea of value-free science. As we saw in chapter 5, many people—lay people as well as health professionals— operated as if they believed that having technical competence alone should lead one to know what was medically indicated or the treatment of choice. When a society wanted to know whether a drug was "safe" or "effective" for a particular condition, it often believed that a scientific question had been raised that competent medical scientists should be able to answer. It was as if science alone could tell us the appropriate treatment for a particular condition.

The Emergence of Values in Modern Medicine

The second manifestation was more open to value considerations. Those working from within the model of modern medicine began to recognize that value-freedom was a gross oversimplification. This led to the first of two shifts within the paradigm of modern medicine. Medical scholars, many of them physicians such as Leon Kass,[3], Eric Cassell,[4] Allen Dyer,[5] and Mark Siegler,[6] began to argue that values were necessary for clinical medicine, but that they were values that could be derived from medicine itself.[7] By careful reflection on the medical role, they argued, certain values "internal to" or "inherent in" medicine itself could be discerned. These included the importance of life, the good of promoting longevity, decreasing morbidity, relieving suffering, and promoting health. While they might have held, perhaps wrongly, to the idea that the basic sciences of medicine—biology, biochemistry, and biophysics—could be value-free, they began to recognize that clinical or applied science could not be.

This acknowledgment of values within the modern medical paradigm was not a serious problem for those who subscribe to the model. The medically correct course could still be determined from within the institution of medicine itself by applying the values inherent in medicine to the medical facts of the case. Soon, however, a second shift, still within the modern medical paradigm, emerged. It was here that bioethics began to record its influence. Good clinicians began to realize that in a number of medical decisions, ethical or other values from outside the institution of medicine were playing an important role. Beginning in the late 1960s and early 1970s, the dominant focus in medicine began to shift from acute illness and infectious disease to chronic illness and more obviously evaluative medical decisions. Our society faced, in rapid succession, organ transplants, debates over the definition of death, abortion, contraception, genetic interventions, and support of patients with cancer, stroke, heart disease, and extensive neurological problems. The Karen Quinlan case, dating from 1975, symbolized the rise in public consciousness of the fact that in at least some cases, the correct medical treatment could not even be determined on the basis of the values inherent in medicine. It was not obvious that it was better to live when it meant living respirator-dependent in a coma, trapped in a cancerous, pain-tormented body, or on an enslaving dialysis machine. Different religious and philosophical systems lead to different clinical choices in oncology (terminally ill patients with metastatic cancer), obstetrics (the patient desiring a midterm abortion for socioeconomic reasons), and surgery (whether to implant an artificial heart).

This shift in consciousness has been pervasive and important. Now clinicians generally acknowledge that when such cases occur, the patient must be consulted in order that his or her value framework can be taken into account when the clinician makes medical decisions. In fact, many sensitive practitioners have begun to express concern that their patients are still operating in the older framework whereby the physician is expected to make all medical decisions based solely on medical science and clinical judgment. Not every physician is cognizant of this value component in medical choices, but such awareness is widespread.

While this shift has irretrievably changed modern medicine, I am convinced that it has not been a serious threat to the basic, underlying conceptual framework of the clinician. Modern medicine is still thought of as an enterprise resting on medical science in which, for the normal case, a set of values inherent in medicine could lead the wise physician to make appropriate choices. Sophisticated modern medical professionals are ready to concede that in certain "ethically exotic cases," religious and philosophical frameworks extrinsic to medicine intervene appropriately.

For these special cases, clinicians still operating in the modern medical paradigm are prepared to call time out from their normal model in order to get the patient's values. For the normal case, however, the physician still thinks of himself or herself as making the medically appropriate decisions based on the facts of medical science, clinical experience, and the values inherent in medicine. A good understanding of technical medicine combined with the values inherent in medicine provides an appropriate basis for doing diagnostic work-ups, taking histories, writing prescriptions, and conducting the day-to-day business of medicine.

BIOETHICS AND POSTMODERN MEDICINE

I suggest, however, that a far more fundamental change is on the horizon, one that begins to question the underlying concepts of modern medicine. The stimulus for this shift, I believe, can be traced to the debate in bioethics in the 1970s and the emergence of the contractual or partnership understanding of the clinical relation. The issues that stimulated debate in the 1970s—the terminal illness cases, Jehovah's Witnesses' blood refusals, abortion choices, the decisions about allocating scarce dialysis machines— did far more than carve out a few special areas where ethical and other values extrinsic to medicine were accepted. Participants in those debates began to examine the basic conceptual framework of modern medicine.

The impact can be seen in efforts to analyze clinical decisions. One way is to try to write a syllogism for such a decision. For example, a simple version of the logic of physicians such as Karen Quinlan's that led to the conclusion that a respirator should be continued is something like the following:

Regardless of the patient's future capacity for consciousness, whenever physicians can preserve the life of a patient, they ought to do so.

Mechanical ventilation of patients in a permanent vegetative state increases the probability that life will be preserved.

Therefore, mechanical ventilation ought to be used.

Bioethicists of the 1970s spent a great deal of time and energy arguing that one cannot conclude that "mechanical ventilation ought to be used" without accepting the major premise that includes the ethical evaluation "whenever physicians can preserve the lives of patients, they ought to do so." They demonstrated that all such arguments for continuing treatment on terminally and critically ill patients contained such an evaluative major premise. The major premise of the clinical judgment contains some evaluative term: *should, ought, must,* or some surrogate. The minor premise, that mechanical ventilation of patients in a permanent vegetative state increases the probability that life will be preserved, was treated as the contribution of modern medical science. It was science that could tell us the medical facts. It was argued, however, that for the ethically exotic cases such as the Karen Quinlans of the world, one could never get to the clinical conclusion solely on the basis of the scientific minor premise. Some evaluative major premise was required. Moreover, they argued, convincingly, that there was no rational reason why persons should necessarily accept the Hippocratic values supposedly inherent in medicine when formulating the evaluative premise. This I take to be, in very simple form, the major contribution of bioethics in the 1970s. It led to the conclusion that ethical and other values, including values not inherent in medicine, were necessarily involved in decisions to continue treatment on terminally ill patients, to perform (or refuse to perform) an abortion, to do a heart transplant, or to manipulate the genetic code.

That was an important, now generally recognized contribution. It, however, is not the only implication of the bioethics debate of the 1970s. It was important for society to recognize that values play a central role in clinical choices in the ethically exotic cases, but inherent in the analysis of clinical choices is something far more important. It is not just for a small number of ethically exotic cases that a supposedly scientific minor premise is combined with a necessarily evaluative major premise in order for a clinical conclusion to follow. The critical shift is in the recognition that in literally every clinical decision, values must penetrate into the major premise, and there is no reason why those values should necessarily come from within the institution of medicine. There is, in short, a ubiquity of values in medical choices. They arise in two ways that stretch the modern medical paradigm beyond its limits.

THE VALUE COMPONENT IN MEDICAL SCIENCE

First, contemporary philosophy of science now generally rejects the notion that the so-called scientific minor premise can ever be value-free. Conceptual and evaluative variables always and necessarily impinge on the formulation of the reported medical science (as well as the evaluation of what ought to be done). For example, the definition-of-death debate during the 1970s often focused on the question whether deciding a person was dead was a scientific or an evaluative enterprise.[8] It was common to argue that science could at least potentially tell us whether a person's brain function was irreversibly lost,[9] but that deciding whether to treat the person as a whole as dead was fundamentally an evaluative or policy question that could never be answered on the basis of neurological science alone. The policy question of when to treat persons as dead was thus separated from the scientific question of when brain function was irreversibly lost.

Now it is increasingly clear that even the question of what criteria to use to determine that brain function is irreversibly lost has elements that extend beyond value-free processes of modern science. The more one considers it morally wrong to treat someone as dead who could, in fact, regain brain function, the longer the period of time one will want to test brain function, while the more one considers it morally wrong to treat someone as alive who has actually irreversibly lost the capacity for brain function, the shorter the time one will want to use. Deciding the "correct" length of time is a function of how one balances the two kinds of moral errors. There is no "scientific" way to solve the problem.

In like manner, it can be shown that all statements of "the medical facts" involve such judgments. They occur in deciding what confidence limits to use in reaching conclusions, deciding which data are "important" enough to transmit, and choosing language and concepts to use in describing findings.

In an early study of the relation between clinical practices and beliefs about the scientific facts regarding pharmacology of oral contraceptives, I found that there was a correlation between beliefs about pharmacology and ethical evaluations.[10] Physicians who believed contraception to be morally acceptable reported the pharmacology of contraceptives differently from those who believed it unacceptable. They thought contraceptives were less likely to cause cancer, for instance. While at first this might be assessed as reflecting biases that one should strive to eliminate, further reflection makes clear that such correlations are inevitable. They have to do with such variables as deciding which data are important, what data have a bearing on the question being asked, and even exactly what question is being asked. Pro-contraception physicians tended to answer the question about cancer with reference to cancer in humans, while anticontraception physicians tended to answer with reference to animal data as well as human studies. In principle, these linkages with evaluative assessment are inescapable even for one who strives to avoid biased presentation.

It could be argued in rebuttal that these are simply pseudo-disagreements. The different scientists are answering different questions. If they were asked if oral contraceptives caused cancer in humans (or in animals), they might well agree. I am not suggesting that there is no "actual reality" underlying the scientific enterprise. I think there is, but that is irrelevant to the issue. What I am suggesting is that the reports of medical and other scientists must always incorporate conceptual and evaluative assumptions, including the rephrasing of the question asked by the nonscientist. So if the patient asked generally whether the pill causes cancer, the scientist must determine whether the question refers to humans or animals. But even if the patient is asked which is intended, further refining will be necessary. The scientist needs to know what counts as evidence for cancer, what probability levels the questioner has in mind, and so forth.

Moreover, since the list of such refinements is virtually infinite, there is no way the scientist can continue to ask the lay person exactly how to reformulate the question. If she did, her very request for reformulation would necessarily incorporate evaluative and conceptual moves that, in principle, cannot be eliminated. The anti–birth control scientist may think precarcinogenic cell changes are "important" or "interesting" and may be stimulated to ask the lay person whether these count as "evidence for cancer." The procontraception physician may find such data so uninteresting that he will fail to comprehend that the lay person could be asked.

Recoding the question into a form that can be processed using scientific method is itself a process that necessarily incorporates conceptual and evaluative moves. Even if there is a "true reality" out there that conscientious scientists are trying to describe, they cannot do the describing without making conceptual assumptions and evaluative decisions at a terribly subtle level, assumptions and decisions so subtle that even good scientists will fail to grasp and convey them to the lay questioner.

The Value Component in Clinical Judgment

The second observation drawn from the clinical judgment syllogism has to do with the more obvious value dimension that occurs in the major premise, the one containing the overt evaluative term. That the evaluative term appears in the syllogism for a clinical judgment is a necessity of any such premise. While the evaluations are more conspicuous and more controversial in the ethically exotic cases, they are necessarily present in every single clinical decision made, no matter how mundane or innocent. One cannot get to a conclusion that contains an ought statement unless the major premise contains a similar "ought."

This means that it is not just the occasional euthanasia or abortion case that requires evaluative assessments, but every move made by the clinician and patient. The fiction that most ordinary medicine can be based exclusively on good science is mistaken in a most fundamental way. Moreover, just as in the ethically exotic cases, there is no reason to assume that the set of values supposedly derived from the concept of medicine itself will be adequate or appropriate for these more mundane clinical choices. Treating a broken arm or a dog bite or a hernia is necessarily contingent on the value system of the one making the choices, and there is no obvious reason why the values of the health care professional are the appropriate ones. In fact, one can assume that health care professionals—or any group of specialists— have atypical values regarding their sphere of interest. This is true whether the specialty is philosophy, aesthetics, warmaking, or medicine.

Moreover, these evaluative choice points arise not just from time to time at critical junctures in clinical care. They arise constantly, hundreds of times a day, every day of the year: when deciding which patients to see, every time a test is "ordered," whenever a visit is made to a patient's room, when a choice is made not to do a physical exam. For every single medical case, there are countless choice points where there is more than one plausible way to proceed: different drugs, different dosages, different lengths of stay in the hospital, different health care institutions, different styles of interacting between professional and lay person.

For the patient with pain, one can use narcotics, because the objective is to do battle with and conquer the evil of pain, or one can intervene more gently with aspirin because one believes that respiratory depression is a serious problem or that suffering builds character. One can use a half grain of morphine or an eighth grain; 300 mgs. of aspirin or 1,000 mgs. It can be administered regularly or only when "indicated." In principle, there is no way to choose among these options without evaluative assessments.

CASE 17: THE TREATMENT OF HERNIA

> To push the argument to a dramatic extreme, consider a routine problem as far from the ethically exotic as possible: routine hernia surgery. A patient following herniotomy was told that it was appropriate for him to leave the hospital; upon leaving, he was told, "Don't drive for a week." Both are inherently evaluative statements.
>
> Consider the innocent-sounding "Don't drive for a week." On what basis can a surgeon make such a statement? Proponents of "modern medicine" might be inclined to say: "It is the technically correct advice." What, however, can it mean for such advice to be technically correct?
>
> Probably what is meant is that most surgery textbook authors or most experienced surgeons would consider a week the right length of time to avoid driving. On what basis, however, can they hold such views?

At best they can be aware of the data regarding the various probabilities of adverse effects of driving after different numbers of days. They might know, for instance, the difference in rates of wound rupture from driving on the sixth and seventh days.

In fact, most surgeons probably do not have such data, but even if they did, on what basis could they say that a week is the right length of time to avoid driving? That is a choice that depends not only on rates of wound rupture, but on such matters as how bad it is for the wound to rupture and, most important, how important it is to drive. The latter question is one about which the surgeon can have no special expertise. In many cases, since he is a specialist to which the patient has been referred quite recently, he is not likely to have knowledge of the patient's need to drive. In fact, he is not nearly as likely to know as the patient is. Yet surely that is the critical question. The millionaire with a chauffeur will have a radically different need to drive than a single parent with a child who needs to be driven to school or to the babysitter. There is no way that the surgeon can be expected to make such assessments.

Similar evaluative choices occur constantly in literally every medical decision; that, at least, is the position of the proponent of a postmodern medicine, who takes the value component in clinical decisions as necessary and important. A decision must be made about whether the various effects of a drug are good or bad and just how good or bad. The advantages and disadvantages of a day of stay in a hospital must be assessed on essentially nonmedical evaluative criteria. In chapter 15 we saw that medical records handling involves similar evaluative choices. The Hippocratic strategy is that information is dangerous in the hands of the lay person.

Clinical decisions in nursing are likewise replete with value trade-offs. Should bed rails be up or down? Should Posey belt restraints be used? These are essentially value trade-offs relating the safety of the patient with the value of freedom. Such judgments cannot possibly be made on the basis of professional experience alone, because professional experience cannot determine the relation between safety and freedom.

IMPLICATIONS

The acceptance of the necessity of evaluation in both the apparently factual minor premise and the more straightforwardly evaluative major premise of a clinical syllogism has radical implications for the ordinary practice of literally every aspect of medical practice and policy. Consider first some of the basic concepts, terminology, and practices of the received modern medicine.

BASIC CONCEPTS, TERMINOLOGY, AND PRACTICES

Medically Indicated Treatments or Procedure

In chapter 5 we saw the difficult conceptual issues raised by the notion of "medical indication," one of the most used notions of modern medicine. The meaning of the term in modern medicine was obvious. Under the unreconstructed value-free medicine, a medically indicated treatment was one that modern science told us as a factual matter to be the best of all things considered. This was based on scientific testing, controlled clinical trials, or at least the combined wisdom of expert clinicians, leaving the postmodern critic to puzzle over how one could reach an evaluative conclusion about what *ought* to be done solely on the basis of medical facts.

When the conception of modern medicine was augmented with the realization that there were value judgments "derived from within medicine itself," the meaning of "medically indicated" was easier to understand. The medically indicated treatment was the one that best promoted the values inherent in medicine: prolongation of life, reduction of morbidity, relief of suffering, and the promotion of health.

In postmodern medicine reconstructed to take into account the inescapability of evaluations even in the scientific aspects of medicine, the necessity of evaluative judgments in literally every move in medicine, and the need to draw on values that come from outside the concepts of medicine, to say a procedure is "medically indicated" means, at most, that it is preferred by practitioners based on their beliefs and values and under the assumption that the patient's views would be similar, an assumption that is surely not always warranted. Consider, for example, what could possibly be meant by an account of chemotherapy for a severely retarded leukemia patient, Joseph Saikewicz, when an author said, "Although chemotherapy was the medically indicated course of treatment, he [a judicial decision-maker] felt it would cause Saikewicz significant adverse side effects and discomfort." If it would cause disproportional adverse effects and discomfort, to the postmodern observer, it is for that reason not "medically indicated."

Treatment of Choice

Likewise, "treatment of choice," which was once thought to be a concept that described something akin to a pharmacological or scientific fact, really can convey only the intervention that is preferred based on the practitioner's particular system of values.

Medically Safe and Effective

While in unreconstructed modern medicine, safety and efficacy were thought to be scientific categories, in postmodern medicine, which is thought to be an evaluative enterprise, these are value terms. In fact, the very notion of whether an effect is a benefit or a harm is part of the evaluative process.

It is told, probably apocryphally, that in a particular Catholic country where contraception was considered morally suspect, the pharmacopoeia reported that estrogen/progesterone combinations were effective for regulating the menstrual cycle, but that there was one serious side effect: they prevented conception. In the postmodern evaluative conception of medicine, to say an intervention is safe is to say nothing more than that the possible outcomes are worth it based on the value system of the one making the judgment.

Likewise, to say an intervention is effective is a judgment based on how important the benefits are as well as exactly which benefits are on the agenda. This is not to deny that the term can, upon occasion, be used to convey nothing more than the claim that an effect is being produced. "Estrogen is effective in preventing pregnancy" could convey nothing more than that it produces that effect at some acceptable level of certainty. Even then, however, some evaluation is taking place. A level of certainty is chosen. More important, that is not normally what we mean when we say a drug is effective. We mean, first, that the effect is a good one, and, second, that it produces the effect at some acceptable level of reliability.

Prescription Writing

If the concepts of medically indicated and treatment of choice are evaluative terms, it would seem to follow that the act of writing a prescription would have to be reassessed. It will be seen in a postmodern conception of medicine as involving making a set of value choices at best on the assumption that the patient's values are similar to those of the one writing the prescription. In fact, if such a judgment is an evaluative enterprise, the entire practice of using the physician as the gatekeeper in limiting access to pharmaceuticals may have to be reassessed. This is not to say that all persons should have unlimited access to all medications. It is to say that the function of limiting access to legend drugs needs to be reformulated.

In an autonomy-loving society, limits on access to drugs that have impact only on the one using them would be hard to defend in the case of the competent lay person. The value judgments are rightfully the lay person's, not some gatekeeper's. On the other hand, it is probably reasonable that some person in society set limits on access to drugs that are dangerous to third parties. Moreover, society has a legitimate interest in protecting incompetents (including children and the mentally ill) from getting access (including access through competents). The question for the proponent of postmodern medicine is why that societal gatekeeping function ought to be vested in the one who holds the particular value profile of the physician. If this is not a pharmacological choice alone, but a choice based on values, then it is much closer to societal decisions to limit access to cigarettes or firearms, decisions not thought appropriately to belong to the physician.

Similarly, the use of the physician as gatekeeper for choices other than medication raises similar problems. For example, deciding that a person should be excused from responsibilities such as work or school becomes an evaluative judgment that the burdens to the individual or risks to others of failing to grant the exemption are too great. The practice of getting a "note from the doctor" implies in postmodern medicine that the physician's assessment of those burdens and risks is the appropriate one. Since that assessment always involves judging how important it is for the person to continue in work or school, this is always a nonmedical determination in addition to one based on evaluation of the medical data. For neither task is the clinician's value system particularly appropriate.

The Language of Medicine

When basic paradigms shift, it is often the case that linguistic shifts are necessary. Feminists were eager to press for avoiding terms such as *girl* and *lady*. Racial rights advocates using terms such as *colored* and *Negro* eventually became signs of life in an outmoded paradigm. The symbolic offense of the use of the wrong language became very significant.

Likewise, in postmodern medicine some of the language inherited from the now-dated conceptual model will require change. In chapter 4, we saw how the notion of "doctor's orders" had lost its original meaning and was beginning to suggest an authoritarianism and legitimacy of physician decisionmaking in areas that are not, in fact, based exclusively on medical knowledge. Consider, as another example, the statement "She is not allowed to have visitors today." There are enormous implications pertaining to the control of another person that may have been appropriate in a world in which it was thought that good science alone or good science combined with a standard set of values could determine what was in a patient's interests. In postmodern medicine, however, deciding whether it is in a patient's interest to have visitors is a process resting more conspicuously on value judgments.

There may still be reasons why certain patients should not be allowed to have visitors. For example, if other patients in close proximity would be exposed to risks or disturbed, one of the rules of the health care institution may appropriately be that visitors be limited. If the patient consents to such rules as a condition for stay within the institution, then imposing them may be reasonable. This is a decision that can no longer be justified in terms of simple medical assessment of the welfare of the patient, however. Saying "She is not allowed to have visitors" is linguistically offensive in the same way that the statement "He won't allow his wife to hold a job" is offensive. In both cases the speaker probably does not actually mean that he has literal control over the autonomy of another person. He probably could reformulate his statement into more acceptable language (such as "I recommend that the patient would be better off if she chose not to have visitors today"). The implied conceptual framework of the statements, however, reveals that the speaker is living in a world that is no longer appropriate. The same can be said for the expression that the patient is being "released" or "discharged" from the hospital. Similarly, terms such as "doctor knows best" are anachronisms something like referring to one's secretary as one's girl.

In one hospitalization of President Reagan, two different reports quoted the president as saying, "I hope the doctors allow me to go home tomorrow" and "The President is under doctor's orders to limit himself to a reduced workload until next week." It is frightening to conjure the implications of these expressions if there were a world crisis needing the president's attention. More important, even as metaphors they fail to recognize that deciding on workload is reasonably a function not only of the medical condition of the president, but also of how important it is for him to work. Especially the latter is clearly beyond the medical realm. Even the former involves value judgments that would be made differently by people who hold different values independent of their knowledge of the medical facts.

INSTITUTIONAL AND POLICY IMPLICATIONS

The new paradigm of medicine as an essentially evaluative enterprise has implications for institutional structures and health policy as well.

The Food and Drug Administration

Under the old model, questions of drug safety and efficacy were essentially scientific questions. Labeling judgments were based on whether the uses were demonstrated scientifically. The task of the FDA was to make sure that quality science was the basis of these determinations.

If, however, safety and efficacy are inherently evaluative choices, then the FDA's role is more complex. It would be a serious mistake to assume that the postmodern conception of medicine should lead to an FDA where science did not count. Presumably scientific method and objectivity are as critical as before. That is why the new paradigm is postmodern, not simply a retreat to the nonscientific world of the woman who wanted vitamins for her cancer. Deciding that an effect is a good one, however, would be seen as requiring more than science. Deciding whether the effect is good enough to label the drug useful or appropriate surely goes beyond science. If even the scientific part of the assessment necessarily involves values, then the FDA's task is a complex combination of scientific and evaluative or political. If, for example, the assessment is contingent upon the values of the ones doing the assessing, then the society ought to be concerned if the ones doing the assessing hold values that are atypical. This means it will be important to evaluate potential FDA employees for their value frameworks as well as their scientific credentials. Staffing the FDA is rightly a political as well as a scientific decision.

In areas outside medicine, we recognize the idea. It would be risky, for example, for a panel of nuclear scientists to make determinations of effects of civilian and military uses of nuclear energy if the scientists held unusual values regarding the economics of energy, militarism, or the dangers of genetic mutation. It is possible that those scientists who have chosen to devote their lives to nuclear energy have atypical views on these subjects. If they do, their science as well as their policy recommendations may be suspect. Edward Teller's and Linus Pauling's science as well as their policy recommendations are different. There is no way they could not be. The same is true for medical assessments at the FDA.

NIH Consensus Development Panels

A similar concern will be manifest in societal scientific consensus development mechanisms such as the NIH consensus development panels. These panels are asked to deal with a combination of scientific and policy questions. One was asked, for example, to determine not only the difference in outcome as a result of critical care units in hospitals, but also whether government ought to be investing in such units.[11] The former question appears scientific. Its precise formulation, however, could easily lead to data showing either they did or did not make a difference. The scientists on an NIH consensus development panel, for example, might have to choose which outcome measures to study. The effect on mortality may not have the same implications as the effect on morbidity, and different morbidity measures may be affected differently. The panelists will have to choose the "important" outcome measures, and that will depend on their values.

If the panelists' values are important even for the scientific tasks, they will be even more important in the policy recommendations. It seems illogical even on its face to ask people who have given their lives to critical care medicine to advise on the question of how important investments in critical care are in comparison to other aspects of medicine, much less investments outside medicine. Yet that is often precisely what is done. In a postmodern conception of medicine as an evaluative enterprise, NIH consensus development panels would be chosen and administered quite differently.

The Organization of Health Care Delivery

If beliefs and values have pervasive impact not only on every clinical decision, but also on the articulation of the science that provides the foundation for clinical judgments, then the organization of health care delivery will be affected dramatically both at the level of the individual lay/professional relationship and at the level of health care institutions.

The Professional/Lay Relationship. If every clinical decision is affected by value frameworks, then the physician/patient relationship as we know it will have to be changed radically. As long as we believed value issues arose only occasionally in the ethically exotic case, we could entreat physicians to solicit their patients' value inputs and incorporate those values into the clinical judgment. Even then occasional problems arose. The patient's values were sometimes so at odds with the professional's that the professional who incorporated those values would be violating his or her own conscience in a morally inappropriate way. The obstetrician who says "Abortion is murder, but if you want one I'll perform it" is morally anemic. Moreover, even referral to someone else who will perform what from the practitioner's point of view is homicide is morally suspect.

As long as these problems were thought to arise only occasionally, however, the physician and patient could each try to be alert to the possibility of a serious value mismatch and, at least for controversial actions, enter into the lay/professional contract accordingly. If, however, every clinical judgment involves evaluations and these evaluations take place countless times a day, then it is impractical to stop and discuss the potential value conflicts at every turn. Moreover, some of the mismatches may be quite subtle. Professionals may unconsciously phrase what they take to be scientific information in subtle ways. Even tone of voice and expression may convey the practitioner's value system.

The only foreseeable solution is to arrange lay/professional interactions so that the parties are purposely paired based on their value frameworks. This will at least require some explicit discussion at the time the relationship is established covering some basic value orientations. Appropriate areas for exploration would include attitudes toward terminal care, the extent of information sharing and consent, and, in the case of women, attitudes about certain obstetrical practices. Perhaps who stand in particular organized systems of belief and value—Orthodox Judaism, Jehovah's Witness, feminist, or fundamentalist Christian as well as liberal secular humanist and conservative Catholic—would appropriately take such commitments into account in creating lay/professional pairings.

Health Care Institutions. This value pairing would appropriately be carried out at the institutional level as well. Health care institutions would begin to announce their own value commitments so that both professional staff and patients could gravitate to them based on their value profiles. At a few sectarian religious institutions, this already happens, as, for example, in Seventh-Day Adventist hospitals, the Oral Roberts Medical Center, and certain feminist health clinics. It also happens in more specialized health care institutions where value commitments are more conspicuously important, as, for example, in abortion clinics, hospices, and aggressive oncology research centers. If a system of beliefs and values is critical for deciding what constitutes good medical practice, then we should expect to see much more institutional expression of the value profiles under which care is delivered. This will benefit not only patients but professional staff, who will be able to follow their convictions with a sense of compatibility with the institutional structures within which they are working. Staff would affiliate with health care institutions on the basis of value compatibility.

A records department of a Protestant hospital organized around the commitment to the lay person as the one who ought to be vested with the critical information ought to look different from a hospital built on Hippocratic notions that information is too dangerous to be in the hands of the lay person. While no patients can be expected to be explicitly committed to the Hippocratic world view (because it is supposed to be a system of beliefs and values for health care professionals), it is possible that some patients may stand in other traditions that would find the Hippocratic view of information appropriate.

If I am correct, medicine as we have come to know it will be radically altered by the recognition that it is essentially an evaluative enterprise. The critical shift from what I have been calling the modern to the postmodern conception is not really the acknowledgment that occasionally values impinge on medicine. That is something most modern health care professionals now readily recognize. It has not dissuaded them from practicing medicine along lines that are, for the most part, quite similar to the practices of the day when medicine was viewed as value-free. It simply requires occasional shifts in framework when the ethically exotic case arises so that patients can be given an opportunity to express and act on their values.

If I am correct, the really important paradigm shift is the one that results when medicine is conceptualized as essentially an evaluative enterprise in the most routine, day-to-day decisions, decisions that must be made countless times a day in the personal clinical relationship as well as in governmental and institutional policy. Postmodern medicine calls for a radical shift in paradigm to one where every move of the health professional as well as the lay person in the medical sphere is an evaluative act. That will mean a way of thinking in medicine that is as different from current practice as the thought patterns of the woman who wanted vitamins to cure her cancer.

The postmodern or contemporary medicine that I have been describing is the medicine of partnership. If medical decisions are viewed as essentially, irretrievably evaluative in character, then the role of the patient in those decisions must be something far different from the one envisioned under the older Hippocratic view. If good medicine and what is good for the patient were thought of as essentially scientific or professional judgments, they could be made by a professional elite. If that professional elite were viewed as having special esoteric and dangerous knowledge, then it would be reasonable to treat the patient as an outsider—as a passive object to be manipulated benevolently by the professional. If, however, medical decisions are essentially evaluative and the appropriate values are not those inherent in medicine but those held by the individual patient, then an entirely new understanding of the patient-physician relation is in order—one in which the basic ethical norms are articulated by an agreement among the members of the moral community and applied at a second level in an agreement between the various professions and the lay public. The result is a contractual understanding of medical ethics and a resulting relationship between lay person and professional that must be viewed as a true partnership.

NOTES

1. MODELS FOR ETHICAL MEDICINE IN A REVOLUTIONARY AGE

1. Robert N. Wilson, *The Sociology of Health: An Introduction* (New York: Random House, 1970), p. 18.

2. Robert M. Veatch, *A Theory of Medical Ethics* (New York: Basic Books, 1981).

3. See William F. May, "Code, Covenant, Contract, or Philanthropy?" *Hastings Center Report* 5 (December 1975):29–38; Robert M. Veatch, "The Case for Contract in Medical Ethics," in *The Clinical Encounter: The Moral Fabric of the Patient-Physician Relationship*, ed. Earl E. Shelp (Dordrecht, Holland: D. Reidel Publishing Co., 1983), pp. 105–112.

2. MEDICAL ETHICS

1. Hippocrates, *The Sacred Disease*, edited by W. H. S. Jones (London: Heineman, 1923–1931), p. 139.

2. Ludwig Edelstein, "The Hippocratic Oath: Text, Translation and Interpretation," in *Ancient Medicine* (Baltimore: Johns Hopkins Press, 1967), pp. 17–20.

3. Max Weber, "Science as a Vocation," in *From Max Weber*, ed. H. H. Gerth and C. Wright Mills (New York: Oxford Press, 1958), pp. 129–156.

4. Paul Ellwood, quoted in "The Health Maintenance Concept in a Nutshell," *Medical World News* (November 6, 1970):32E.

5. For a fuller discussion see Robert M. Veatch, "Value Freedom in Science and Technology" (unpublished dissertation, Harvard University, 1971), especially pp. 173–187.

6. I am not suggesting that the philosophical debate over the nature of the "system of evaluation" is closed. One very important and plausible position, known as philosophical empiricism or naturalism, holds that the system of evaluation itself may have an empirical basis, being rooted in "moral facts." See Ralph Barton Perry, *The General Theory of Value* (Cambridge, Mass.: Harvard University Press, 1926); C. O. Broad, "Is Goodness the Name of a Simple, Non-Natural Quality," *Proceedings of the Aristotelian Society* 34 (1933–34):249–268; and Roderick Firth, "Ethical Absolutism and the Ideal Observer," *Philosophy and Phenomenological Research* 12 (1952):317–345, for various examples.

7. American Medical Association. "Report of the Ad Hoc Committee on the Principles of Medical Ethics," unpublished report, 1979, p. 3.

8. Neh. 10:28.

9. Firth, "Ethical Absolutism and the Ideal Observer Theory."

10. John Rawls, *A Theory of Justice* (Cambridge, Mass.: Harvard University Press, 1971).

3. THE PHYSICIAN AS STRANGER

1. Talcott Parsons, *The Social System* (New York: The Free Press, 1964), pp. 171–177.

2. Renee C. Fox and H. Lief, "Training for 'Detached Concern' in Medical Students," in *The Psychological Basis of Medical Practice*, ed. H. Lief et al. (New York: Harper and Row, 1963), pp. 12–35.

3. Richard Flathman, "Power, Authority, and Rights in the Practice of Medicine," in *Responsibility in Health Care*, ed. George Agich (Dordrecht: D. Reidel Publishing Co., 1982), p. 108.

4. Manfred Bleuler, "Let Us Stay Near Our Patients," *Diseases of the Nervous System* 34 (1973):73.

5. Thomas P. Almy, "The Healing Bond," *The American Journal of Gastroenterology* 73 (1980):403–407.

6. Samuel W. Bloom and Pamela Summey, "Physician-Patient Expectations in Primary Care," *Bulletin of the New York Academy of Medicine* 53 (1977):75–82.

7. Edmund D. Pellegrino, "Protection of Patients' Rights and the Doctor-Patient Relationship," *Preventive Medicine* 4 (1975):44.

8. Robert M. Veatch, *A Theory of Medical Ethics* (New York: Basic Books, Inc., 1981).

9. See Charles E. Curran, "Roman Catholicism," in *Encyclopedia of Bioethics*, ed. Warren T. Reich (New York: The Free Press, 1979), pp. 1526–1530; Gerald Kelly, *Medico-Moral Problems* (St. Louis: The Catholic Hospital Association of the U.S. and Canada, 1958), pp. 1–16; Richard A. McCormick, *How Brave a New World: Dilemmas in Bioethics* (Garden City, N.Y.: Doubleday and Co., 1981); and Charles J. McFadden, *Medical Ethics* (Philadelphia: F. A. Davis Co., 1967), for a variety of examples of medical ethical scholarship from within this tradition.

10. See J. David Bleich, "The Obligation to Heal in the Judaic Tradition: A Comparative Analysis," in *Jewish Bioethics*, ed. Fred Rosner and J. David Bleich (New York: Sanhedrin Press, 1979), pp. 1–44; Immanuel Jakobovits, *Jewish Medical Ethics* (New York: Bloch, 1975); Seymour Siegel, "Medical Ethics, History of: Contemporary Israel," in *Encyclopedia of Bioethics*, ed. Warren T. Reich (New York: The Free Press, 1978), pp. 895–896, for examples of Jewish medical ethics.

11. Ludwig Edelstein, *American Medicine: Selected Papers of Ludwig Edelstein* (Baltimore: Johns Hopkins University Press, 1967), p. 6.

12. Thomas Percival, *Percival's Medical Ethics*, edited by Chauncey D. Leake (Baltimore: Williams and Wilkins, 1927), p. 7.

13. American Medical Association, "Principles of Medical Ethics," in *Current Opinions* (Chicago: Judicial Council, American Medical Association, 1981), p. ix.

14. Howard Brody, "The Physician-Patient Contract: Legal and Ethical Aspects," *The Journal of Legal Medicine* 4 (July–August 1976):25–29; Richard A. Epstein, "Contracting Out of the Medical Malpractice Crisis," *Perspectives in Biology and Medicine* 20 (Winter 1977):228–245; Richard M. Magraw, "Social and Medical Contracts, Explicit and Implicit," in *Hippocrates Revisited: A Search for Meaning*, ed. Roger J. Bulger (New York: Medcom Press, 1973), pp. 148–157; William F. May, "Code, Covenant, Contract, or Philanthropy," *Hastings Center Report* 5 (December 1975):33; Edmund D. Pellegrino, "Toward an Expanded Medical Ethics: The Hippocratic Ethic Revisited," in *Hippocrates Revisited: A Search for Meaning*, ed. Roger J. Bulger (New York: Medcom Press, 1973), pp. 133–147; Robert M. Veatch, *Value-Freedom in Science and Technology*, Doctoral Dissertation, Harvard University, Cambridge, Mass. (1971); Robert M. Veatch, "Models for Ethical Medicine in a Revolutionary Age," *Hastings Center Report* 2 (June 1972):5–7 (chapter 1 in this volume); Veatch, *A Theory of Medical Ethics*.

15. Albert R. Jonsen, "Do No Harm: Axiom of Medical Ethics," in *Philosophical Medical Ethics: Its Nature and Significance*, ed. Stuart F. Spicker and H. Tristram Engelhardt, Jr. (Dordrecht: D. Reidel Publishing Co., 1977), pp. 27–41; C. Sandulescu, "Primum non nocere: Philological commentaries on a Medical Aphorism," *Acta-Antiqua Hungarica* 13 (1965):359–388; Veatch, *A Theory of Medical Ethics*.

16. Paul Ramsey, *Ethics and the Edges of Life* (New Haven: Yale University Press, 1978), p. 178.

17. Roger Masters, "Is Contract an Adequate Basis for Medical Care?" *Hastings Center Report* 5 (December 1975):33.

18. Hunter v. Brown, 484 P. 2d 1162 (Wash. 1971); Robert M. Veatch, "Federal Regulation of Medicine and Biomedical Research: Power, Authority, and Legitimacy," in *The Law-Medicine Relation: A Philosophical Exploration*, ed. Stuart F. Spicker et al. (Boston: D. Reidel Publishing Co., 1981), pp. 75–91; Robert M. Veatch, "Professional Medical Ethics: The Grounding of Its Principles," *The Journal of Medicine and Philosophy* 4 (March 1979):1–19; Veatch, *A Theory of Medical Ethics*.

19. U.S. Department of Health and Human Services, "Use of Ambulatory Care by the Poor and Nonpoor," *Health: United States*, 1980 National Center for Health Statistics Publication No. 81–232 (December 1980):168.

20. U.S. Department of Health and Human Services, *1797 Summary, National Ambulatory Medical Care Survey, U.S., Jan.–Dec. 1979*, edited by T. McLemore, Vital and Health Statistics, National Center for Health Statistics, Advanced Data Report No. 66, Publication No. (PhS) 81–2150 (March 1981).

21. John Rogers and Peter Curtis, "The Achievement of Continuity of Care in a Primary Care Training Program," *American Journal of Public Health* 70 (1980):528.

22. Josephine Kasteler et al., "Issues Underlying Prevalence of Doctor-Shopping Behavior," *Journal of Health and Social Behavior* 17 (1976):328.

23. Alan Meisel, "The 'Exceptions' to the Informed Consent Doctrine: Striking a Balance between Competing Values in Medical Decisionmaking," *Wisconsin Law Review* 2 (1979):460–470; Robert M. Veatch, "When Should the Patient Know?" *Barrister* 8 (1981): 6–8, 17–20 (chapter 12 in this volume).

24. Berkey v. Anderson, 1 Cal. App. 3d 790, 805, 82 Cal. Rptr. 67, 78; Canterbury v. Spence, 464 F2d 772 (D.C. Cir.), cert. denied, 409 U.S. 1064 (1972); Cobbs v. Grant, 502 P. 2d 1 (Cal. 1972); Cooper v. Roberts, 286 A. 2b 647 (Pa. 1971); Dow v. Kaiser Foundation, 90 Cal. Rptr. 747 (Cal. 1970); Hunter v. Brown, 484 P. 2d 1162 (Wash. 1971); Wilkenson v. Vesey, 295 A. 2d 676 (R.I. 1972); Ruth Faden and Tom L. Beauchamp in collaboration with Nancy M. P. King, *A History and Theory of Informed Consent* (New York: Oxford University Press, 1986), pp. 32–33.

25. Alan Meisel et al., "Toward a Model of the Legal Doctrine of Informed Consent," *American Journal of Psychiatry* 135 (1977):287–288.

26. Robert Lifton, "Protean Man," *Archives of General Psychiatry* 24 (1971): 298–304.

4. VALUES IN ROUTINE MEDICAL DECISIONS

1. Stuart J. Youngner, Wendy Lewandowski, Donna K. McClish, Barbara W. Juknialis, Claudia Coulton, and Edward T. Bartlett, "Do Not Resuscitate Orders," *Journal of the American Medical Association* 285 (1985): 54–57; and Susanna E. Bedell and Thomas L. Delbanco, "Choices about Cardiopulmonary Resuscitation in the Hospital: When Do Physicians Talk with Patients?" *New England Journal of Medicine* 310 (1984):1080–1093.

2. Robert J. Levine, "Do Not Resuscitate Decisions and Their Implementation," in *Dilemmas of Dying: Policies and Procedures for Decisions Not to Treat*, ed. Cynthia B. Wong and Judith P. Swazey (Boston: G. K. Hall Medical Publishers, 1981), pp. 23–41; and Steven H. Miles, Ronald Cranford, and Alvin L. Schultz, "The Do-Not-Resuscitate Order in a Teaching Hospital," *Annals of Internal Medicine* 96 (1982):660–664.

3. President's Commission for the Study of Ethical Problems in Medicine and Biomedical and Behavioral Research, *Deciding to Forego Life-Sustaining Treatment:*

Ethical, Medical, and Legal Issues in Treatment Decisions (Washington, D.C.: U.S. Government Printing Office, 1983).

5. THE CONCEPT OF "MEDICAL INDICATIONS"

1. National Conference on Standards and Guidelines for Cardiopulmonary Resuscitation and Emerging Cardiac Care, "Standards and Guidelines for Cardiopulmonary (CPR) and Emergency Cardiac Care (ECC)," *Journal of the American Medical Association* 255 (June 6, 1986):2905–2984.

2. U.S. Department of Health and Human Services, "Child Abuse and Neglect Prevention and Treatment Program: Final Rule: 45 CFR 1340," *Federal Register: Rules and Regulations* 50 (No. 72, April 15, 1985):14880.

3. W. D. Hudson, *The Is/Ought Question* (London: Macmillan, 1969).

4. Alasdair MacIntyre, *After Virtue* (Notre Dame, Ind.: University of Notre Dame Press, 1981).

5. Darrel W. Amundsen, "The Physician's Obligation to Prolong Life: A Medical Duty without Classical Roots," *The Hastings Center Report* 8 (August 1978):23–30.

6. U.S. Department of Health and Human Services, "Child Abuse and Neglect Prevention and Treatment Program: Final Rule: 45 CFR 1340," p. 14887.

7. Court of Appeal of the State of California, Second Appellate District, Division Two, *Neil Barber and Robert Nejdl v. Superior Court of the State of California for the County of Los Angeles,* October 12, 1983. See also In re Conroy, No. A-108 (N.J. Sup. Ct., Jan. 17, 1985); Joanne Lynn and James F. Childress, "Must Patients Always Be Given Food and Water?" *The Hastings Center Report* 13 (October 1983):17-21.

6. THE PRINCIPLES FOR MEDICAL ETHICS

1. "The Hippocratic Oath," in *Ancient Medicine: Selected Papers of Ludwig Edelstein,* ed. Owsei Temkin and C. Lilian Temkin (Baltimore: The Johns Hopkins Press, 1967), p. 6.

2. General Medical Council: Disciplinary Committee," *British Medical Journal Supplement* no. 3542 (March 20, 1971):79-80. See also Robert M. Veatch, *Case Studies in Medical Ethics.* (Cambridge, Mass.: Harvard University Press, 1977), pp. 131–135.

3. "The Hippocratic Oath," in Edelstein, p. 6.

4. British Medical Association, *Medical Ethics* (London: British Medical Association, 1970). American Medical Association, *Judicial Council Opinions and Reports* (Chicago: American Medical Association, 1971).

5. Donald Oken, "What to Tell Cancer Patients: A Study of Medical Attitudes," *Journal of the American Medical Association* 175 (1961): 1120–1128.

6. "The Hippocratic Oath," in Edelstein, p. 23.

7. In reaching this conclusion, we should not overlook the difficult conceptual and evaluative problems raised by a notion of "objective medical welfare." While the medical profession has tended in the past to presume that the notion of an objective medical interest of a patient is a coherent concept, it is increasingly doubtful that it is. In order for there to be an objectively determined medical interest for a patient, there must be some agreement that there is an unequivocal objectively good end to be pursued medically. When one realizes that the end of preserving life can sometimes conflict with the end of relieving suffering, one begins to encounter the difficulties of determining objective medical welfare. In fact there are even more complex choices to be made among potential medical ends, no one of which is

obviously correct. In later chapters, particularly the last chapter, we shall explore further the notion of objective medical welfare. At this point we need to acknowledge that even if there is an objectively derivable medical good for a patient, it seems clear that knowledge of medical science alone will not lead one to it.

8. "Declaration of Geneva," in *Encyclopedia of Bioethics*, 4 vols., ed. Warren T. Reich (New York: The Free Press, 1978), vol. 4, p. 1749.

9. Immanuel Kant, *Groundwork of the Metaphysics of Morals*, trans. H. J. Paton (New York: Harper and Row, 1964); W. D. Ross, *The Right and the Good* (Oxford: Oxford University Press, 1930); John Rawls, *A Theory of Justice* (Cambridge, Mass.: Harvard University Press, 1971); Robert Nozick, *Anarchy, State, and Utopia* (New York: Basic Books, 1974).

10. Ruth Macklin, "Moral Concerns and Appeals to Right and Duties: Grounding Claims in a Theory of Justice," *The Hastings Center Report* 6 (1976):31–38.

11. It is further debated whether such a principle, if it exists, applies only to humans or to all sentient beings including animals. For purposes of most issues in medical ethics, we can take the following discussion to apply to humans, leaving open the question whether the same consideration applies to animals. Of course, for certain issues such as medical research, xenograft transplantation, and the use of animals in other therapies, the question of whether animals are included in the prohibition on killing would have to be settled.

12. W. D. Ross, *The Right and the Good* (Oxford: Oxford University Press, 1939), p. 21.

13. Ibid., p. 41.

14. Baruch Brody, *Life and Death Decision Making* (New York: Oxford University Press, 1988), pp. 75–79; p. 51.

7. INFORMED CONSENT

1. L. C. Epstein and L. Lasagna, "Obtaining Informed Consent: Form or Substance," *Arch Intern Med* 123 (1969):682; R. Winer, Robert M. Veatch, V. W. Sidel, and M. Spivack, "Informed Consent: The Use of Lay Surrogates to Determine How Much Information Should Be Transmitted," in Robert M. Veatch, *The Patient as Partner* (Bloomington, Ind.: Indiana University Press, 1987), pp. 153–168.

2. Epstein and Lasagna, "Obtaining Informed Consent."

3. William Beaumont's Code, 1883, in Henry K. Beecher, *Research and the Individual: Human Studies* (Boston: Little-Brown and Co., 1970), p. 219.

4. Robert M. Veatch, "Three Theories of Informed Consent: Philosophical Foundations and Policy Implications," in the *Belmont Report: Ethical Principles and Guidelines for the Protection of Human Subjects of Research*, edited by the National Commission for the Protection of Human Subjects of Biomedical and Behavioral Research (Washington, D.C.: U.S. Government Printing Office), U.S. Dept. of HEW, DHEW Publication no. (OS) 78-0014, pp. 26-1 through 26-66; and "The Principle of Autonomy: The Foundation for Informed Consent," in *The Patient as Partner*, pp. 36–65.

5. Schloendorff v. New York Hospital, 211 N.Y. 127, 129, 105 N.E. 92, 93 (1914).

6. Natanson v. Kline, 186 Kansas. 393, 350 p. 2d. 1093 (1960).

7. Halushka v. Saskatchewan, 52 W.W.R. 608–09 (Sask. 1965).

8. U.S. Department of Health and Human Services, "Final Regulations Amending Basic HHS Policy for the Protection of Human Research Subjects: Final Rule: 45 CFR 46," *Federal Register: Rules and Regulations* 46 (No. 16, January 26, 1981):8390.

9. Natanson v. Kline, 186 Kansas. 393, 350 p. 2d. 1093 (1960).

10. California, Idaho, New York, Ohio, Oregon, Pennsylvania, Rhode Island, Washington, Wisconsin, and Tennessee.

11. See, for example, L. L. Riskin, "Informed Consent: Looking for the Action," *U Ill Law For* 1975 (1975):580.

12. Berkey v. Anderson, 1 Cal. App. 3d 790, 805. 82 Cal. Rptr. 67, 78 (1969).

13. Cobbs v. Grant, 502 p. 2d 1 (Cal. 1972).

14. L. A. Fox, "Medical and Prescription Records: Patient Access and Confidentiality," *U.S. Pharmacist* 4 (No. 2, 1979):15; G. Tucker, "Patient Access to Medical Records," *Legal Aspects of Medical Practice* 6 (1978):45.

8. MALPRACTICE IN THE CONTRACT MODE

1. James S. Todd, "Report of the Ad Hoc Committee on the Principles of Medical Ethics [of the American Medical Association]," unpublished report [1980].

2. James F. Childress, *Moral Responsibility in Conflicts* (Baton Rouge and London: Louisiana State University Press, 1982).

3. Donald Oken, "What to Tell Cancer Patients: A Study of Medical Attitudes," *Journal of the American Medical Association* 175 (April 1, 1961): 1120–1128; Daniel Cappon, "Attitudes of and towards the Dying," *Canadian Medical Association Journal* 87 (September 29, 1962):693–700.

4. Dennis H. Novack, Robin Plumer, Raymond L. Smith, Herbert Ochitil, Gary R. Morrow, and John M. Bennett, "Changes in Physicians' Attitudes toward Telling the Cancer Patient," *Journal of the American Medical Association* 241 (March 2, 1979):897–900.

5. Berkey v. Anderson, 1 Cal. App. 3d 790. 82 Cal. Rptr. 67 (1969).

6. Todd, "Report of the Ad Hoc Committee on the Principles of Medical Ethics [of the American Medical Association]."

7. Judicial Council, American Medical Association, *Current Opinions of the Council on Ethical and Judicial Affairs of the American Medical Association—1986: Including the Principles of Medical Ethics and Rules of the Council on Ethical and Judicial Affairs* (Chicago: American Medical Association, 1986), pp. 31–32.

8. Ruth R. Faden, Catherine Becker, Carol Lewis, John Freeman, and Alan I. Faden, "Disclosure of Information to Patients in Medical Care," *Medical Care* 19 (No. 7, July 19, 1981):718–733.

9. THE ETHICS OF GENERIC DRUG USE

1. Robert M. Veatch, *Case Studies in Medical Ethics* (Cambridge, Mass.: Harvard University Press, 1977), pp. 32–33.

2. "Generic Drug Substitutes Can Save $20 Million," *Modern Health Care* 9 (1979):16.

3. Igor Francetic et al., "Prescription Prices under the New York Generic Substitution Law," *Annals of Internal Medicine* 92 (1980):419.

4. Ibid.

5. George J. Annas, Leonard H. Glantz, and Barbara Katz, "Legal Control of Drugs and Generic Drugs," *Nursing Law and Ethics* 1 (1980):4.

6. A. A. Angrist, "Comments," *New York State Journal of Medicine* 79 (1979):1243.

7. Michael Weintraub et al., "Digoxin-Prescribing: Mostly Good News," *Journal of the American Medical Association* 242 (1979):445.

8. Sheldon S. Stoffer and Walter E. Szpunar, "Potency of Brand Name and Generic Levothyroxine Products," *Journal of the American Medical Association* 244 (1980):1704.

9. Angrist, "Comments."

10. George Dunea, "Generic Acrimony," *British Medical Journal* 2 (1979, 6181):31.

11. Annas, Glantz, and Katz, "Legal Control."

12. D. Craig Brater and William A. Pettinger, "The Generic Prescribing Issue," *Annals of Internal Medicine* 92 (1980):427.

13. Gina Bari Kolata, "Large Drug Firms Fight Generic Substitution," *Science* 206 (1979):1054.

14. Brater and Pettinger, "The Generic Prescribing Issue."

10. TREATMENT INDS

1. Investigational New Drug, Antibiotic, and Biological Drug Product Regulations: Treatment Use and Sale; Final Rule," *Federal Register* 52 (May 22, 1987):19466–19477; Frank E. Young, John A. Norris, Joseph A. Levitt, and Stuart L. Nightingale, "The FDA's New Procedures for the Use of Investigational Drugs in Treatment," *Journal of the American Medical Association* 259 (April 15, 1988):2267–2270.

2. Stuart L. Nightingale, "From the Food and Drug Administration," *Journal of the American Medical Association* 260 (November 25, 1988):2980.

3. Robert M. Veatch, "Case Study: Risk-Taking in Cancer Chemotherapy," *IRB* 1 (No. 5, August/September, 1979):4–6.

4. H. O. Conn, "Therapeutic Portacaval Anastomosis: To Shunt or Not to Shunt," *Gastroenterology* 67 (1974):1065–1073.

11. ETHICS OF DRUGS FOR NONAPPROVED USES

1. Steven H. Erikson, et al., "The Use of Drugs for Unlabeled Indications," *Journal of the American Medical Association* 243 (1980):1543.

2. G. R. Mundy et al., "Current Medical Practice and the Food and Drug Administration: Some Evidence for the Existing Gap," *Journal of the American Medical Association* 229 (1974):1744.

3. Erikson et al., "The Use of Drugs for Unlabeled Indications."

4. "Use of Approved Drugs for Unlabeled Indications," *FDA Drug Bulletin* 12 (No. 1, 1982):4.

5. Stuart L. Nightingale, "FDA's Role in Appropriate Drug Use," unpublished manuscript, 1981, p. 11.

6. Murray Weiner, "Should the Public Have the Legal Right to Use Unproven Remedies? Yes," in *Controversies in Therapeutics*, ed. Louis Lasagna (Philadelphia, Penn.: W. B. Sanders, 1980), pp. 483–493.

7. Peter Barton Hutt, "The Legal Requirement That Drugs Be Proved Safe and Effective before Their Use," in *Controversies in Therapeutics*, ed. Louis Lasagna (Philadelphia, Penn.: W. B. Sanders, 1980), pp. 495–505.

8. Hearings before the Intergovernmental Relations Subcommittee, U.S. House of Representatives, 92nd Congress, July 29, 30, 1971, "New Drugs for Nonapproved Purposes" (Washington, D.C., 1971), p. 59. In J. T. Gibson, *Medication Law and Behavior* (New York: Wiley Interscience, 1976), p. 321.

9. N. Dorsen et al., "Review Panel on New Drug Regulation" (Washington, D.C.: Department of Health, Education, and Welfare, 1977), p. 100.

12. WHEN SHOULD THE PATIENT KNOW?

1. Herman Feifel et al., "Physicians Consider Death," *Proceedings of the American Psychological Association*, 1967, pp. 201–202.

2. Hubert W. Smith, "Therapeutic Privilege to Withhold Specific Prognosis from Patient Sick with Serious or Fatal Illness," *Tennessee Law Review* 19 (No. 3, April 1946):349–357.

3. See generally Jay Katz, *Experimentation with Human Beings* (New York: Russell Sage Foundation, 1972), pp. 9–65.

4. Nishi v. Hartwell, 473 P. 2d 116, 119 (Haw. 1970).

5. Williams v. Menehan, 379 P.2d 292 (Kans. Supreme Court, 1963); Ferrara v. Galluchio, 152 N.E. 2d 249 (N.Y. 1958); Kraus v. Spielberg, 236 N.Y.S. 2d 143 (Sup. Ct. 1962); Stauffer v. Karabin, Colo. App., 492 P.2d 862 (1971); Di Filippo v. Preston, 53 Del. 539, 173 A.2d 333 (1961).

6. Bernard C. Meyer, "Truth and the Physician," in *Ethical Issues in Medicine,* ed. E. F. Torrey (Boston: Little, Brown, 1968), p. 172.

7. Natanson v. Kline, 350 P.2d 1093 *(Kans.), rehearing denied,* 354 P.2d 670 *(Kans.* 1960).

8. Ibid. p. 1106.

9. Ibid. p. 1107.

10. Paul S. Appelbaum, Charles W. Lidz, and Alan Meisel, *Informed Consent: Legal Theory and Clinical Practice* (New York: Oxford University Press, 1987). Also see Ruth Faden and Tom L. Beauchamp in collaboration with Nancy M. P. King, *A History and Theory of Informed Consent* (New York: Oxford University Press, 1986), p. 37; and Alan Meisel, "The 'Expectations' to the Informed Consent Doctrine: Striking a Balance between Competing Values in Medical Decisionmaking," *Wisconsin Law Review* 1979(1979):413–488.

11. Canterbury v. Spence, 464 F.2d 772 (D.C. Cir. 1972); see also Cobbs v. Grant 502 P.2d 1 (Cal. 1972).

12. Ibid., p. 789.

13. Ibid.

14. Ibid. See also Barclay v. Campbell, 704 S.W.2d 8 (Tex. 1986).

15. Robert M. Veatch, *Death, Dying, and the Biological Revolution* (New Haven, Conn.: Yale University Press, 1989).

16. See G. P. Fletcher, "Prolonging Life," *Washington Law Review* 42(1967):999–1016.

14. THE ETHICS OF DISPENSING PLACEBOS

1. A. K. Shapiro, "The Placebo Response," in *Modern Perspectives in World Psychiatry,* ed. J. G. Howells (Edinburgh: Oliver and Boyd, 1968).

2. Howard Brody, *Placebos and the Philosophy of Medicine* (Chicago: The University of Chicago Press, 1980), p. 11.

3. Ibid.

4. Norman Cousins, *Anatomy of an Illness as Perceived by the Patient* (New York: W. W. Norton, 1979).

5. Jon Levine, Newton C. Gordon, and Howard L. Fields, "The Mechanism of Placebo Analgesia," *The Lancet* 2 (1978):654–657.

6. Brody, *Placebos,* p. 97.

7. Sissela Bok, "The Ethics of Giving Placebos," *Scientific American* 231 (1974): 17.

8. Brody, *Placebos,* p. 107.

9. Lee C. Park and Lino Covi, "An Exploration of Neurotic Outpatients' Responses to Placebo When Its Inert Content Is Disclosed," *Archives of General Psychiatry* 12 (1965):336.

15. THE PATIENT'S RIGHT OF ACCESS TO MEDICAL RECORDS

1. Greg Tucker, "Patient Access to Medical Records," *Legal Aspects of Medical Practice* 6 (October 1978):45–50; John Hayes, "The Patient's Right of Access to His Hospital and Medical Records," *Medical Trial Technique Quarterly*, Winter 1978, pp. 295–305; Barbara L. Kaiser, "Patients' Rights of Access to Their Own Medical Records: The Need for New Law," *Buffalo Law Review* 24 (1974):317–330; Tucker, "Patient Access to Medical Records"; George J. Annas, Daryl B. Matthews, and Leonard H. Glantz, "Patient Access to Medical Records," *Medicolegal News* 8 (No. 2, April 1980):17–18.

2. See, for example, Georgia Code Annotated, sections 38–717 to 38–721 (1974).

3. Public Citizen Health Research Group, *Medical Records: Getting Yours* (Washington, D.C.: Public Citizen Health Research Group, 1986), p. 33; Eugene J. Stein, Ronald L. Furedy, Mary Jane Simonton, and Cynthia H. Neuffer, "Patient Access to Medical Records on a Psychiatric Inpatient Unit," *American Journal of Psychiatry* 136 (March 1979):327–329; "Summary of Selected Statutes concerning Confidentiality of and Patient Access to Medical Records," *State Health Legislation Report* 9 (No. 1, May 1981):13–23.

4. Hugh I. Schade, "My Patients Take Their Medical Records with Them," *Medical Economics*, March 8, 1976, pp. 75–81; R. Giglio, B. Spears, David Rumpf, and Nancy Eddy, "Encouraging Behavior Changes by Use of Client-Held Health Records," *Medical Care* 16 (1978):757–764; Budd N. Shenkin and David C. Warner, "Giving the Patient His Medical Record: A Proposal to Improve the System," *New England Journal of Medicine* 289 (1973): 688–692.

16. THE LIMITS OF CONFIDENTIALITY

1. Ludwig Edelstein, "The Hippocratic Oath: Text, Translation and Interpretation," in *Ancient Medicine: Selected Papers of Ludwig Edelstein*, ed. Owsei Temkin and C. Lilian Temkin (Baltimore, Md.: The Johns Hopkins Press, 1967), p. 6.

2. World Medical Association, "Declaration of Geneva," *World Medical Journal* 3 (1956), supplement, pp. 10–12. Reprinted in *Encyclopedia of Bioethics*, Vol. 4, ed. Warren T. Reich (New York: The Free Press, 1978), p. 1749.

3. American Medical Association, *Judicial Council Opinions and Reports* (Chicago: American Medical Association, 1971), p. vii.

4. Tarasoff v. Regents of University of California. 17C.3d 425, 131 Cal. Rptr. 14, 551 P.2d 334, in Thomas A. Shannon and Jo Ann Manfra, ed., *Law and Bioethics: Texts with Commentary on Major U.S. Court Decisions* (New York: Paulist Press, 1982), pp. 293–319.

5. Judicial Council, American Medical Association, *Current Opinions of the Council on Ethical and Judicial Affairs of the American Medical Association—1986: Including the Principles of Medical Ethics and Rules of the Council on Ethical and Judicial Affairs* (Chicago: American Medical Association, 1986), p. ix.

6. Ibid., p. 21.

17. PATIENTS' DUTIES AND PHYSICIANS' RIGHTS

1. Claude Bernard, *An Introduction to the Study of Experimental Medicine*, translated by Henry Copley Greene, A.M. (New York: Dover Publications, Inc., 1957), pp. 428–479.

2. Robert N. Wilson, *The Sociology of Health: An Introduction* (New York: Random House, 1970), p. 18.

3. Eric J. Cassell, *The Healer's Art* (Philadelphia: J. B. Lippincott, 1976), pp. 44–46.

4. Thomas Percival, *Percival's Medical Ethics, 1803*, reprint, edited by Chauncey D. Leake (Baltimore: Williams and Wilkins, 1927).

5. American Medical Association, *Code of Medical Ethics: Adopted by the American Medical Association at Philadelphia, May, 1847, and by the New York Academy of Medicine in October, 1847* (New York: H. Ludwig and Co., 1848), pp. 14–16.

6. Bouvia v. County of Riverside, No. 159780 (Cal. Super. Ct. Dec. 16, 1983).

7. Ibid.

8. Bouvia v. Superior Court of Los Angeles County, California Court of Appeal, Second District, 1986, 179 Cal. App. 3d 1127, 225 Cal. Rptr. 297 (Ct. App.), *review denied* (June 5, 1986).

9. Roe v. Wade, 410 U.S. 113, 93 S.Ct. 705, 1973.

18. AUTONOMY'S TEMPORARY TRIUMPH

1. Robert M. Veatch, *A Theory of Medical Ethics* (New York: Basic Books, 1981).

2. Paul Ramsey, *Ethics at the Edges of Life* (New Haven, Conn.: Yale University Press, 1978), p. 273, n. 10.

3. Gordon Rich, Norman J. Glass, and J. B. Selkon, "Cost-effectiveness of Two Methods of Screening for Asymptomatic Bacteriuria," *British Journal of Preventive and Social Medicine* 30 (1976):54–59.

4. I develop this thesis in detail in chapter 4 of Robert M. Veatch, *The Foundations of Justice: Why the Retarded and the Rest of Us Have Claims to Equality* (New York: Oxford University Press, 1986).

19. DRGS AND THE ETHICS OF COST CONTAINMENT

1. The FY 1987 figures are 500.3 billion. HHS News, U.S. Department of Health and Human Services, November 17, 1988, p. 6.

2. See Mark S. Freeland and Carol E. Schendler, "Health Spending in the 1980's: Integration of Clinical Practice Patterns with Management," *Health Care Financing Review* 5 (Spring 1984):4.

3. United States Department of Health and Human Services, Health Care Financing Administration, "Medicare Program: Prospective Payment for Medicare In-patient Hospital Services: Final Rule," *Federal Register* 49 (January 3, 1984):234–334; Group on Health Service Policy Division of Health Policy and Program Evaluation Department of Health Care Resources, "DRGs and the Prospective Payment System: A Guide for Physicians" (Chicago: American Medical Association, 1983).

4. Center for Health Affairs, *Case Approach to DRG Assignment: A Guide for Physicians* (Cleveland: Greater Cleveland Hospital Association, 1984).

5. Steve Holman, "DRGs: Forcing Physicians into a Business Role?" *Hospital Physician* 20 (5):102–111.

6. The Hastings Center, Institute of Society, Ethics and the Life Sciences, "Values, Ethics, and CBA in Health Care," in *The Implications of Cost-Effectiveness Analysis of Medical Technology*, Office of Technology Assessment, Congress of the United States (Washington, D.C.: Office of Technology Assessment, 1980), p. 170; Michael S. Baram, "Cost-Benefit Analysis: An Inadequate Basis for Health, Safety,

and Environmental Regulatory Decisionmaking," *Ecology Law Quarterly* 8 (No. 3, 1980):474.

7. John Rawls, *A Theory of Justice* (Cambridge: Harvard University Press, 1971).

8. For a fuller discussion of the infinite demand problem, see chapter 6 of Robert M. Veatch, *The Foundations of Justice: Why the Retarded and the Rest of Us Have Claims to Equality* (New York: Oxford University Press, 1986).

9. Robert M. Veatch, *A Theory of Medical Ethics* (New York: Basic Books, 1981), pp. 250–287.

20. JUSTICE AND ECONOMICS

1. S. J. Mushkin, ed., *Consumer Incentives for Health Care* (New York: Prodist, 1974), pp. 183–216; B. S. Cooper and D. P. Rice, "The Economic Cost of Illness Revisited," *Social Security Bulletin* 39 (No. 2, 1976): 21; P. A. Piro and T. Lutins, *Utilization and Reimbursement under Medicare for Persons Who Died in 1967 and 1968* (Washington, D.C.: Social Security Administration, 1973), DHEW Publication No. (SSA) 74-11702; A. A. Scitovsky and A. M. Capron, "Medical Care at the End of Life: The Interaction of Economics and Ethics," *Annual Review of Public Health* 7 (1986):59–75; Anne A. Scitovsky, "The High Cost of Dying: What Do the Data Show?" *Milbank Memorial Fund Quarterly* 62 (No. 4, 1984):591–608; Allan S. Detsky, Steven C. Stricker, Albert G. Mulley, and George E. Thibault, "Prognosis, Survival, and the Expenditure of Hospital Resources for Patients in an Intensive-Care Unit," *New England Journal of Medicine* 305 (1981):667–672.

2. J. Lubitz and R. Prihoda, "The Use and Costs of Medicare Services in the Last Two Years of Life," *Health Care Financing Review* 5 (1984):117–31.

3. Ronald Bayer, Daniel Callahan, John Fletcher, Thomas Hodgson, Bruce Jennings, David Monsees, Steven Sieverts, and Robert Veatch, "The Care of the Terminally Ill: Morality and Economics," *New England Journal of Medicine* 309 (December 15, 1983): 1491.

4. Clark C. Havighurst and James F. Blumstein, "Coping with Quality/Cost Trade-offs in Medical Care: The Role of PSROs" *Northwestern University Law Review* 70 (No. 1, March/April 1975): 55.

5. Stephen E. Rhoads, ed., *Valuing Life: Public Policy Dilemmas* (Boulder, Colo.: Westview Press, Inc., 1980); Dorothy P. Rice and Barbara S. Cooper, "The Economic Value of Human Life," *American Journal of Public Health* 57 (November 1967): 1954–1966.

6. T. C. Schelling, "The Life You Save May Be Your Own," in *Problems of Public Expenditure Analysis*, ed. Samuel B. Chase (Washington, D.C.: Brookings Institution, 1966).

7. Ronald Dworkin, "What Is Equality? Part 1: Equality of Welfare," *Philosophy and Public Affairs* 10 (Summer 1981):185–246; Ronald Dworkin, "What Is Equality? Part 2: Equality of Resources," *Philosophy and Public Affairs* 10 (Fall 1981): 283–345; cf. Robert M. Veatch, *The Foundations of Justice: Why the Retarded and the Rest of Us Have Claims to Equality* (New York: Oxford University Press, 1986).

8. John Rawls, *A Theory of Justice* (Cambridge, Mass.: Harvard University Press, 1971), pp. 136ff.

9. Norman Daniels, *Just Health Care* (Cambridge: Cambridge University Press, 1985); Norman Daniels, *Am I My Parents' Keeper?: An Essay on Justice between the Young and the Old* (New York: Oxford University Press, 1988).

10. Kurt Baier, *The Moral View* (New York: Random House, 1965).

11. Ronald E. Cranford and Harmon L. Smith, "Some Critical Distinctions

between Brain Death and the Persistent Vegetative State," *Ethics in Science and Medicine* 6 (Winter 1979):199–209.

12. Jeffrey Prottas, Mark Segal, and Harvey M. Sapolsky, "Cross-National Differences in Dialysis Rates," *Health Care Financing Review* 4 (No. 3, March 1983):91–103.

13. Robert M. Veatch, "Distributive Justice and the Allocation of Technological Resources to the Elderly," in *Life Sustaining Technologies and the Elderly: Working Papers, Volume 3: Legal and Ethical Issues, Manpower and Training, and Classification Systems for Decisionmaking* (Washington, D.C.: U.S. Congress, Office of Technology Assessment, 1987), pp. 87–189.

14. Jerry Avorn, "Benefit and Cost Analysis in Geriatric Care: Turning Age Discrimination into Health Policy," *New England Journal of Medicine* 310 (May 17, 1984):1294–1300.

15. James Childress, "Ensuring Care, Respect, and Fairness for the Elderly," *Hastings Center Report* 14 (No. 5, 1984):27–31.

16. Harry Moody, "Is It Right to Allocate Health Care Resources on Grounds of Age?" in *Bioethics and Human Rights*, ed. Bertram and Elsie Bandman (Boston: Little, Brown, Inc., 1978), pp. 197–201.

17. Daniel Callahan, *Setting Limits: Medical Goals in an Aging Society* (New York: Simon and Schuster, 1987), pp. 137, 138.

18. Norman Daniels, "Am I My Parents' Keeper?" in President's Commission for the Study of Ethical Problems in Medicine and Biomedical and Behavioral Research, *Securing Access to Health Care*, Vol. 2 (Washington, D.C.: U.S. Government Printing Office, 1983), pp. 265–291; Norman Daniels, *Am I My Parents' Keeper? An Essay on Justice between the Young and the Old* (New York: Oxford University Press, 1988).

21. VOLUNTARY RISKS TO HEALTH

1. Talcott Parsons, *The Social System* (New York: The Free Press, 1951), p. 437.

2. Robert S. Morison, "Rights and Responsibilities: Redressing the Uneasy Balance," *Hastings Center Report* 4 (1974):1–4; Eugene Vayda, "Keeping People Well: A New Approach to Medicine," *Human Nature* 1 (1978):64–71; Anne R. Somers and Mary C. Hayden, "Rights and Responsibilities in Prevention," *Health Education* 9 (1978):37–39; Leon Kass, "Regarding the End of Medicine and the Pursuit of Health," *Public Interest* 40 (1975):11–42.

3. Nedra B. Belloc and Lester Breslow, "Relationship of Physical Status Health and Health Practices," *Preventive Medicine* 1 (1972):409–421; Nedra B. Belloc, "Relationship of Health Practices and Mortality," *Preventive Medicine* 2 (1973):67–81; Lester Breslow, "Prospects for Improving Health through Reducing Risk Factors," *Preventive Medicine* 7 (1978):449–458.

4. Morison, "Rights and Responsibilities"; Daniel Wikler, "Coercive Measures in Health Promotion: Can They Be Justified?" *Health Education Monographs* 6 (1978):223–241; Daniel Wikler, "Persuasion and Coercion for Health: Ethical Issues in Government Efforts to Change Life-styles," *Milbank Memorial Fund Quarterly* 56 (1978):303–338.

5. Robert M. Veatch, *A Theory of Medical Ethics* (New York: Basic Books, 1981).

6. Tom L. Beauchamp, "The Regulation of Hazards and Hazardous Behaviors," *Health Education Monographs* 6 (1978):242–257.

7. Robert M. Veatch, "The Medical Model: Its Nature and Problems," *Hastings Center Report* 1 (1973):59–76.

8. J. N. Morris, "Social Inequalities Undiminished," *Lancet* 1 (1979):87–90.

9. W. Ryan, *Blaming the Victim* (New York: Vintage Books, 1971); R. Crawford,

"Sickness as Sin," *Health Policy Advisory Center Bulletin* 80 (1978):10–16; R. Crawford, "You Are Dangerous to Your Health," *Social Policy* 8 (1978):11–20; Dan E. Beauchamp, "Public Health as Social Justice," *Inquiry* 13 (1976):3–14.

10. L. Syme and I. Berkman, "Social Class, Susceptibility and Sickness," *American Journal of Epidemiology* 104 (1976):1–8; P. W. Conover, "Social Class and Chronic Illness," *International Journal of Health Services* 3 (1973):357–368; *Health of the Disadvantaged: Chart Book,* Publication (HRA) 77-628 (Hyattsville, Md.: U.S. Department of Health, Education, and Welfare, Public Health Service, Health Resources Administration, 1977).

11. Dan E. Beauchamp, "Alcoholism Is Blaming the Alcoholic," *International Journal of Addiction* 11 (1976):41–52.

12. Beauchamp, "The Regulation of Hazards and Hazardous Behaviors."

22. THE ETHICS OF ORGAN TRANSPLANTATION

1. Oscar Salvatierra, in United States House of Representatives, *Procurement and Allocation of Human Organs for Transplantation: Hearings before the Subcommittee on Investigations and Oversights of the Committee on Science and Technology,* 98th Congress, 1st Session, November 7, 9, 1983 (Washington, D.C.: U.S. Government Printing Office, 1984), pp. 274–283.

2. Michael R. Harrison, "The Anencephalic Newborn as Organ Donor," *Hastings Center Report* 16 (April 1986):21–23; Ethics and Social Impact Committee, Transplant Policy Center, Ann Arbor, Mich., "Anencephalic Infants as Sources of Transplantable Organs," *Hastings Center Report* 18 (October/November 1988):28–30.

3. J. David Bleich, "Neurological Death and Time of Death Statutes," *Jewish Bioethics,* ed. Fred Rosner and J. David Bleich (New York: Sanhedrin Press, 1979), p. 310.

4. Fred Rosner, "Organ Transplants: The Jewish Viewpoint," *Journal of Thanatology* 3 (1975):233–241.

5. Pius XII, "The Prolongation of Life," An Address to an International Congress of Anesthesiologists on November 24, 1957, *The Pope Speaks* 4 (Spring 1958):396.

6. Paul Byrne, Sean O'Reilly, and Paul M. Quay, "Brain Death—An Opposing Viewpoint," *Journal of the American Medical Association* 242 (November 2, 1979):1985–1990.

7. Paul Ramsey, "On Updating Procedures for Stating That a Man Has Died," *The Patient as a Person* (New Haven, Conn.: Yale University Press, 1970), pp. 59–112.

8. Joseph Fletcher, "Cerebration," in *Humanhood: Essays in Biomedical Ethics* (Buffalo, N.Y.: Prometheus Books, 1979), pp. 159–65.

9. Paul Ramsey, "Giving or Taking Cadaver Organs for Transplants," in *The Patient as Person,* esp. pp. 205–209; *Ethical and Religious Directives for Catholic Health Facilities,* Directive 30 (Washington, D.C.: Department of Health Affairs, United States Catholic Conference, 1971), p. 8; Benedict M. Ashley and Kevin D. O'Rourke, *Health Care Ethics: A Theological Analysis,* 2nd ed. (St. Louis, Mo.: The Catholic Health Association of the United States, 1982), pp. 308–312.

10. Paul Freund, "Organ Transplants: Ethical and Legal Problems," *Proceedings of the American Philosophical Society* 15 (August 1971):276; Fred Rosner, "Organ Transplantation in Jewish Law," in *Jewish Bioethics,* esp. p. 360.

11. Jesse Dukeminier and David Sanders, "Organ Transplantation: A Proposal for Routine Salvaging of Cadaver Organs," *New England Journal of Medicine* 279 (1968):413–419.

12. Robert M. Veatch, *Death, Dying, and the Biological Revolution* (New Haven, Conn.: Yale University Press, 1978), pp. 211–216.

13. Fred Rosner, "Autopsy in Jewish Law and the Israeli Autopsy Controversy," in *Jewish Bioethics*, p. 343.

14. "France Widens Authority for Transplants from Dead," *New York Times*, April 16, 1978, p. 11. Cited in *Medical Care Review* 35 (May 1978):512.

15. *The Removal of Cadaveric Organs for Transplantation: A Code of Practice*, Document drawn up by a Working Party on Behalf of the Health Departments of Great Britain and Northern Ireland, October 1979.

16. U.S. Health Care Financing Administration, "Exclusion of Heart Transplantation Procedures from Medicare Coverage," *Federal Register* 45 (August 6, 1980):52296–52297.

17. President's Commission for the Study of Ethical Problems in Medicine and Biomedical and Behavioral Research, *Securing Access to Health Care: The Ethical Implications of Differences in the Availability of Health Services*, Vol. 1: Report (Washington, D.C.: U.S. Government Printing Office, March 1983), p. 4.

18. "Report of the National Institutes of Health," *Spectrum* 16 (1):19–26.

19. President's Commission for the Study of Ethical Problems in Medicine and Biomedical and Behavioral Research, *Deciding to Forego Life-Sustaining Treatment: Ethical, Medical, and Legal Issues in Treatment Decisions* (Washington, D.C.: U.S. Government Printing Office, 1983), p. 212. See chapter 24 for a full discussion of the limits on parental decisionmaking.

20. See Norman Daniels, *Am I My Parents' Keeper? An Essay on Justice between the Young and the Old* (New York: Oxford University Press, 1988), and Daniel Callahan, *Setting Limits: Medical Goals in an Aging Society* (New York: Simon and Schuster, 1987), for further discussions of age-based allocation.

23. THE TECHNICAL CRITERIA FALLACY

1. John Lorber, "Results of Treatment of Myelomeningocele," *Developmental Medicine and Child Neurology* 13 (1971):279–303.

2. John Lorber, "Selective Treatment of Myelomeningocele: To Treat or Not to Treat?" *Pediatrics* 53 (March 1974):307–08.

3. John Lorber, "Early Results of Selective Treatment of Spina Bifida Cystica," *British Medical Journal* 4 (October 27, 1973):201–204.

4. G. Keys Smith and E. Durham Smith, "Selection for Treatment in Spina Bifida," *British Medical Journal* 4 (October 27, 1974):189–97.

5. Sherman C. Stein, Luis Schut, and Mary D. Ames, "Selection for Early Treatment in Myelomeningocele: A Retrospective Analysis of Various Selection Procedures," *Pediatrics* 54 (November 1974):556.

6. Richard C. Cook, "Spina Bifida and Hydrocephalus," *British Medical Journal* 4 (December 25, 1971):795–99; R. B. Zachary, "Ethical and Social Aspects of Treatment of Spina Bifida," *Lancet* 2 (1968):274; John M. Freeman, "The Short-sighted Treatment of Myelomeningocele: A Long-Term Case Report," *Pediatrics* 53 (March 1974):311–313.

7. Report by a Working Party, "Ethics of Selective Treatment of Spina Bifida," *Lancet* (January 11, 1975):88.

8. Herbert B. Eckstein, "Severely Malformed Children: The Problem of Selection," *British Medical Journal* (May 5, 1973):284. For a fuller discussion of the generalizing of expertise from ability to make technical measures to the ability to make moral and other value choices, see Robert M. Veatch, "Generalization of Expertise," *Hastings Center Studies* 1 (No. 2, 1973):29–40.

9. Raymond S. Duff and A. G. M. Campbell. "Moral and Ethical Dilemmas in the Special-Care Nursery," *New England Journal of Medicine* 289 (October 25, 1973):894. For another paper reaching a similar conclusion, see Anthony Shaw,

"Dilemmas of Informed Consent in Children," *New England Journal of Medicine* 289 (October 25, 1973):885–894.

24. LIMITS OF GUARDIAN TREATMENT REFUSAL

1. Superintendent of Belchertown State School v. Saikewicz, 373 Mass. 728, 370 NE 2d 417 (1977).

2. See generally Note, "Decisionmaking for the Incompetent Terminally Ill Patient: A Compromise in a Solution Eliminates a Compromise of Patients' Rights," *Indiana Law Journal* 57 (1982):325–348.

3. See generally Charles H. Baron, "Assuring 'Detached but Passionate Investigation and Decision': The Role of Guardians Ad Litem in *Saikewicz*-type Cases," *American Journal of Law and Medicine* 4 (1978):111–130; Charles H. Baron, "Medical Paternalism and the Rule of Law," *American Journal of Law and Medicine* 4 (Winter 1979):337–365.

4. See generally Arnold S. Relman, "The Saikewicz Decision: Judges as Physicians," *New England Journal of Medicine* 298 (1978):508–509; Arnold S. Relman, "The *Saikewicz* Decision: A Medical Viewpoint," *Journal of Law and Medicine* 4 (1978):233–242. See also Allen Buchanan, "Medical Paternalism or Legal Imperialism: Not the Only Alternatives for Handling *Saikewicz*-type Cases," *American Journal of Law and Medicine* 5 (Summer 1979):97–117.

5. In re Quinlan, 70 N.J. 10, 355 A. 2d 647 (1976), cert. denied sub nom., Garger v. New Jersey, 429 U.S. 922 (1976), overruled in part, In re Conroy, 98 NJ 321, 486 A. 2d 1209 (1985).

6. Superintendent of Belchertown State School v. Saikewicz.

7. In re Dinnerstein, 6 Mass. App. Ct. 466, 380 N.E. 2d 134 (App. Ct. 1978).

8. See, e.g., Norman Cantor, "Quinlan, Privacy, and the Handling of Incompetent Dying Patients," *Rutgers Law Review* 30 (1977):243–266; Note, "Family Law—Guardians of Incompetent Persons Can Refuse Life-Prolonging Treatment for Their Wards," *Suffolk University Law Review* 12 (1978):1039–1057; Buchanan, "Medical Paternalism."

9. See In re Osborne, 294 A. 2d 372 (D.C. 1972); In re Brooks Estate, 32 Ill. 2d 361, 205 N.E. 2d 435 (1965); Satz v. Perlmutter, 362 So. 2d 160 (Fla. Dist. Ct. App. 1978), aff'd, 379 So. 2d 359 (Fla. Sup. Ct. 1980); Lane v. Candura, 6 Mass. App. Ct. 377, 376 N.E. 2d 1232 (1978); In re Quackenbush, 156 N.J. Super. 282, 383 A. 2d 785 (1978); Erickson v. Dilgard, 44 Misc 2d 27, 252 N.Y.S. 2d 705 (Sup. Ct. 1962). See generally Robert N. Veatch, *Death, Dying, and the Biological Revolution* (New Haven: Yale University Press, 1989), pp. 91–93.

10. The constitutional right of privacy was developed in a series of cases concerning marriage and procreation. See Griswold v. Connecticut, 381 U.S. 479 (1965); Eisenstadt v. Baird, 405 U.S. 438 (1972); Roe v. Wade, 410 U.S. 113, 93 S.Ct. 705, 1973. The right of privacy has also been applied to refusal of treatment cases. E.g., In re Quinlan, 70 N.J. 10, 355 A. 2d 647 (1976), cert. denied sub nom., Garger v. New Jersey, 429 U.S. 922 (1976), overruled in part, In re Conroy, 98 N.J. 321, 486 A 2d 1209 (1985):40.

11. The right to control one's body has long been recognized by the judiciary. See, e.g., Schloendorff v. Society of N.Y. Hosp., 211 N.Y. 125, 129, 105 N.E. 92, 93 (1914); see also Union Pacific Railroad v. Botsford, 141 U.S. 250 (1891). See generally Jonathan Brant, "Last Rights: An Analysis of Refusal and Withholding of Treatment Cases," *Missouri Law Review* 46 (No. 2, 1981):337–370.

12. See Whalen v. Roe, 429 U.S. 589, 599–600 (1977) (suggesting that the right of privacy includes "an interest in independence in making certain kinds of important decisions.").

13. In re Brooks Estate, 32 Ill. 2d 361, 205 N.E. 2d 435 (1965); see also In re Osborne, 294 A. 2d 372 (D.C. 1972); Lane v. Candura, 6 Mass. App. Ct. 377 376 N.E. 2d 1232 (1978); In re Quackenbush, 156 N.J. Super. 282, 383 A. 2d 785 (1978); In re Melideo, 88 Misc. 2d 974, 390 N.Y.S. 2d 523 (1976); In re Maida Yetter, 62 Pa.D. and C. 2d 619 (1973).

14. A third exception to the general right of competent patients to refuse treatment appears to arise in the prison context. But upon close examination, these cases also fall within the two traditional exceptions. In some cases, the prisoner was de facto incompetent, even though he was never formally adjudged to be incompetent; Peek v. Ciccone, 288 F. Supp. 329 (W. D. Mo. 1968); in others the treatment was ordered to protect the welfare of others. See, e.g., Commissioner of Correction v. Myers, 379 Mass. 255, 264, 399 N.E. 2d 452, 457 (1979).

15. See Fred Rosner, *Modern Medicine and Jewish Law* (New York: Yeshiva University, 1972), pp. 115–123; Rabbi Immanuel Jakobovits, "Some Recent Jewish Views on Death and Euthanasia," in *Jewish Medical Ethics* (New York: Bloch Publishing Co., 1975), pp. 275–276.

16. Franklin H. Epstein, "No, It's Our Duty to Keep Patients Alive," *Medical Economics* 50 (April 2, 1973):97.

17. See, e.g., Strunk v. Strunk, 445 S.W. 2d 145 (Ky. 1969).

18. See Jeremy Bentham, "An Introduction to the Principles of Morals and Legislation," in *Ethical Theories: A Book of Readings*, ed. A. I. Melden (Englewood Cliffs, N.J.: Prentice-Hall, Inc., 1967), pp. 367–390; J. S. Mill, *Utilitarianism and Other Writings* (1962); Henry Sidgwick, *The Methods of Ethics* (New York: Dover Publications, Inc., 1966 [1874]).

19. Richard A. McCormick, "Proxy Consent in the Experimentation Situation," *Perspectives in Biology and Medicine* 18 (1974):2–20.

20. See President's Commission for the Study of Ethical Problems in Medicine and Biomedical and Behavioral Research, *Deciding to Forego Life-Sustaining Treatment* (Washington, D.C.: U.S. Government Printing Office, 1981), pp. 132–134.

21. Ibid., pp. 134–136.

22. In re Spring, 380 Mass. 629, 405 N.E. 2d 115 (1980); In re Quinlan, 70 N.J. 10, 355 A. 2d 647 (1976), *cert. denied* sub nom., Garger v. New Jersey, 429 U.S. 922 (1976), overruled in part, In re Conroy, 98 N.J. 321, 486 A. 2d 1209 (1985); In re Colyer, 99 Wash. 2d 114, 660 P. 2d 738 (1983).

23. In re Spring, 380 Mass. 629, 405 N.E. 2d 115 (1980), p. 40; Superintendent of Belchertown State School v. Saikewicz, 373 Mass. 728, 370 NE 2d 417 (1977), pp. 424–425; In re Quinlan, 70 N.J. 10, 355 A. 2d 647 (1976), *cert. denied* sub nom., Garger v. New Jersey, 429 U.S. 922 (1976), overruled in part, In re Conroy, 98 N.J. 321, 486 A. 2d 1209 (1985), p. 40; "Artificial Feeding Dominates: Beverly Requena (New Jersey)," *Society for the Right to Die Newsletter* (Fall 1986); In re Colyer, 99 Wash. 2d 114, 660 P. 2d 738 (1983), In re Quinlan, 70 N.J. 10, 355 A. 2d 647 (1976), *cert. denied* sub nom., Garger v. New Jersey, 429 U.S. 922 (1976), overruled in part, In re Conroy, 98 N.J. 321, 486 A. 2d 1209 (1985).

24. Wisconsin v. Yoder, 406 U.S. 205 (1972); Pierce v. Society of Sisters, 268 U.S. 510 (1925).

25. President's Commission Report, pp. 34, 35, n. 68.

26. Arnold S. Relman, "The *Saikewicz* Decision: A Medical Viewpoint," *Journal of Law and Medicine* 4 (1978):241–242.

27. Ibid., p. 236.

28. Ibid., p. 237.

29. Baron, "Assuring 'Detached but Passionate Investigation and Decision,'" "Medical Paternalism and the Rule of Law."

30. Relman, "The *Saikewicz* Decision," p. 236.

31. Ibid., p. 240. In attempting to rebut the interpretation that sees him as excessively paternalistic, he has said, "whenever possible, physicians should act only with the informed consent of their patient or, if the patient is legally incompetent, of the family or legal guardian." Arnold S. Relman, "Correspondence: A Response to Allen Buchanan's Views on Decision Making for Terminally Ill Incompetents," *American Journal of Law and Medicine* 5 (1979):119. He says the judicial role is acceptable when there are "disputes, requests for help, or complaints of wrongdoing" (p. 120). Even then, however, he seems to work with a model of "family and physician" rather than one of the family (or other appropriate guardians) as the primary decisionmaker with the physician serving as one among many potential advisors in a capacity similar to a minister, a lawyer, or other relatives, and close, trusted friends. For some reason, the physician is given much more of a primary role.

32. Physicians might also be authorized to make a temporary but definitive determination of incompetency and to designate themselves guardians. Even physicians committed to the preservation of patient autonomy are concerned about such situations. David Jackson, and Stuart Youngner, "Patient Autonomy and 'Death with Dignity,'" *New England Journal of Medicine* 301 (August 23, 1979):404–408.

At this time, however, there are no statutory guidelines for such action on the part of physicians. If Jackson and Youngner are to sustain their position to give physicians authority in such truly emergency situations, they will have to provide some assurance that emergency treatment without court order is carefully confined to the limited situation where (1) the patient obviously would be declared incompetent, (2) the patient needs treatment so badly that a guardian refusal would be beyond the limits of tolerance, (3) taking the time to get judicial authorization to treat would seriously harm the patient, and (4) the patient has not previously refused the needed treatment while competent. The burden of proof should fall on any physician treating in emergencies against the expressed wishes of the patient to establish that all of these conditions were satisfied.

It is troublesome that many of the examples given in defense of emergency unauthorized presumptions of guardianship do not meet all of these criteria. None of Jackson and Youngner's six reported cases of potentially legitimate physician decision-making for patients of the sort discussed here clearly meets all these criteria. Only one, a case of a woman suffering an asthmatic attack, may meet the third condition. Even if one accepts the emergency condition for recognizing the physician as temporary primary decisionmaker, it seems unlikely that she should use that temporary role to make definitive treatment refusals of life-sustaining treatment.

33. In re Dinnerstein, 6 Mass. App. Ct. 466, 380 N.E. 2d 134 (App. Ct. 1978).

34. Relman, "The *Saikewicz* Decision," p. 241.

25. "DO NOT RESUSCITATE" ORDERS

1. Standards for Cardiopulmonary Resuscitation (CPR) and Emergency Cardiac Care (ECC)," *Journal of the American Medical Association* 227 (1974):839.

2. Supreme Court of the State of New York, Queens County: Criminal Term, "Report of the Special January Third Additional 1983 Grand Jury concerning 'Do Not Resuscitate' Procedures at a Certain Hospital in Queens County," February 8, 1984.

3. Susanne E. Bedell, and Thomas L. Delbanco, "Choices about Cardiopulmonary Resuscitation in the Hospital: When Do Physicians Talk with Patients?" *New England Journal of Medicine* 310 (1984):1089–1093.

4. No Code Subcommittee, Medical-Legal Interprofessional Committee, Bar Association of San Francisco Medical Society, in President's Commission for the Study of Ethical Problems in Medicine and Biomedical and Behavioral Research, *Deciding to Forego Life-Sustaining Treatment: Ethical, Medical, and Legal Issues in*

Treatment Decisions (Washington, D.C.: U.S. Government Printing Office, 1983), p. 496.

5. City of Boston Department of Health and Hospitals, "Guidelines: Do Not Resuscitate Orders," in President's Commission for the Study of Ethical Problems in Medicine and Biomedical and Behavioral Research, *Deciding to Forego Life-Sustaining Treatment: Ethical, Medical, and Legal Issues in Treatment Decisions* (Washington, D.C.: U.S. Government Printing Office, 1983), p. 505.

6. New York State Task Force on Life and the Law, *Do Not Resuscitate Orders: The Proposed Legislation and Report of the New York State Task Force on Life and the Law* (N.p.: The New York State Task Force on Life and the Law, 1986), pp. 62–63.

7. Steven H. Miles, Ronald Cranford, and Alvin L. Schultz, "The Do-Not-Resuscitate Order in a Teaching Hospital," *Annals of Internal Medicine* 96 (1982):660–664.

8. Northwestern Memorial Hospital, "Do Not Resuscitate Orders," in President's Commission for the Study of Ethical Problems in Medicine and Biomedical and Behavioral Research, *Deciding to Forego Life-Sustaining Treatment: Ethical, Medical, and Legal Issues in Treatment Decisions* (Washington, D.C.: U.S. Government Printing Office, 1983), p. 512.

9. "Principles and Guidelines for the Treatment of a Patient for Whom a No-Code Order Has Been Written, St. Joseph Hospital, Orange," in *Legal and Ethical Aspects of Treating Critically and Terminally Ill Patients*, ed. A. E. Doudera and J. D. Peters (Ann Arbor, Mich: AUPHA Press, 1982), p. 97.

10. Richard F. Uhlman, Christine K. Cassel, and Walter J. McDonald, "Some Treatment-Withholding Implications of No-Code Orders in an Academic Hospital," *Critical Care Medicine* 12 (1984):879–881.

11. Andrew L. Evans and Baruch A. Brody, "The Do-Not-Resuscitate Order in Teaching Hospitals," *JAMA* 53 (1985):2236–2239: Stuart J. Youngner, "Do-Not-Resuscitate Orders: No Longer Secret, but Still a Problem," *Hastings Center Report* 17 (1987):24–33.

12. Alan Meisel, Ake Grenvik, Rosa L. Pinkus, and James V. Snyder, "Hospital Guidelines for Deciding about Life-Sustaining Treatment: Dealing with Health 'Limbo,'" *Critical Care Medicine* 14 (1986):246.

13. Marney Halligan and Ronald P. Hamel, "Ethics Committee Develops Supportive Care Guidelines," *Health Progress* 66 (1985):29.

14. Standards and Guidelines for Cardiopulmonary Resuscitation (CPR) and Emergency Cardiac Care (ECC)," *Journal of the American Medical Association* 255 (1986):2981.

15. Bedell and Delbanco, "Choices about Cardiopulmonary Resuscitation," p. 1091.

16. Susanna E. Bedell, Denise Pelle, Patricia L. Maher, and Paul D. Cleary, "Do-Not-Resuscitate Orders for Critically Ill Patients in the Hospital: How Are They Used and What Is Their Impact?" *JAMA* 256 (1986):233–237.

17. Ronald L. Stephens, "'Do Not Resuscitate' Orders: Ensuring the Patient's Participation," *JAMA* 255 (1986):240–241.

18. Mary E. Charlson, Frederic L. Sax, C. Ronald MacKenzie, et. al., "Resusciation: How Do We Decide? A Prospective Study of Physicians' Preferences and the Clinical Course of Hospitalized Patients," *JAMA* 255 (1986):1316–1322.

19. "Guidelines for 'No-Code' Orders in Los Angeles County Department of Health Services' Hospitals," in President's Commission for the Study of Ethical Problems in Medicine and Biomedical and Behavioral Research, *Deciding to Forego Life-Sustaining Treatment: Ethical, Medical, and Legal Issues in Treatment Decisions* (Washington, D.C.: U.S. Government Printing Office, 1983), p. 511.

20. Veterans' Administration, "Chief Medical Director's Letter on 'No Code' and Other Similar Orders," in President's Commission for the Study of Ethical

Problems in Medicine and Biomedical and Behavioral Research, *Deciding to Forego Life-Sustaining Treatment: Ethical, Medical, and Legal Issues in Treatment Decisions* (Washington, D.C.: U.S. Government Printing Office, 1983), p. 519.

21. "Statement on 'Do Not Resuscitate Orders,'" *Medical Staff Bulletin of the Washington Hospital Center*, Special Supplement, July 1984, p. 1.

22. Minnesota Medical Association, "Do Not Resuscitate (DNR) Guidelines," in President's Commission for the Study of Ethical Problems in Medicine and Biomedical and Behavioral Research, *Deciding to Forego Life-Sustaining Treatment: Ethical, Medical, and Legal Issues in Treatment Decisions* (Washington, D.C.: U.S. Government Printing Office, 1983), p. 500.

23. American Hospital Association, General Council Special Committee on Biomedical Ethics, *Values in Conflict: Ethical Issues in Hospital Care* (Chicago: American Hospital Association, 1985), p. 27.

24. Ad Hoc Committee on Medical Ethics, *American College of Physicians Ethics Manual* (Philadelphia: American College of Physicians, 1984), p. 27.

25. Ibid., p. 28.

26. "Standards and Guidelines," p. 2980.

27. Miles, Cranford, and Schultz, "The Do-Not-Resuscitate Order," p. 663.

28. Ibid., p. 660.

29. Ibid., p. 662.

30. Beth Israel Hospital, "Guidelines: Orders Not to Resuscitate," in President's Commission for the Study of Ethical Problems in Medicine and Biomedical and Behavioral Research, *Deciding to Forego Life-Sustaining Treatment: Ethical, Medical, and Legal Issues in Treatment Decisions* (Washington, D.C.: U.S. Government Printing Office, 1983), p. 503.

31. New York State Task Force, *Do Not Resuscitate Orders*, p. 63.

32. Meisel, Pinkus, and Snyder, "Hospital Guidelines," p. 244.

33. "Guidelines for 'No-Code' Orders in Los Angeles County," p. 511.

34. Committee on Policy for DNR Decisions, Yale New Haven Hospital, "Report on Do Not Resuscitate Decisions," *Connecticut Medicine* 47 (1983):481.

35. American Hospital Association, *Values in Conflict*, p. 28.

36. "A CMA Position: Resuscitation of the Terminally Ill," *Canadian Medical Association Journal* 136 (1987):424A.

37. Department of the Navy, National Naval Medical Center, "Guidelines for Orders Not to Resuscitate NHBETH INSTRUCTION 6320.37," in President's Commission for the Study of Ethical Problems in Medicine and Biomedical and Behavioral Research, *Deciding to Forego Life-Sustaining Treatment: Ethical, Medical, and Legal Issues in Treatment Decisions* (Washington, D.C.: U.S. Government Printing Office, 1983), pp. 530.

38. See also Allen Buchanan, "The Limits of Proxy Decision Making for Incompetents," *U.C.L.A. Law Review* 29 (393):1981.

39. Standards for Cardiopulmonary Resuscitation, p. 864.

40. Massachusetts General Hospital Clinical Care Committee, "Optimum Care for Hopelessly Ill Patients," *New England Journal of Medicine* 295 (1976):362–364.

41. Merian Kirchner, "How Far to Go Prolonging Life: One Hospital's System," *Medical Economics*, July 12, 1976, pp. 69–75.

42. New York State Task Force, *Do Not Resuscitate Orders*, p. 65.

43. Miles, Cranford, and Schultz, "The Do-Not-Resuscitate Order," pp. 660–661.

44. Ronald B. Schram, John C. Kane, Jr., and Daniel T. Roble, "'No Code' Orders: Clarification in the Aftermath of *Saikewicz*," *New England Journal of Medicine* 299 (1978):875–878; Judith Areen, "The Legal Status of Consent Obtained from Families of Adult Patients to Withhold or Withdraw Treatment," *JAMA* 258 (1987):229–235.

26. THE ETHICS OF INSTITUTIONAL ETHICS COMMITTEES

1. Robert M. Veatch, "Choosing Not to Prolong Dying," *Medical Dimensions* (December 1972): 10; *Death, Dying and the Biological Revolution: Our Last Quest for Responsibility* (New Haven: Yale University Press, 1976), especially pp. 60–61; 173–176; "Hospital Ethics Committees: Is There a Role?" *Hastings Center Report* 7 (June 1977):22–25.

2. Karen Teel, "The Physician's Dilemma—A Doctor's View: What the Law Should Be," *Baylor Law Review* 27 (Winter 1975); 6–9.

3. Robert M. Veatch, *A Theory of Medical Ethics* (New York: Basic Books, 1981), especially pp. 184–189. "Text of AMA's New Principles of Ethics," *American Medical News* 23 (August 1980):9; World Medical Association, Declaration of Geneva, reprinted in *Encyclopedia of Bioethics* vol. 4, ed. Warren T. Reich (New York: The Free Press, 1978), p. 1749; British Medical Association, *Medical Ethics* (London: British Medical Association House, 1974), p. 3.

4. Final Regulations Amending Basic Health and Human Services Policy for the Protection of Human Research Subjects, Section 46.103, *Federal Register* 46 (January 26, 1981):8837.

5. Robert Nozick's formulation of this idea is as follows: "Individuals have rights, and there are things no person or group may do to them (without violating their rights)." *Anarchy, State, and Utopia* (New York: Basic Books, 1974), p. ix.

6. The Massachusetts General Hospital criteria are discussed by Henning et al. in "Optimum Care for Hopelessly Ill Patients," *New England Journal of Medicine* 295 (No. 7, 1976):362–364. See also Merian Kirchner, "How Far to Go Prolonging Life: One Hospital's System," *Medical Economics* 53 (July 12, 1976):70, for similar criteria of New York's Mt. Sinai Hospital.

7. Kathi Esqueda, "Hospital Ethics Committees: Four Case Studies," *Hospital Medical Staff* 7 (November 1978):30.

8. "Natural Death Act of Virginia," House Bill No. 329, signed into law by Governor Robb on March 28, 1983. Article 7.1, section 54-325.8:1 states: "the General Assembly hereby declares that the laws of the Commonwealth of Virginia shall recognize the right of a competent adult to make an oral or written declaration instructing his physician to withhold or withdraw life-prolonging procedures or to designate another to make the treatment decision for him, in the event such a person is diagnosed as suffering from a terminal condition."

9. See chapter 24 for further elaboration.

27. CONTEMPORARY BIOETHICS AND THE DEMISE OF MODERN MEDICINE

1. Thomas S. Kuhn, *The Structure of Scientific Revolutions* (Chicago: University of Chicago Press, 1962).

2. H. Tristram Engelhardt, Stuart F. Spicker, and Bernard Towers, eds., *Clinical Judgment: A Critical Appraisal* (Dordrecht, Holland: D. Reidel Publishing Co., 1979).

3. Leon R. Kass, *Toward a More Natural Science* (New York: The Free Press, 1985).

4. Eric J. Cassell, *The Healer's Art* (Cambridge, Mass.: MIT Press, 1985).

5. Allen R. Dyer, "Virtue and Medicine: A Physician's Analysis," in *Virtue and Medicine: Exploration in the Character of Medicine*, ed. Earl E. Shelp (Dordrecht, Holland: D. Reidel Publishing Co., 1985), pp. 223–235.

6. Mark Siegler, "Clinical Ethics and Clinical Medicine" *Archives of Internal Medicine* 139 (No. 8, August 1979):914–915.

7. Also see philosophers who take this approach, such as John Ladd in "The Internal Morality of Medicine: An Essential Dimension of the Patient-Physician Relationship," in *The Clinical Encounter: The Moral Fabric of the Patient-Physician Relationship,* ed. Earl E. Shelp (Dordrecht, Holland: Reidel, 1983), pp. 209–231. Alasdair MacIntyre implies a similar notion of an internal morality to the practice of medicine in *After Virtue* (Notre Dame, Ind.: University of Notre Dame Press, 1981), when he holds that practices have virtues internal to them and that medicine is one such practice. See pp. 180–181.

8. President's Commission for the Study of Ethical Problems in Medicine and Biomedical and Behavioral Research, *Defining Death: Medical, Legal and Ethical Issues in the Definition of Death* (Washington, D.C.: U.S. Government Printing Office, 1981).

9. Harvard Medical School, "A Definition of Irreversible Coma: Report of the Ad Hoc Committee of the Harvard Medical School to Examine the Definition of Brain Death," *Journal of the American Medical Association* 205 (1968):337–340.

10. Robert M. Veatch, *Value-Freedom in Science and Technology* (Missoula, Mont.: Scholars Press, 1976).

11. National Institutes of Health Consensus Development Panel, "Critical Care Medicine," *Journal of the American Medical Association* 250 (1983):798–804.

INDEX

ROBERT M. VEATCH is Professor of Medical Ethics and Director of the Kennedy Institute of Ethics
at Georgetown University. He is the author of several books in the field of ethics, including *Death,
Dying, and the Biological Revolution; A Theory of
Medical Ethics;* and *The Patient as Partner: A Theory of Human-Experimentation Ethics.*

$27.50